Exploring the Thalamus and Its Role in Cortical Function

Exploring the Thalamus and Its Role in Cortical Function

Second Edition

S. Murray Sherman and R. W. Guillery

The MIT Press
Cambridge, Massachusetts
London, England

MIT Press books may be purchased at special quantity discounts for business or sales promotional use. For information, please email special_sales@mitpress. mit.edu or write to Special Sales Department, The MIT Press, 55 Hayward Street, Cambridge, MA 02142-1315.

This book was set in 10/13 Sabon by SNP Best-set Typesetter Ltd., Hong Kong. Printed and bound in the United States of America.

Library of Congress Cataloging-in-Publication Data

Sherman, S. Murray.
Exploring the thalamus and its role in cortical function / S. Murray Sherman and R. W. Guillery.—2nd ed.
    p. ; cm.
Rev. ed. of: Exploring the thalamus. © 2001
Includes bibliographical references and index.
ISBN 0-262-19532-1 (alk. paper)
1. Thalamus. I. Guillery, R. W. II. Sherman, S. Murray. Exploring the thalamus. III. Title.
[DNLM: 1. Thalamus—physiology. 2. Cerebral Cortex—physiology.
WL 312 S553e 2006]
QP383.5.S53 2006   612.8′262—dc22   2005052120

10 9 8 7 6 5 4 3 2 1

Brief Contents

Preface to the First Edition

The title of this book, *Exploring the Thalamus*, is intended to convey the sense that there is a great deal still unknown about the thalamus and that our aim in writing has been to show some of the major and minor roads, the footpaths, and the frank wildernesses that still need to be explored. The thalamus, in terms of its detailed connectivity patterns, the functioning of its circuitry, and, perhaps most interestingly, its functional relationship to the cerebral cortex, is largely *terra incognita*. The cortex depends critically on the messages it receives from the thalamus. It receives very little else. Understanding cortical functioning will depend on understanding the thalamic inputs that are the necessary first step in cortical processing. There is a serious sense in which one can regard the thalamus as the deepest layer of the cortex. That is, cortex and thalamus depend very closely on each other; neither would amount to much without the other, and if we are to understand the workings of either, we must, as we try to show in what follows, be able to understand the messages that each is sending to the other. Our main focus on the thalamus in this book will be on its relation to cortical function. Perhaps this focus on thalamocortical interrelationships should have been a part of our title, but we wanted a brief title and we had in mind a book on the thalamus, not one on the cortex. We are looking at ways to explore how thalamic organization should influence our views of cortical function; we are not looking to provide a general account of the thalamus as an entity in itself.

In a preface, authors are expected to say for whom the book has been written. We hope that this book will serve to introduce graduate students, postdoctoral fellows, and investigators who need to learn about the thalamus to some of the interesting aspects of the subject. Also, since many view the thalamus as an uninteresting, mechanical relay of peripheral messages to cortex that is already well understood, we have tried to explain that this view is far too simplistic and that there are many important problems about the function and the structure of thalamus that remain unrecognized and unresolved. One of our aims has been to persuade colleagues that these problems are of interest and worth significant research investment. We have tried to make each chapter more or less independent, so that perhaps one or another can be assigned as course reading for graduate students. This entails some repetition from one chapter to another; we trust that it is not excessive for those who are motivated to read the whole thing.

Our thoughts about who would read the book were not our main focus when we first started discussions and rough drafts almost 10 years ago. Rather, we undertook the task initially because we found that the thoughts, the discussions, and the arguments that have accompanied the job of writing were sufficient stimulus in themselves. As we wrote, exchanged drafts, sent each chapter back and forth many times to be annotated, corrected, reannotated, and recorrected, we gradually learned a great deal about our subject (and about each other). The real truth is that we wrote the book for ourselves, and once we had that aspect of the writing fairly in hand, we worked hard to make it accessible to others.

We have not attempted to present a complete and coherent view of everything that is known about the thalamus. We have instead followed arguments and lines of inquiry that can lead to new questions, interesting thoughts, or new experimental approaches. Knowledge of the thalamus is extraordinarily patchy. The thalamus is divided into many different "nuclei." There are some thalamic nuclei that have been studied in considerable detail, and others about which we know almost nothing. Our plan in writing the book has been to assume that there is a basic ground plan for the thalamus. Although there are often important differences between one thalamic nucleus and another, in one species or between species, there is yet a common pattern of organization seen over and again in essentially all thalamic nuclei. We have tried to explore the nature of this common pattern and to ask questions about its functional significance.

We have both spent the greater part of our careers studying the visual pathways, and it won't take a very subtle reading of the book to recognize this. We turn to the visual relay in the thalamus repeatedly not only because this is the part we know best but also because in our readings and in our discussions with colleagues we find that the visual relay has, time and again, received more detailed experimental study than other thalamic relays. The visual relay may well have some special characteristics that distinguish it from other relays. In some instances this is clear, and we recognize it. However, in many instances it is reasonable to treat the visual relay as an exemplar of thalamic relays in general, and in many parts of the book, that is how we have approached the analysis of thalamic functions. This approach raises important questions about non-visual parts of the thalamus, and our expectation is that the comparisons will stimulate further study of these questions.

We have stressed that this book is not a complete inventory of all that is known about the thalamus. There are many important references we have not cited, and there are several lines of inquiry that we have not included. We say virtually nothing about the development or the comparative anatomy of the thalamus even though each is an extremely interesting subject in its own right. They should perhaps form the nucleus of another book. Nor do we cover the clinical aspects of thalamic dysfunction, another potentially interesting area, although it seems likely to us that this will become of greater interest once we know more about some of the basic ground rules of thalamic function and connectivity that are still missing from our current knowledge. For instance, the thalamus has long been implicated in epilepsy and certain sleep disorders, it is related to the production of pathological pain, and there is new interest in the thalamus as a particularly interesting site of pathology in schizophrenia and other cognitive problems. The complexity of the two-way links between thalamus and cortex and the limited nature of our knowledge about these links, especially in the human brain, make interpretations of clinical conditions extremely difficult and often rather tenuous, and we have not addressed them in this book.

We have tried to achieve two major aims in the book. The first is to look at many of the outstanding puzzles and unanswered questions that arise as one studies the structural and functional organization of the thalamus. The second aim, growing out of a small proportion of these questions, is to move toward an understanding of the possible role(s) of the thalamus in cortical functions, so that some coherent suggestions about this role could be presented as the book proceeds. The first aim is summarized to a limited extent by a short list of "Unresolved Questions" that appears at the end of each chapter. These are not questions to which a student can find answers in the text. They are, rather, designed to focus on some of the issues that need to be resolved if we are to advance our understanding of the thalamus. They do not represent an exhaustive list, and the interested reader is likely to find a number of other questions that are currently unanswered and often unasked. The listed questions should be seen as representing a state of mind, and they are an important part of the book as a whole. They should lead to more questions, and they should point to paths that have perhaps never been explored or along which our predecessors have been lost in the past. We hope that by stimulating a questioning attitude to thalamic organization we will encourage a view of the thalamus as far more mysterious than is commonly taught. This clearly implies that our second aim, to understand the role of the thalamus, which we present in detail in the later chapters, can at best be only partially achieved. We present a view of the thalamus that is based on the classical view of it as a relay of ascending messages to cortex. However, we see it as a continually active relay, serving sometimes as a "lookout" for significant new inputs and at other times as an accurate relay that allows detailed analysis of input content in the cortex. This is based on the recognition of two distinct types of input to the thalamus, the "drivers" that carry the message and the "modulators" that determine how the message is transmitted to cortex. The former can carry ascending messages from the periphery as well as descending messages from cortex itself. These messages are generally mapped, giving them a definite locus in the environment or in some other part of the brain. In contrast, the latter either can be mapped and thus act locally like the drivers or can lack a mapped organization and then act globally. Recognizing that drivers can take origin in the cortex leads to an interesting new view of corticocortical communication because it stresses that messages that pass from one cortical area to another may be under the same set of modulatory controls in the thalamus as are the inputs that are passed to the cortex from the peripheral senses.

It is probable that many of the ideas we present in this book will prove wrong. Whether they are right or wrong, we have tried to make them stimulating. To quote Kuhn (1963) quoting Francis Bacon, "Truth emerges more readily from error than from confusion," which provides our best justification for writing this book about a subject that in terms of the currently available literature is often extremely confusing.

Finally, both authors owe thanks and the book itself owes its existence to many people and organizations. A number of colleagues read an early draft of the book, and the comments and critical points that they raised have helped us to reorganize and correct a great deal of the book in terms of style, order of presentation, and content. We thank Paul Adams, Joe Fetcho, Sherry Feig, Lew Haberly, Carsten Hohnke, Jon Levitt, John Mitrofanis, and Phil Smith for their helpful comments. We recognize the amount of time and effort that they have contributed; we are most grateful for it and for the significant improvements that their careful readings have produced. The final version of this book is, of course, entirely our responsibility. All of our colleagues will likely find many places where they can write further instructive comments in the margins, and perhaps some of these will lead to useful explorations of the thalamus in the future. Marjorie Sherman helped with the proof-reading. Sherry Feig helped one of us (R.W.G.) learn how to draw on a computer. Both authors received support from the NIH while this book was being written (Grants EY03038, EY11409, and EY11494), and at the early stages R.W.G., while in the Department of Human Anatomy at Oxford, was supported by the Wellcome Trust. The initial stimulus for planning the book came from the year S.M.S. spent as a Newton-Abraham Visting Professor at Oxford in 1985–1986.

S. Murray Sherman
R. W. Guillery

Abbreviations

We have, as far as possible, avoided the use of abbreviations, except for a few that are commonly used and widely recognized for complex names. They are the following: AMPA, (R,S)-α-amino-3-hydroxy-5-methyl-4-isoxazolepropionic acid; EPSP, excitatory postsynaptic potential; GABA, γ-aminobutyric acid; GAD, glutamic acid decarboxylase; IPSP, inhibitory postsynaptic potential; NMDA, N-methyl-D-aspartate.

1 Introduction

1.A. Thalamic Functions: What Is the Thalamus, and What Does It Do?

1.A.1. The Classical View of the Thalamus

The thalamus is the major relay to the cerebral cortex. It has been described as the gateway to the cortex. Almost everything we can know about the outside world or about ourselves is based on messages that have had to pass through the thalamus. The thalamus forms a relatively small structure on each side of the midline (figure 1.1) and can be divided into several distinct cell groups, or "nuclei," each concerned with transmitting a characteristic type of afferent signal (visual, auditory, somatosensory, cerebellar, etc.) to a structurally and functionally distinct, corresponding area or group of areas of the cerebral cortex (figures 1.2 and 1.3) on the same side of the brain. The thalamus relates to the largest part of the cortex, the neocortex, and it is the relationships between thalamus and neocortex that are explored in this book. Other areas of cortex, olfactory cortex and hippocampal cortex, are not neocortex and do not receive comparable thalamic afferents. Olfactory afferents represent the only pathway of a sensory system that does not have to go through the thalamus before it can reach the cortex.

This view of the thalamus was developed during the 70-plus years up to about 1950. It has served us well, and is still the view presented in most textbooks. It was based on clinical observations related to post-mortem study of the brain and on relatively crude experimental neuroanatomical methods: the Nissl method, which shows the distinct nuclei in normal material and shows them undergoing degenerative changes after their axons in the cortex have been cut, and the Marchi method, which stains degenerating myelin in pathways that have been cut or injured. These methods give results in terms of large populations

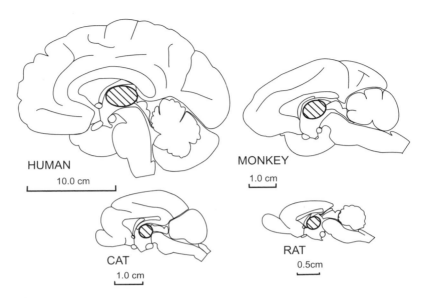

HUMAN
10.0 cm

MONKEY
1.0 cm

CAT
1.0 cm

RAT
0.5cm

Figure 1.1
Midsagittal view of the cerebral hemisphere of a human, a monkey, a cat, and a rat (in inverse size order) to show the position and relative size of the thalamus, which is indicated by diagonal hatching.

of cells or axons and large areas of thalamus or cortex. Perhaps it was fortunate that modern methods for studying detailed connectivity patterns of single cells or small groups of cells were not available when the thalamic connections were first being defined. If they had been, it is probable that no one would have been able to see the larger thalamic forest for the details of the connectional trees. We shall start with the forest.

The schematic view of thalamocortical relationships, summarized in Walker's great book (Walker, 1938) and in Le Gros Clark's earlier review (Le Gros Clark, 1932), provided a powerful approach to understanding thalamic function. Even though it was heavily dependent on relatively gross methods, this schematic view showed how to divide up the thalamus and how to relate each of the resulting major thalamic nuclei or nuclear groups to one or another part of the cerebral cortex (see figures 1.2 and 1.3). Above all, this classical view of the thalamus showed how the functions of any one part of the neocortex depend on thalamocortical inputs. We present the basic structure of the classical view of the thalamus in the next section, where we provide an abbreviated account

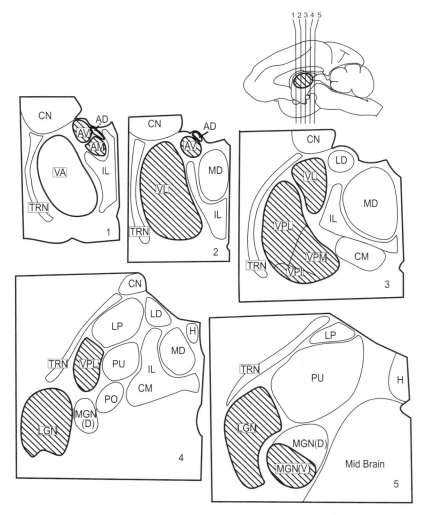

Figure 1.2

Schematic view of five sections through the thalamus of a monkey. The sections are numbered 1 through 5 and were cut in the coronal planes indicated by the arrows in the upper right midsagittal view of the monkey brain from figure 1.1. The major thalamic nuclei in one hemisphere are shown for a generalized primate. The nuclei that are outlined by a heavier line and filled by diagonal hatching are described as first order nuclei (see text), and the major functional connections of these, in terms of their afferent (input) and efferent (output) pathways to cortex, are indicated in figure 1.3. Abbreviations: AD, anterior dorsal nucleus; AM, anterior medial nucleus; AV, anterior ventral nucleus; CM, center median nucleus; CN, caudate nucleus (not a part of the thalamus); H, habenular nucleus (part of the epithalamus); IL, intralaminar (and midline) nuclei; LD, lateral dorsal nucleus; LGN, lateral geniculate nucleus; LP, lateral posterior nucleus; MD, medial dorsal nucleus; MGN, medial geniculate nucleus; PO, posterior nucleus; PU, pulvinar; TRN, thalamic reticular nucleus; VA, ventral anterior nucleus; VL, ventral lateral nucleus; VPI, VPL, and VPM, inferior, lateral, and medial parts of the ventral posterior nucleus.

Note: The ventral anterior nucleus, although in receipt of some cerebellar afferents, receives significant driver inputs from cortex and is therefore not shown as a first order nucleus.

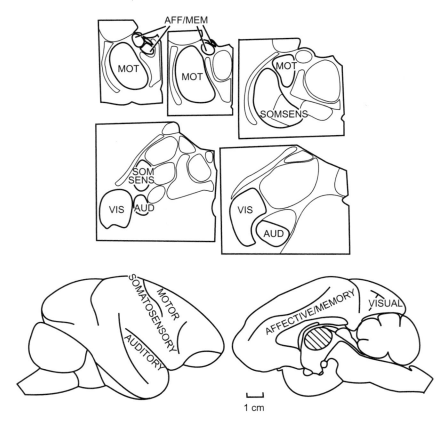

Figure 1.3
The upper part of the figure shows the nuclei illustrated in figure 1.2 and the lower part shows a lateral (left) and a medial view of the hemisphere in a monkey to indicate the functional connections of the major first order thalamic nuclei.

of the major thalamic nuclei, their functions, and their afferent and efferent connections.

Although this classical view of thalamic nuclei provides a useful practical guide, it is, after more than 70 years of refinement, added detail, new terminology, and the demonstration of ever more complex connectivity patterns, which will be introduced in the later parts of this book, beginning to be less useful than it was in the past.

1.A.2. Defining Thalamic Nuclei

The concept of the thalamic nucleus as a single structural, functional, and connectional entity has barely survived advancing techniques and new information. We stay with the thalamic nuclei as one of our prime analytical tools because, as yet, we have little to use in its place. Almost any one of the classical thalamic nuclei can be shown to be made up of several functionally and connectionally distinct cell types; many recent staining methods reveal functionally distinct cell groupings or scattered cell types that cut right across classical nuclear borders. There are cells scattered through the nuclei that simply do not fit the classical rules, and there are puzzling borders between nuclei where one has learned to be on the lookout for novel and surprising connections. It is probable that eventually we will have to treat the pathways that go through the thalamus to cortex in terms of many functionally distinct parallel pathways, several of which may often share a single nucleus, even though they may show no significant interactions within the shared nucleus.

We stress these exceptions as a warning, not because we devote a significant part of the book to them, and not because we have insights that allow us to fit them into new interpretative views of the thalamus, but because we recognize, and think it important for the reader to recognize, that the schematic representation of the thalamus presented in the next section in terms of its nuclei is inadequate. However, it is the best we have at present. This book is not planned to present the thalamus in classical terms, nor is it planned to explore the inadequacies of the classical nuclei in any detail. We start with the classical picture of the thalamic nuclei and their connections because that is still the best starting point, but we have other aims for the book. There follows a brief outline of these aims to orient the reader and to provide a rough guide that will explain the nature of and the need for the rather detailed analysis provided in the rest of the book.

1.A.3. Major Topics Addressed in This Book

A key question concerns the thalamic circuitry that acts on messages arriving along the input pathways and sends them on as outputs to cortex, giving each recipient cortical area particular and characteristic functional properties. Although we recognize that there are differences between the parts of the thalamus (and between species) in the detailed circuitry, we stress that the thalamus is a developmental and a functional unit and that there is a common, basic plan, from one nucleus to another, made plain especially by physiological recordings from thalamic cells and by studies of the morphological detail of the cells and their interconnections. This basic plan allows us not only to trace how messages pass through the thalamus, but also to look at how thalamic circuitry allows transmission to be modified in relation to current behavioral needs or constraints. This requires a close examination of the cells in the thalamus, the relay cells that send their axon to the cortex, and also the local interneurons that act on the relay cells. The circuitry is complex and depends not only on the precise connections that are established but also on the transmitters, the receptors, and the membrane properties that are involved in the synaptic interactions in the thalamus. Further, understanding thalamic circuits requires identification of the functionally significant input.

It may seem surprising that, for a large part of the thalamus, we know little about what the crucial input for transmission to cortex actually is. It is important to distinguish the functional input that carries the messages for transmission to the cortex, which we call the driver, from the many other inputs, the modulators, which can modify the way in which the message is transmitted without significantly changing the basic functional characteristics of the message that reaches cortex. Thus, for the main sensory relays of the thalamus (visual, auditory, somatosensory), the drivers bring messages about the relevant sensory events. Identifying functional and morphological criteria that will help to distinguish drivers from modulators becomes of prime importance. One such criterion, which in terms of classical views of the thalamus is surprising, is that in the thalamus, where neurons do not fire at very high rates, inhibitory axons cannot, for reasons outlined in chapter 7, be drivers.

Throughout the thalamus, modulators far outnumber drivers in terms of the numbers of synaptic connections, and once rules for recognizing drivers are established, then it becomes clear that much of the thalamus, whose connections were largely undefined in the past, receives its drivers not from subcortical centers but from cerebral cortex and is therefore concerned with sending messages from one cortical area to another. The importance of this pathway, which allows one cortical area to receive inputs from another cortical area through a thalamic relay that can be modulated in accordance with behavioral constraints, is not widely appreciated and has been but poorly explored.

Once we think of the thalamus in terms of the functionally distinct driver pathways that pass through it, we can begin to see one alternative to the classical nucleus. That is, we can start to think of the thalamus, or of any one part of the thalamus, often one of the classical nuclei, as a relay for transmitting information to cerebral cortex along functionally parallel driver pathways. Where such pathways lie in close relationship to each other, we have to ask about the nature of possible interactions. We also have to consider interactions between the parts of any one such pathway.

Many of the functional pathways through the thalamus, possibly all of them, are mapped. That is, there is a topographic order to the inputs, the thalamic circuits, and the thalamocortical outputs that we refer to as *local sign*. Understanding the maps in any one pathway allows for an investigation of how the parts relate to each other, and knowing the maps in two or more related parallel pathways provides clues as to how these may interact. Currently there is little evidence for such interactions between functionally distinct parallel pathways within a thalamic nucleus, but critical evidence is lacking for most of the thalamus. However, for any one functional mapped pathway, lateral interactions occur, either in the thalamus itself or on the way to the cortex.

One important feature that becomes apparent once one identifies the functional drivers for the many distinct parallel pathways that pass through the thalamus is that many of the drivers, possibly all, give off branches to centers in the spinal cord or brainstem concerned directly or indirectly with the control of movement. This branching pattern leads us to consider the thalamus not just as a sensory relay in the classical sense but rather as also bringing to cortex information about current motor instructions. We apply this view not only to the ascending pathways going to primary cortical sensory areas but also to the transthalamic corticocortical pathways (described earlier), which are then seen as carrying to higher cortical areas information about the current outputs of lower cortical areas.

When it is recognized that the classical "sensory" functions are intimately linked to instructions that are on their way to motor centers even before the sensory messages can reach the cerebral cortex, it becomes necessary to look at a conundrum long discussed by philosophers—how perceptual processes may be linked to action. In the final chapter we consider this problem. We cannot address all of the issues that have been discussed on this subject, but we can cast a new light on them by showing that there are anatomical connections that speak directly to the often puzzlingly close link between action and perception.

1.B. Thalamic Nuclei and Their Connections: The Classical View

Figure 1.1 shows the thalamus in relation to the rest of the cerebral hemisphere. The thalamus is small relative to the whole cerebral hemisphere in all mammals. There are a great many more neocortical cells than there are thalamic cells, even though the neocortex depends on the thalamus for its major inputs.[1] Each major neocortical area depends on a well-defined thalamic nucleus or group of nuclei, and these nuclei in turn receive their input from a well-defined path into the thalamus. In the evolutionary history of mammals, an increase in the size of any one part of cortex generally corresponds to an increase in the related thalamic nuclei. The functionally best-defined cortical areas (visual, auditory, motor, etc.) depend for their functional properties on the messages to that cortical area from the thalamus. The visual cortex is visual because it receives visual messages from the retina through its thalamic relay, and this relationship holds for the other thalamic nuclei outlined in bold and hatched in figure 1.2, which shows some of the major thalamic nuclei in a simplified, schematic form for a generalized primate.

Details concerning the thalamic nuclei differ for each species, and there are a number of nuclei that are not included in figure 1.2 because they play no significant role in the rest of this book. However, the general relationships shown apply to all mammals. Figure 1.3 shows how some of these major thalamic nuclei are linked to specific, functionally or structurally defined cortical areas. Further details on individual thalamic nuclei and their connections can be found in Berman (1982) and Jones (1985).

Figures 1.2 and 1.3 show that for some, but by no means all, of the thalamic nuclei, we can identify the dominant or functionally "driving" afferents. That is, figure 1.3 shows that the lateral geniculate nucleus is visual, the medial geniculate nucleus is auditory, and the

---

1. From the evidence available for the geniculocortical pathway to the primary visual cortex (variously called V1, area 17, or striate cortex) it appears that there are about $350–460 \times 10^6$ cortical nerve cells in V1 of each hemisphere in the monkey, and about $55–70 \times 10^6$ in the cat. The numbers of nerve cells for one lateral geniculate nucleus are about 1.6×10^6 and 0.45×10^6, respectively. Since not all geniculate cells project to V1, the projecting geniculate cells represent 0.5% or less of the total number of cortical cells in the area receiving the projection. See Rockel et al. (1980) for cell densities in cortex, Duffy et al. (1998) for area V1, Matthews (1964) for cell numbers in the monkey lateral geniculate nucleus, and Bishop et al. (1953) for the cat.

ventral posterior nucleus[2] is somatosensory, which is to say that the ascending pathways concerned with tactile stimuli and with stimuli related to body position and movements (kinesthesis) go to this nucleus, as do pathways concerned with pain and temperature. We treat these several sensory pathways as the "drivers," because they are the afferents that determine the receptive field properties of the thalamic relay cells that pass the messages on to cortex. Other afferents, which we treat as "modulators," can modify the way that the message is transmitted, but they are not responsible for the main qualitative nature of the message conveyed to cortex. Each thalamic nucleus has drivers and modulators, and identifying the drivers for thalamic nuclei whose function is still poorly defined is likely to be a key to understanding their functions. For reasons detailed in chapter 3, we treat the afferents from the cerebellum to the ventral lateral and ventral anterior nuclei as drivers related to movement control, and axons of the mamillothalamic tract as drivers sending information to the anterior thalamic nuclei about ongoing activity in the mamillary bodies. These, and the main sensory afferents mentioned earlier, represent the major known ascending driver inputs to the thalamus. Afferents to the other main thalamic nuclei, indicated with lighter outlines and no hatching in figure 1.2 and unlabeled in figure 1.3, are less straightforward; they are considered in more detail in chapters 3 and 8. These nuclei receive their major driving afferents from the cerebral cortex itself and therefore act as relays on corticocortical pathways, not as relays of subcortical afferents to cortex (Sherman & Guillery, 1996; Guillery & Sherman, 2002a). They are "higher order" relays (figure 1.4). First order relays are defined as those that send messages to the cortex about events in the subcortical parts of the brain, higher order relays as those that provide a transthalamic relay from one part of cortex to another. In primates, the nuclei that contain higher order circuits form more than half the thalamus. The relationship of these transthalamic corticocortical relays to the more widely studied direct corticocortical connections is a challenging question considered in chapters 8 and 10. It is

---

2. The lateral and medial parts of the ventral posterior nucleus are often referred to as part of the ventrobasal complex, and a distinction is made between a nuclear complex, or group of nuclei, and a thalamic nucleus that has no further subdivisions. The term "complex" has been rather inconsistently applied in the past and is difficult to apply rigorously; the same is true when the term "nucleus" is used to apply to a cell grouping and to its subdivisions. For the purposes of this book, these problems are not important, and we will stay with the term nucleus throughout.

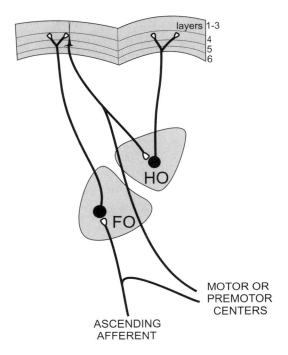

Figure 1.4
Schematic representation of first order (FO) and higher order (HO) thalamic relays. The first order relay receives driving afferents from ascending pathways, whereas the higher order relay receives driving afferents from layer 5 of the cortex. Both of these driving afferents send branches to subcortical motor or premotor centers.

important to stress that some of the nuclei shown without hatching in figure 1.2 are likely to contain a mixture of first and higher order relays (see chapter 8), so that it may not be appropriate to speak of higher order *nuclei* but instead to consider specific *relays*.

Although for many of the thalamic nuclei we can show how they serve to connect different cortical areas to sensory surfaces of the body or to other parts of the brain, we cannot readily demonstrate what it is that the thalamus does for the messages that are passed from ascending pathways to the cerebral cortex. Why don't the ascending pathways go straight to the cortex? This question was always present, but was brought into striking focus in the 1960s when electron microscopists showed the complexities of the synaptic relationships in the thalamus (Szentágothai, 1963; Colonnier & Guillery, 1964; Peters & Palay, 1966).

Only about 20% of the synapses in the major relay nuclei, such as the lateral geniculate or the ventral posterior nucleus, were then seen to come from the major ascending pathways (Guillery, 1969a), and recent figures are significantly lower (Van Horn et al., 2000). Complex synaptic formations involving serial synapses and connections from local or distant inhibitory cells characterize all of the thalamic nuclei (e.g., Jones & Powell, 1969; Ralston & Herman, 1969; Morest, 1975; Jones, 1985), and most thalamic nuclei, in accordance with their shared developmental origin, have more or less the same general organizational plan.

The complexity of thalamocortical pathways was further increased by the demonstration of the connections shown in figure 1.5. Not only is there a massive input from the deeper layers of the cerebral cortex back to the thalamus, but there is a specialized cell group adjacent to the thalamus, the thalamic reticular nucleus, which receives excitatory branches from the corticothalamic and thalamocortical axons and sends inhibitory axons back to the thalamus (Jones, 1985).

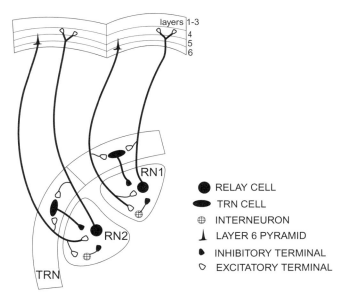

Figure 1.5
Schematic view of the interconnections of two thalamic relay nuclei (RN1, RN2) layer 6 of the cerebral cortex, and the thalamic reticular nucleus. Thalamic nuclei RN1 and RN2 are connected with distinct sectors of the reticular nucleus and with distinct cortical areas. Details of the connections within the nuclei are discussed in chapter 3 (see figure 3.16).

The functional role of the reticular connections and of the complex synaptic arrangements found in the thalamus represented (and still represents) a challenging puzzle, a challenge that was greatly increased in recent years by the discovery of diverse transmitters, voltage and ligand gated ion channels, and receptors that contribute to the synaptic organization in the thalamic relay (see Sherman & Guillery, 1996, and chapters 4 through 6). The functional control of membrane conductances depends on a highly complex interplay of afferent activity and local conditions that will be considered in chapter 4. These conditions in turn determine the way in which a thalamic cell responds to its inputs, and thus determines how messages that come into the thalamus are passed on to cortex. This, the manner in which a thalamic cell passes messages on to cortex, is not constant but depends on the attentive state of the whole animal (awake, drowsy, or sleeping), and probably on the local salience of a particular stimulus or group of stimuli, as well; are the stimuli new, threatening, interesting, or merely a continuation of prior conditions? This question is addressed in chapter 6.

When one considers the factors relevant to how the transfer of messages is controlled or gated in the thalamus, it is probable that more than one functionally significant mechanism will become apparent once we have a clear understanding of these aspects of thalamic organization. That is, there are likely to be several more or less distinct functional roles for the synaptic arrangements present in the thalamus. Particular patterns may be active at different times, or they may have concurrent effects. Two that have received significant attention in the recent past occur in sleep and in the production of epileptic discharges (Steriade et al., 1993b; McCormick & Bal, 1997). A third aspect that has come into focus recently and is addressed in chapter 6 concerns how the role of the relays may change in relation to different behavioral states, and relate to attentional mechanisms. All three involve the circuit going through the thalamic reticular nucleus that was mentioned earlier (figure 1.5; see also Jones, 1985). We anticipate that the role of first and higher order thalamic circuits in passing messages to the cortex will follow the same basic ground rules. That is, whatever it is that the thalamus does for the major ascending pathways, it is likely to be doing something very similar for corticocortical communication. Understanding what it is that the thalamus does should help us to understand not only the functional organization of sensory pathways in relation to perception but should also throw new light on perceptual and cognitive functions that in the past were largely or entirely ascribed to corticocortical interconnections

(Zeki & Shipp, 1988; Felleman & Van Essen, 1991; Salin & Bullier, 1995).

There is one interesting corollary to the above. If the thalamus acts to control the way that information is relayed to the cortex, then it may be a mistake to expect it to act as an integrator of distinctive inputs as well. At present, the most detailed information available on thalamic relays shows that information from the ascending pathways is passed to cortex without a significant change in "content." That is, there are thalamic nuclei that receive afferents from more than one source, but currently there is no evidence that the multiple inputs in such nuclei interact on single relay neurons to produce a significant change in the content of the input messages. The multiple pathways appear to run in parallel, with little or no interaction.

In this book we explore the way in which thalamic functions relate to cortical functions. Outputs of the thalamus that link it to other cerebral centers, particularly the striatum and the amygdala, represent a relatively small though important part of the thalamic relay. They play no role or only a very indirect role in influencing neocortical activity, and for this reason we will not explore them further. We shall argue that there is likely to be a basic thalamic ground plan that represents the way in which the thalamus transmits messages from its input to its output channels. It seems probable that this ground plan will apply to all thalamic relays, and possibly, when we understand how the thalamus relates to the cortex, the nature of the thalamic relay to other cerebral centers will help us understand the function of these currently even more mysterious pathways.

1.C. The Thalamus as a Part of the Diencephalon: The Dorsal Thalamus and the Ventral Thalamus

The term "thalamus" is commonly used to refer to the largest part of the mammalian diencephalon, the dorsal thalamus, and we generally use it in this sense in this book. However, there are several subdivisions of the diencephalon, and it is important to look briefly at all of them before focusing on just two subdivisions, the large dorsal thalamus and the smaller but closely related ventral thalamus.

Figure 1.6 shows relationships in the diencephalon at a relatively early stage of development. On the left is a view of a parasagittal section of the brain early in development, which shows that the most dorsal part of the diencephalon is the epithalamus. In the adult the epithalamus is

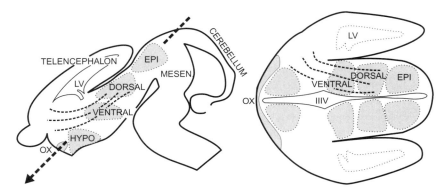

Figure 1.6
Schematic views of two sections through a 14-day postconception fetal mouse brain, based on photographs in Schambra et al. (1992). At left is a parasagittal section in which the position of the epithalamus, the dorsal thalamus, the ventral thalamus, and the hypothalamus within the diencephalon is shown (EPI, DORSAL, VENTRAL, HYPO). At right is a section cut transversely in the oblique plane (indicated by the arrow) that includes these four diencephalic parts and the optic chiasm (OX). The subthalamus is not included in these figures. The interrupted lines show the course of the fibers that link the dorsal thalamus to the telencephalon. LV, lateral ventricle; IIIV, third ventricle.

made up of the habenular nuclei, a few other small, dorsally placed nuclei, and the related pineal body. These structures will not be of further concern to us, nor will two more ventral cell groups, the subthalamus, which is not shown in figure 1.6 and is involved with motor pathways, and the hypothalamus, which plays a vital role in neuroendocrine and visceral functions. In this book we are concerned solely with the dorsal thalamus and with a major derivative of the ventral thalamus, the thalamic reticular nucleus.[3] These two are closely connected by the two-way links shown in figure 1.5, and it is reasonable to argue that neither can function adequately without the other. Figure 1.6 shows that originally, during development, the ventral thalamus lies ahead of (rostral to) the dorsal thalamus. The thick dotted lines in the schematic views in figure 1.6 stress an important relationship between the dorsal and the ventral

---

3. The ventral lateral geniculate nucleus is also developmentally a part of the ventral thalamus but will not play a significant role in this book. Although, like the thalamic reticular nucleus, it receives cortical afferents and does not send axons to cortex, it does not have the important connections with the dorsal thalamus that make the reticular nucleus a key part of the thalamocortical system as a whole.

thalamus, because they show that lines of communication between the dorsal thalamus and the telencephalon, which includes the cerebral cortex, must pass through the ventral thalamus. This is a key relationship and is maintained even when the ventral thalamic derivative, the thalamic reticular nucleus, moves into its adult position lateral to the dorsal thalamus, as shown in figures 1.2 and 1.3.

1.C.1. *The Dorsal Thalamus*

In most mammalian brains, and most strikingly in the primate brain, the dorsal thalamus is by far the largest part of the diencephalon. In size and complexity it is closely related to the development of the cerebral cortex. It can be defined as the part of the diencephalon that develops from the region between the epithalamus and the ventral thalamus. More significantly, it is the part of the diencephalon that has its major efferent connections with telencephalic structures, either striatal or neocortical. In mammals, the neocortical connections dominate, and all dorsal thalamic nuclei project to neocortex. Connections to the striatum are seen for only a few of the nuclei (primarily the intralaminar nuclei) in mammalian brains. All thalamic nuclei have relay cells, which send their axons to the telencephalon, and, with the curious exception of many nuclei in rats and mice,[4] all have interneurons with locally ramifying axons.

1.C.1.a. The Afferents

We have seen that the first order nuclei of the dorsal thalamus receive a significant part of their afferent connections from ascending pathways. Some bring information about the environment to many of the major thalamic nuclei through sensory pathways, such as the visual, auditory, somatosensory, or taste pathways. Others bring information about activity in lower, subthalamic centers of the brain, such as the cerebellum for the ventral anterior and ventral lateral nuclei or the mamillary bodies for the anterior thalamic nuclei (figures 1.2 and 1.3). We shall argue that these afferents can be regarded as the driving inputs for their thalamic nuclei, determining the qualitative characteristics of the receptive fields

---

4. In a typical mammalian thalamic nucleus, roughly 15%–25% of the cells are interneurons, the remainder being relay cells. Thalamic nuclei in mice and rats appear to lack interneurons or to have only a few (Arcelli et al., 1997; but see Figure 12 of Li et al., 2003b, which shows a significant number of interneurons in the lateral posterior nucleus of a rat). The lateral geniculate nucleus of rats and mice has a normal share of interneurons, as do the thalamic nuclei of other rodent species that have been studied.

of the thalamic cells, where these can be defined. Other inputs, including all inhibitory inputs to first order nuclei, are best regarded as modulatory. These can change the way in which the message is transmitted and can affect quantitative aspects of the receptive field, but not its essential character or its qualitative structure.[5] The modulators come from the brainstem, the thalamic reticular nucleus, the hypothalamus, the cerebral cortex itself, and the thalamic interneurons.

The thalamic nuclei not outlined in bold in figure 1.2 contain higher order circuits and appear to receive most or all of their driving afferents from the cerebral cortex itself, so that the qualitative aspects of their receptive field properties, insofar as they can be defined, depend directly on cortical, not ascending, inputs. This distinction is discussed further in later chapters, particularly chapter 8. Here it is to be noted that the higher order thalamic relays, in addition to the driving afferents that they receive from cortex, also receive modulatory afferents from cortex and from the other structures noted previously for the first order nuclei.

The distinction between corticothalamic axons that are drivers and those that are modulators can be made on the basis of the cortical layer from which they arise: current evidence suggests that corticothalamic afferents arising in cortical layer 5 are drivers, whereas those arising in layer 6 are modulators (Sherman & Guillery, 1996, 1998; see also chapter 3). In a few instances, discussed in more detail in chapter 9, this distinction between drivers and modulators can be demonstrated in functional terms by recording how inactivation of the cortical afferents affects the receptive field properties of thalamic cells, but so far these instances are regrettably rare. Silencing a cortical driver produces a loss of the receptive field, whereas after a modulator is silenced the receptive field survives. The difference between these two groups, the drivers and modulators, is seen not only in terms of their origin and their action on receptive field properties of dorsal thalamic cells, but also in terms of the structure of the terminals that are formed in the thalamus and the synaptic properties they display. This relationship is discussed in chapters 3 and 5.

---

5. To clarify the distinction between qualitative and quantitative receptive field properties, consider the receptive field of a relay cell of the lateral geniculate nucleus. Its classical visual properties, mainly the ocular input and the center/surround configuration, are what we would term the qualitative receptive field. Quantitative features include overall firing rate or pattern, size of the center or surround, relative strength of center or surround, etc. These quantitative features can be altered without changing the qualitative organization of the receptive field.

In summary, the thalamus can be regarded as a group of cells concerned, directly or indirectly, with passing on to the cerebral cortex information about almost everything that is happening in the central or peripheral nervous system. This includes passing information about one cortical area on to another. This relay of information is subject to a variety of modulatory inputs that modify the way the information is passed to the cortex without significantly altering the nature of that information, except where, as during slow wave sleep, it essentially prevents such information from reaching the cortex (see chapter 6).

We have seen that inhibitory inputs reach thalamic relay cells from the local interneurons and from cells in the thalamic reticular nucleus. In addition, there are some other, GABA[6] immunoreactive, inhibitory afferents going to certain thalamic nuclei. The medial geniculate nucleus receives ascending GABAergic afferents from the inferior colliculus (Peruzzi et al., 1997), the lateral geniculate receives such afferents from the pretectum, there are GABAergic afferents from the zona incerta to higher order thalamic relays (Barthó et al., 2002; but see Power & Mitrofanis, 2002), and the globus pallidus and substantia nigra and zona incerta send GABAergic axons to the ventral anterior and the center median nucleus (Balercia et al., 1996; Ilinsky et al., 1997). The precise role of the GABAergic afferents is not well defined and is discussed further in chapter 7.

1.C.1.b. Topographic Maps
There is another basic feature of the organization of the dorsal thalamus that needs to be understood: most, possibly all, thalamocortical pathways are topographically organized. This organization is most easily seen in the visual, auditory, or somatosensory pathways, where the sensory surfaces (retina, cochlea, body surface) are represented or mapped in an orderly way in the thalamus and in the cortex, so that the pathways linking thalamus and cortex must carry these orderly maps. Even where it is not clear what is being mapped, or where the map appears not to be very accurate, as in many higher order circuits, we shall speak of mapped projections as having "local sign."[7] For example, there is

---

6. Gamma-aminobutyric acid (GABA) is the most common inhibitory neurotransmitter in the thalamus.

7. Mapped projections that represent a sensory or cortical surface have been widely described and discussed in the past. The implication is that such maps are representations that can be interpreted in terms of the detailed topography of their source, and the expectation has been that such maps, to be useful,

evidence for local sign for the whole of the pathways from the mamillary bodies through the anterior thalamus and to the cingulate cortex (Cowan & Powell, 1954), although it is not clear exactly what function is being mapped for most of this pathway.

Strictly speaking, a connection that shows no local sign can be regarded as a "diffuse" projection, but this term is often used rather loosely. Quite often the term is used (see Jones, 1998) to refer to a pathway that shows local sign but has significant overlap of terminal arbors or relatively large receptive fields. It is better to keep the term diffuse for a pathway that demonstrably lacks local sign. This means that the relationship between the cells of origin and the terminal arbors is essentially random in topographic terms, a relationship that is not easy to demonstrate. Mostly the term has been used where experiments based on relatively large lesions or injections of tracers fail to show topography for terminals or cells of origin, or where large receptive fields have been recorded and their topographic ordering has been difficult to discern. Any organization with large receptive fields and a crude local sign must be regarded as topographic rather than diffuse. It is probable that all driver afferents and many modulatory afferents have local sign. Some of the modulatory afferents coming from the brainstem will prove to be truly diffuse, but it is likely that others have local sign (Uhlrich et al., 1988).

A further distinction has to be made between an afferent system that is diffuse and relatively global, terminating throughout the thalamus, and one that is diffuse but has terminals that are limited to a single thalamic nucleus or a few specific terminal zones. Those that terminate throughout the thalamus can be regarded as global from the point of view of thalamic organization in general, whereas others that are limited to a few parts of the thalamus, possibly associated with one sensory modality, are to be seen as specific, although they may prove to be diffuse in the sense of lacking local sign within their specifically localized terminal sites.

It should be clear that within a diffuse projection any one afferent fiber may be limited to a small part of the total terminal zone of that

---

must have relatively small receptive fields. Large receptive fields have been represented as evidence for the lack of a map in a pathway. However, so long as receptive fields do not match the total projection, if they are arranged in a topographic order, then, no matter what their size, we shall treat them as a part of a projection that has local sign. We could refer to "crude maps" and "accurate maps," but we stress the importance of "local sign" because there often is a reluctance to recognize a mapping in a pathway that simply allows a distinction between up and down, left and right.

projection without this revealing anything about the nature of the projection as a whole. It could be a part of a diffuse global pathway, or it could be a part of a mapped projection to a specific terminal region. In contrast, a single cell that sends axonal branches to different parts of a single established map should be regarded as a part of a diffusely organized projection. As the role of the modulatory pathways in the control of thalamic functions becomes defined, these perhaps arcane distinctions are likely to prove functionally highly significant.

The mapped projections between the thalamus and the cortex are of interest not only because they show how a group of thalamic cells relates to a group of cortical cells, but also because they impose important constraints on the pathways that link thalamus and cortex, and these constraints are likely to influence the connections made in the thalamic reticular nucleus as the fibers pass through it on the way to or from the cortex. If the thalamocortical and corticothalamic connections were both simple one-to-one relationships between a single thalamic nucleus and a corresponding single cortical field, then the topographic mapping of the pathways could be carried out by two simple sets of radiating connections, one coming from the thalamus and the other going to the thalamus, meeting each other on the way, as has been proposed by Molnár et al. (1998). The connections of the reticular nucleus lying on this pathway would then relate to this simple radiating pattern, with little interaction between adjacent sectors. However, the real-life situation is far more complex. Single thalamic nuclei can connect to several cortical areas, and vice versa, for both the driving and the modulatory connections. And many of the cortical maps are mirror reversals of each other, as are some of the thalamic maps. Figure 1.7 shows two adjacent cortical areas carrying mirror-reversed topographic maps (represented by 3, 2, 1 and 1, 2, 3 in the cortex) and connected to a single thalamic nucleus. In the cat, relationships in the visual pathways between areas 17 and 18 and the lateral geniculate nucleus show precisely this arrangement. In figure 1.7, the modulatory corticothalamic axons going from layer 6 of the cortex to the thalamus show that the mapping between thalamus and cortex requires complex crossing of the axon pathways. It should be clear that if all of the thalamocortical and corticothalamic pathways, which for any one modality often include several thalamic nuclei or subdivisions and several cortical areas, had been included in the figure, the result would show a complex system of crossing and interweaving axon pathways between the thalamus and the cortex. In the adult, some of this crossing occurs in the region of the thalamic reticular nucleus, as shown

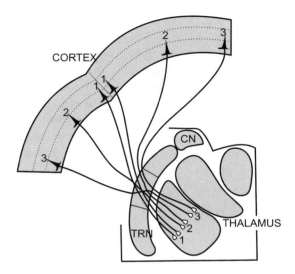

Figure 1.7
Schematic views of a coronal section through thalamus and cortex to show a
single thalamic nucleus such as the lateral geniculate nucleus receiving corticothalamic afferents from two cortical areas. The topographic order of the projections is indicated by the numbers 1–3, and the two cortical representations
are shown, as they often are, as mirror reversals of each other. The axons cross
in the thalamic reticular nucleus, which is not labeled.

in the figure (Adams et al., 1997), and some occurs just below the cerebral cortex (Nelson & LeVay, 1985). The complex crossings are of interest because they establish a potential for connections in the reticular
nucleus between the several maps present in the thalamocortical pathways of any one modality.

To summarize the main points presented so far, the dorsal thalamus can be subdivided into nuclei. Each nucleus sends its outputs to neocortex, and each nucleus receives different types of afferents, some
classifiable as drivers, others as modulators. Many of these connections
are mapped, and the multiplicity of maps leads to complex interconnections in the thalamic reticular nucleus, the major part of the ventral
thalamus.

1.C.2. *The Ventral Thalamus*

The main part of the ventral thalamus lies directly on the pathways that
link the dorsal thalamus to the telencephalon, either the striatum or the

neocortex. Figure 1.6 shows that axons do not pass in either direction between thalamus and telencephalon without going through the ventral thalamus. One important difference between the ventral and the dorsal thalamus is that the ventral thalamus sends no axons to the cortex. In mammals, the major part of the ventral thalamus forms the thalamic reticular nucleus, which was briefly introduced earlier. A smaller part forms the ventral lateral geniculate nucleus, which appears to have specialized roles related to eye movements but is of no further concern here.

As pointed out earlier and shown in figures 1.5 and 1.6, the thalamic reticular nucleus is strategically placed in the course of the axons that are going in both directions between the cerebral cortex and the thalamus. Although the positions of ventral relative to dorsal thalamus change as development proceeds, both sets of axons continue to relate to the ventral thalamic cells, and in the adult, many of them give off collateral branches to the cells of the reticular nucleus. The reticular cells in turn send axons back to the thalamus, roughly to the same region from which they receive inputs. The cortical and thalamic afferents to the reticular nucleus are predominantly excitatory (but see Cox & Sherman, 1999), and the axons that go back from the reticular nucleus to the thalamus are inhibitory (summarized in Jones, 1985). Through these connections the reticular nucleus can play a crucial role in the transmission of information through the thalamic relay to the cerebral cortex.

Although the reticular nucleus has a relatively homogeneous structure, it can be divided into sectors that connect to particular thalamic nuclei or groups of thalamic nuclei and the cortical area to which they connect. Thus, visual, somatosensory, auditory, and motor sectors can be identified, as well as a sector related to the cingulate cortex. Not only do the cells within each of the functionally distinct sectors of the reticular nucleus lie in a key position in terms of their connections, with pathways going in both directions between cortex and thalamus, they also lie in a region where many of these axons undergo some of the complex interweaving discussed earlier. Major changes in the topographic organization of thalamocortical interconnections occur in and just adjacent to the region of the thalamic reticular nucleus, and this pattern of interweaving axons gives the reticular nucleus its characteristic reticulated structure. This structure also contributes to important aspects of the function of the reticular nucleus, because we shall see that within any one sector of the nucleus, connections from more than one thalamic nucleus (first and higher order) and from more than one functionally related cortical area are established. Kölliker (1896), more than 100 years ago, recognized the crossing bundles and called the nucleus the *Gitterkern*, from the German word *Gitter*, for lattice. These axonal crossings and interweavings put the reticular nucleus in a position where the cells within any one sector can serve as a nexus, relating several different but functionally related thalamocortical and corticothalamic pathways to each other.

The thalamic reticular nucleus was for many years considered to have a diffuse organization and to lack the well-defined maps seen in the dorsal thalamus. More recent evidence has shown that in spite of the complex network that characterizes the nucleus, there are maps of peripheral sensory surfaces and of cortical areas within the reticular nucleus (Montero et al., 1977; Crabtree & Killackey, 1989; Conley et al., 1991; Crabtree, 1996). Understanding these maps and how they relate to each other and to the maps within the main thalamocortical pathways is likely to prove a key issue in future studies of the thalamic reticular nucleus.

There is one nucleus that is generally treated as part of the thalamic reticular nucleus and that has a distinct name and may have a distinct developmental origin. This is the perigeniculate nucleus, present in dogs, cats, ferrets, and other members of the order Carnivora. It lies between the reticular nucleus and the dorsal lateral geniculate nucleus, and many of the observations reported for reticular cells and connections have in fact been made in cats or ferrets on the perigeniculate nucleus. Perigeniculate cells show many of the same connections and functional properties as do reticular cells in rodents or primates, and throughout this book we treat the perigeniculate nucleus as a part of the reticular nucleus. However, there are some reasons for thinking that this generally accepted identity may be an oversimplification. This issue is considered in more detail in chapter 9.

1.D. The Overall Plan of the Next Ten Chapters

There are many (more than 30) individually identifiable nuclei in the thalamus, and it is probable that in any one species, each one has a more or less distinctive organization. Further, it is well established, and not surprising, that there are significant differences between species for any pair of homologous nuclei. For example, we noted that the perigeniculate nucleus characterizes members of the order Carnivora, and that some rodents lack interneurons. Some nuclei may receive their primary afferents from just one set or group of axons, whereas other nuclei receive afferents from more than one functionally distinct set of primary afferent or driver pathways. Details of transmitters, receptors, and calcium-binding proteins differ to a significant extent from one nucleus to another, so that it may seem that a book on the thalamus must necessarily be a compendium of details about many individual nuclei. Even if such an account of the many differences among thalamic nuclei were to be limited to commonly used experimental animals, it would form a very heavy and singularly boring volume.

In the following chapters we present accounts of some of the major known structural and functional features of the thalamus. In the early chapters we introduce many of the relevant facts and start to look at interpretations, but our major interpretations are presented in detail in the later parts of the book. We have planned this book to be focused on questions about the functional organization of the thalamic relay in general, and we are especially interested in how this relay operates during normal, active behavioral states. As far as we can, we shall be looking for a common plan of thalamic organization that can serve as a basis for understanding any of the thalamic nuclei. Differences between nuclei can then be seen as opportunities for looking at the possible functional significance of one type of organization relative to another. Much of our discussion is focused on the visual relay through the lateral geniculate nucleus and will extend to other sensory relays, particularly the somatosensory and the auditory relays, as we look for common patterns and detailed differences. These nuclei are, at present, the best-studied thalamic nuclei, and details available for these sensory relays are often not available for the majority of thalamic nuclei.

The visual relay through the lateral geniculate nucleus has received very considerable attention over the years. In part this relates to the fact that we know a great deal about the organization of its input in the retina and about its cortical recipient area, the visual cortex (Hubel & Wiesel, 1977; Martin, 1985; Dowling, 1991; Rodieck, 1998; for more recent overviews see Callaway, 2004; Copenhagen, 2004; Ferster, 2004; Freeman, 2004; Nelson & Kolb, 2004; Sterling, 2004), so that it has been of particular interest to study the thalamic cell group that links these two. Not only has the intrinsic organization of the nucleus received detailed attention, but its reaction to varying, complex regimes of visual deprivation has taught us a great deal about the plasticity and development of thalamocortical connections (Wiesel & Hubel, 1963; Sherman & Spear, 1982; Shatz, 1994; Rittenhouse et al., 1999; Berardi et al., 2003; Heynen et al., 2003). In part the interest in the visual relay relates to the intrinsic beauty of the lateral geniculate nucleus, most evident in primates and carnivores, where mapped inputs from the two eyes are brought into precise register in distinct but accurately aligned layers (Walls, 1953; Kaas et al., 1972a; Casagrande & Xu, 2004). We explore this arrangement in later chapters to a limited extent. Primarily, we use current knowledge of the visual relay in the thalamus to lead to general questions about thalamic organization, first in other sensory pathways and then in thalamic relays more generally.

In the next two chapters we first consider the nerve cells of the thalamus (chapter 2), distinguishing the relay neurons from the local interneurons and reticular cells and looking at the different ways in which distinct classes can be recognized within each of these major cell groups. Then in chapter 3 we look at the afferents that provide inputs to the thalamus, distinguishing them in terms of their structure, origin, and possible functional role as drivers or modulators. In chapter 4 we consider the intrinsic membrane properties of thalamic cells and outline the properties of the several distinctive conductances that determine how a thalamic nerve cell is likely to react to its inputs. In chapter 5 we consider the distinct actions of different types of synaptic input, focusing on the variety of transmitters and receptors that play a role in determining how activity in any one particular group of afferents is likely to influence the cells of the thalamus.

For each of these topics, only some of the available information can at present be readily related to the functional organization of the thalamus, which we consider in the later chapters. Many of the points presented raise key questions about the thalamus that are as yet unanswered. We have listed some of these questions at the end of each chapter, but the reader is likely to find a great many other that are interesting and deserve attention. In these four chapters (2–5) we present evidence in some detail to indicate the range of problems that still need to be considered before anyone can claim to understand the thalamus. As new investigators are attracted to the thalamus, as we hope they will be, they will be able to look at some of these problems anew, and where we see only puzzles and unanswered questions, they are likely to look at the problems from a fresh angle and have new insights. At present, only a limited part of the knowledge that we have about thalamic cells and their functional connections can be interpreted in functional terms.

In the second part of the book we introduce some of the features that are relevant to our view of what it is the thalamus may be doing. Chapter 6 explores the fact that the thalamic relay cells have two distinct response modes, which depend on the intrinsic properties and synaptic inputs discussed in chapters 4 and 5. One is the tonic mode, which allows an essentially linear transfer of information through the thalamus to the cortex, and the other is the burst mode, which does not convey an accurate representation of the afferent signal to cortex but instead has a high signal-to-noise ratio, so that it is well adapted for spotting new signals. Chapter 7 considers the two types of afferent to thalamic relay cells. The drivers serve to bring the information to the relay cells and the modulators determine the mode, burst or tonic, of the relay cell response. Distinguishing drivers from modulators is relatively simple in a few instances, but in many relays the distinction cannot be readily made, and we look at ways in which one may be able to classify afferents as either drivers or modulators. In chapter 8 the distinction between first order and higher order thalamic relays is explored. The former receive their driving afferents from ascending (subcortical) pathways; the latter receive their driving afferents from cortex and so serve as a relay in corticocortical communication, and insert essential thalamic functions into cortical communication. For any one ascending afferent to thalamus, as, for example, for any one sensory modality, there are several higher order circuits and several cortical areas. There are consequently many mapped pathways that relate to each other as they pass through the thalamus and the thalamic reticular nucleus. Chapter 9 considers some of the connectional relationships that are produced by a multiplicity of interconnected topographic maps in first and higher order thalamocortical circuits, showing how the functions of distinct cortical areas are brought into relation with each other in the thalamus and reticular nucleus. Chapter 10 presents evidence that many, possibly all, of the pathways that serve to innervate the thalamus are made up of axons that have branches innervating motor or premotor[8] centers at levels below cortex and thalamus. That is, the pathways that are relayed in the thalamus, first order as well as higher order, carry not just the sensory messages represented by the classical model but also copies of motor commands that have already been sent out to the motor periphery before any messages can reach the cortex. The implication of these connections for understanding how action and perception may be intimately linked

---

8. *Premotor* is used here and in the rest of the book to refer to centers with significant connections to lower motor pathways, as opposed to ascending pathways that pass through the thalamus to the cortex. Examples include the pontine nuclei, the superior colliculus, the inferior olive, and some of the reticular nuclei of the brainstem.

is explored, and we conclude that this close link between action and perception, which has long puzzled philosophers, psychologists, and psychophysicists, may be understood to a significant extent in terms of the close, indeed inexorable, anatomical links that exist at the earliest stages of sensory processing but that have been largely ignored in the past. Chapter 11 presents an overview of some our major conclusions, but we stress that this represents a relatively small slice of what is known about the thalamus. Many of the problems and issues raised as questions or currently unsolved problems in each of the chapters deserve close attention if we are to arrive at a more profound understanding of what it is that the thalamus does.

2   The Nerve Cells of the Thalamus

This chapter is concerned with the different nerve cell types that can be distinguished in the thalamus on the basis of their position, their connections, and their morphology. These features relate closely to each other and to the function of the cells. The position of the cells in a thalamic nucleus or a part of a nucleus, such as a layer, often relates to their connections, and knowledge of these, that is, of the inputs and outputs, is essential for understanding the functional pathway within which any one cell plays a role. The particular functional role of a thalamic cell within a relay pathway, however, is more elusive and relates to the morphology of a cell. That is, the morphology relates to the electrical properties of a cell (see chapter 4) and to the distribution of the afferents on the surface of the cell (discussed in chapter 3). Beyond that, where it is possible to recognize distinct cell types on the basis of their perikaryal size and dendritic arbor, one expects to find that distinct cell types play distinctive roles in the transfer of information through the thalamus.

One basic and simple classification of cells in the dorsal thalamus distinguishes cells with axons that project to the telencephalon from those that have locally ramifying axons. These are the relay cells and the interneurons, respectively. The former have axons that mostly go through the reticular nucleus and the internal capsule to the neocortex, and we consider them first; a minority go to the striatum or amygdala. The interneurons are defined as having axons that stay in the thalamus, generally quite close to the cell body. These two cell types also differ in the pattern of their dendritic arbors and in the transmitters produced, so that even where the axon is not identifiable they are readily distinguishable. The cells of the thalamic reticular nucleus form a distinct third population. They have axons that terminate primarily in the dorsal thalamus, with some evidence for locally ramifying axons within the reticular nucleus itself. Whereas the interneurons and reticular cells are

GABAergic, producing inhibitory actions at the presynaptic terminals of their axons, the relay neurons are glutamatergic and produce excitatory actions.

2.A. On Classifying Relay Cells

2.A.1. Early Methods of Identifying and Classifying Thalamic Relay Cells

Most, probably all, dorsal thalamic nuclei in mammals have cells that project to neocortex. We shall treat the main function of the thalamus as the transmission of messages to the neocortex. From this point of view, thalamocortical cells are self-evidently the most important cells. They also represent the great majority of thalamic cells, from about 70% to 99% in mammals, depending on the nucleus and the species. Cells in the relatively small group of intralaminar and midline nuclei have long been recognized as sending a more significant axonal component to the striatum, as do scattered cells in other thalamic nuclei (Cowan & Powell, 1954; Powell & Cowan, 1956; Macchi et al., 1984; Francois et al., 1991; Giménez-Amaya et al., 1995; Harting et al., 2001; Cheatwood et al., 2003), some connecting to cortex and striatum by branching axons (Macchi et al., 1984). Here we are primarily concerned with the pathway to the cortex, and the pathways to the striatum will not concern us further.

We saw in chapter 1 that an early method of demonstrating the cortical connections of the relay cells was to study the severe and rapid retrograde degeneration that thalamic cells undergo when their cortical terminals are damaged by local lesions (in particular, see Walker, 1938), and it was this degenerative change that proved most useful for early studies of thalamocortical connections. Although the method has now been superceded by others that rely on the identification of axonally transported marker molecules, it is useful to look at the way the earlier method was used and interpreted. This is of interest primarily because interpretations of the degenerative changes have had a profound and longlasting effect on contemporary views of thalamic organization. Further, the degenerative changes that characterize most of the thalamocortical pathways provide an insight into the heavy dependence of thalamic cells on an intact cortical connection.

Small cortical lesions produce well-defined, limited segments of rapid neuronal degeneration and death, with associated gliosis in a corresponding small segment of the relevant thalamic relay nucleus (figure 2.1);

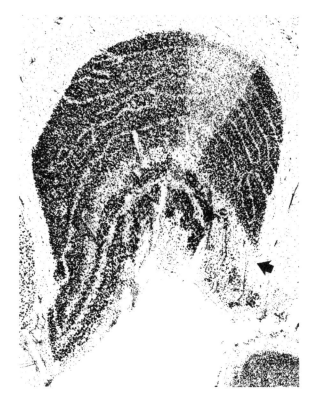

Figure 2.1
Photograph of retrograde degeneration in monkey lateral geniculate nucleus
(from Kaas et al., 1972b). A coronal, Nissl-stained section through the lateral
geniculate nucleus of a mandrill (*Mandrillus sphinx*) shows a sector of retrograde
cell degeneration produced by a restricted lesion in the visual cortex (area 17).
In this animal there were several localized cortical lesions and, correspondingly,
several sectors of retrograde geniculate degeneration. Dorsal is up, medial to the
left. The main sector of degeneration in this section passes through the dorsal,
parvocellular geniculate layers and just includes the dorsal of the ventral two
magnocellular layers. Another sector of degeneration is seen in the magnocellular layers to the right (arrow). A complete serial reconstruction would show each
sector going through all of the geniculate layers.

larger lesions produce more extensive retrograde degeneration in more of the thalamus. Early investigators, particularly von Monakow (1895) and Nissl (1913), used the method of retrograde degeneration to define relationships between the major subdivisions of the thalamus and large areas of cortex and to show that most of the thalamus is "dependent" on the neocortex in this sense. That is, destruction of all of the cerebral cortex, specifically of neocortex, produces retrograde degeneration in all of the thalamic nuclei, sparing only the thalamic reticular nucleus, the cells of the epithalamus, and, to a significant extent, the cells of the midline and intralaminar nuclei (Jones, 1985).

The very dramatic retrograde changes that occur in the thalamus after cortical lesions represent an extreme form of the reaction of a nerve cell to damage of its axon. Cells in many other parts of the nervous system undergo only a mild reaction or no reaction at all after their axons are cut (Bielschowsky, 1928; Geist, 1933; Brodal, 1940). The interpretation of such sparing of damaged cells is generally attributed to axon branches that are not damaged,[1] and on this interpretation one has to regard the relatively modest branches that thalamocortical cells give off before they reach the cortex, mainly to the thalamic reticular nucleus and to local interneurons (Friedlander et al., 1981; Cox et al., 2003), as unable to sustain the thalamic cells damaged by cortical lesions. However, figure 2.2 also shows that it is no longer appropriate to interpret the thalamic degeneration such as that shown in figure 2.1 simply in terms of damage done to the fibers that pass from the thalamus to the cortex. Most, probably all, thalamic nuclei receive afferents back from the cortical area that they innervate, so that one is seeing a combination of transneuronal and retrograde degeneration in the thalamus. We know that often the thalamic cell loss is rapid and severe. It was this that provided such a useful tool for studying the connections between the thalamus and the cortex and fixed attention on the close link between individual thalamic nuclei and functionally or architectonically definable cortical areas (see, e.g., Rose & Woolsey, 1948, 1949). The close link revealed by the lesion studies was interpreted as a "dependence" of thalamus on cortex (see particularly Nissl, 1913; Hassler, 1964). This dependence is evidence for a trophic interaction, but it has often been

---

1. The argument about such "sustaining" collaterals clearly has an unfortunate circular structure, because currently we are unable to define independent criteria by which sustaining branches could be distinguished from nonsustaining branches. Possibly their ability to take up and transport adequate amounts of growth factors could provide the needed criterion.

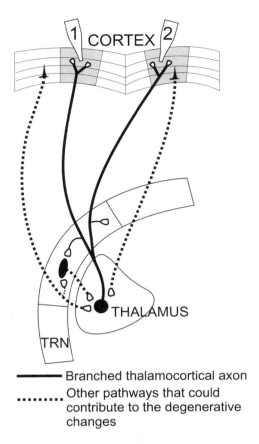

Figure 2.2
Schema to show a single thalamic cell projecting to two cortical areas. Damage to either of the two cortical areas (grey boxes) produced little or no retrograde change in the thalamus, whereas damage to both areas produced severe retrograde cell degeneration. In later experiments, injection of two distinct retrogradely transported markers (1 and 2) demonstrated that single thalamic cells have branching axons, suggesting that these connections play a significant role in the production of the cell changes. For further details see text.

interpreted mainly as a functional link (e.g., Macchi, 1993), which of course it is, as well. And in a sense this link between the degenerative change and the functional role of the pathway was the strength of the method of retrograde degeneration. However, it was also a weakness, because we now know that a mild retrograde reaction, or the absence of a retrograde reaction, does not signify the absence of a functional link (Rose & Woolsey, 1958). As so often, the negative evidence is far less compelling than the positive. It should be stressed that the nature of the functional link, whether driver or modulator (see chapter 7), is important for evaluating the functional significance of thalamocortical pathways generally, far more important than the numerical strength, which is relevant for the degenerative change but is generally undefined.

This last point becomes particularly important where a thalamic relay cell in a major thalamic nucleus sends axonal branches to more than one cortical area (Geisert, 1980; Tong & Spear, 1986; Miceli et al., 1991), or, as do some of the cells of the intralaminar nuclei, sends branches to the striatum and to a cortical area (Macchi et al., 1984). Then damage to one axon branch may not be sufficient to produce a marked retrograde change, whereas damage to both branches is (figure 2.2). This interpretation was first explicitly proposed by Rose and Woolsey in 1958. On the basis of the retrograde reactions visible in Nissl preparations of the medial geniculate nucleus after localized lesions of more than one area of auditory cortex, they proposed that there are "sustaining" projections passing from the medial geniculate nucleus to the auditory cortex. A sustaining projection was defined as one whose cortical terminals could be destroyed without producing any significant thalamic degeneration but, when cut in combination with damage to another cortical area, produced severe retrograde changes in the thalamus that the second lesion alone did not produce. This was interpreted as evidence for single thalamic cells having axons that branched to innervate more than one cortical area. Although this did not represent the only interpretation of the evidence at the time, it is now reasonably regarded as the best interpretation, and it was a critical step forward in our understanding of thalamocortical relationships. Subsequently such branched axons were demonstrated for several thalamocortical pathways by the use of two distinguishable retrogradely transported markers such as those used in the studies cited earlier in this paragraph.

The method of retrograde degeneration thus allows us to categorize relay cells in terms of the thalamic nucleus they belong to and the cortical area they connect to, and on occasion the method can show cells that send their axons to more than one cortical area. On the whole, the method was not very good at revealing the interneurons that fail to degenerate after a cortical lesion, generally because these are small and tend to get lost among the heavy glial changes that accompany the retrograde neuronal degeneration. Initially the interneurons were recognized on the basis of Golgi preparations (see below), although incontrovertible evidence that these small cells did not send an axonal branch to the cortex had to await the advent of two techniques: reliable retrograde markers like horseradish peroxidase, and the demonstration that cells not labeled retrogradely when injections of such markers are made into cortex are immunoreactive for GABA or GAD[2] (Penny et al., 1983; Montero, 1986). For the thalamocortical projections, horseradish peroxidase allows the ready distinction between relay cells and interneurons, provided that the retrograde marker has labeled a sufficiently extensive area of cortex to include all candidate relay cell axons for that sector of the thalamocortical projection. Since the interneurons of the thalamus are GABAergic whereas the relay neurons are glutamatergic, the GABA immunoreactivity of the cells that are not labeled by the horseradish peroxidase provides strong evidence about the distinction between interneurons and relay cells and has now gained sufficient acceptability that in the thalamus, the identification of interneurons can be made on the basis of immunohistochemical methods that reveal the presence of GABA, by staining either for GABA itself or for GAD, an enzyme involved in its synthesis. Other features that distinguish interneurons from relay cells are considered in sections 4.A.3, 4.B.3, 5.B, and 5.C.

2.A.2. General Problems of Cell Classification

Often in the past, relay cells were classified on the basis of a single variable, such as cell size, type of axonal or dendritic arbor, axon diameter or conduction velocity, receptive field properties, or on the basis of two apparently loosely linked variables. Because each quantifiable parameter can vary continuously, it is important to ensure that one is dealing with two distinguishable populations rather than two parts of one continuous population, or (worse still) a continuous population whose extremes are described, measured, and stressed while intermediate values are ignored or arbitrarily assigned to the "populations" represented by

---

2. Glutamic acid decarboxylase (GAD) is critical for the production of GABA and is often used as a marker for GABAergic processes.

one or the other extreme, as has happened with earlier studies of thalamus.[3]

If a classification is based on only one variable (such as size), and if this variable can be represented as a single bell-shaped function, then one should generally reject claims for distinct classes, even though cells at the high and low ends of the distribution may play somewhat different functional roles. If the relevant parameter shows two quite distinct peaks in a population histogram, or if it is a characteristic that shows no intermediate forms, such as having a particular calcium-binding protein or not having it, having terminals in layer IV of cortex or not having them, then of course one is on surer ground. Also, it is possible that two or more single parameters vary continuously, but when they are plotted against each other clear clustering can be seen, indicating two or more distinct classes.

An excellent demonstration of such clustering is the morphological study of retinal ganglion cells by Boycott and Wässle (1974) that was reanalyzed by Rodieck and Brening (1983), who found that soma size forms a single continuum, but when this was plotted against retinal position there was a clear separation of the data points into two clusters, which correspond to the retinal Y and X cells, respectively (see legend for figure 2.5 for the functional distinction between X cells and Y cells). Figure 2.3 shows their results, and figure 2.4 shows a comparable study of cells in the lateral geniculate nucleus. In figure 2.4 the dendritic arbors are analyzed in terms of dendritic intersections with "Sholl" circles (see caption). It is clear that when the distribution of these intersections is plotted against cell body size, cells that have receptive field properties characteristic of X cells are readily distinguished from those that have the properties of Y cells. As we shall see, it is entirely reasonable to expect that for thalamic nuclei in general, when appropriate sets of variables are studied, dendritic arbors will contribute significantly to defining functionally distinguishable relay cell classes, but exactly how the shape of dendritic arbors relates to the function of thalamic cells is still not defined. For any proposed classification, the more independent parameters one can measure and plot in n-dimensional space, the more likely one is to find evidence for discontinuities in their distribution and, thus, a justification for distinct classes, if they exist.

Whereas it is possible to demonstrate that two or more classes exist within a population if the parameters measured form clusters of values,

---

3. Walshe's (1948) discussion of the giant cells of Betz in motor cortex is entertaining, instructive, and pertinent to this point.

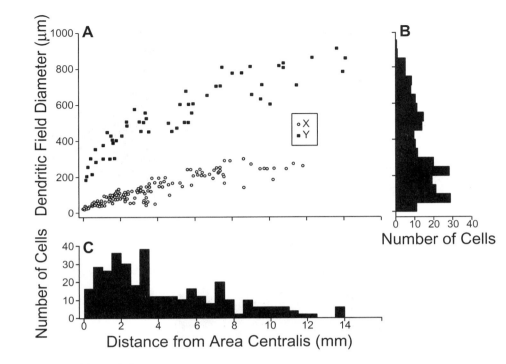

Figure 2.3
Measures of distance from the area centralis within retina and diameter of dendritic arbor for X and Y retinal ganglion cells of the cat. *A.* Relationship of the two variables. Note the clear separation of the X and Y classes within this scatterplot. *B.* Histogram of dendritic arbor diameters for cells in *A. C.* Histogram of distances from the area centralis for cells in *A.* Note that with the single parameters of *B* and *C,* it is not possible to discern more than a single cell population. (Redrawn from Rodieck and Brening, 1983, and based on the data of Boycott and Wässle, 1974, with permission). For the functional distinction between the X and Y cells, see the legend for figure 2.5.

one cannot use such a method to prove that a cell population forms a single class, because the *appropriate* parameters may not have been studied. Again, the negative evidence can say nothing about the possible presence of important distinctions. In general, when one is dealing with distinct populations, one expects to find that several parameters vary independently, and such independent variation will not only strengthen the logical basis of a classification but may also make it more interesting in terms of the functional implications.

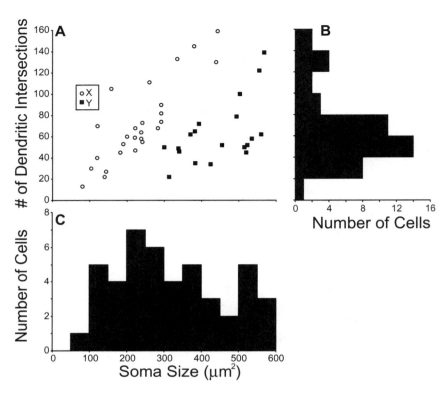

Figure 2.4
Measures of soma size and number of dendritic intersections for X and Y relay cells of the cat's lateral geniculate nucleus; conventions as in figure 2.3. Dendritic intersections derive from Sholl ring analysis as follows. A two-dimensional reconstruction was made of the neuron on tracing paper, and a series of concentric circles spaced at 50-µm intervals was centered on the soma. The number of intersections made by the dendrites with these rings was counted. Note again that the clear separation of the X and Y classes that could, in separate experiments, be shown to have the functional properties of X and Y cells is seen in A, with two variables, but is lost when a single variable is measured (B and C).

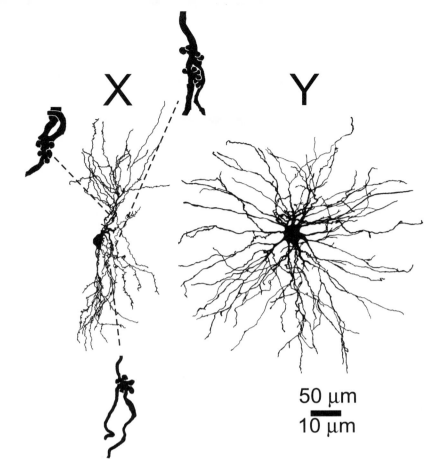

Figure 2.5
Tracings of an X cell and a Y cell from the A-laminae of the cat's lateral geniculate nucleus. The cells were identified physiologically during in vivo intracellular recording, and then horseradish peroxidase was passed from the recording pipette into the cell bodies. With minor, subtle changes, the receptive field properties of these thalamic neurons are the same as those of their retinal afferents, and thus the X/Y differences are established in the retina. Compared to X cells, Y cells have larger receptive fields at matched retinal eccentricities, faster conducting axons, better responses to visual stimuli of low spatial and high temporal frequencies, but poorer responses to low temporal and high spatial frequencies; also, Y cells respond to higher spatial frequencies with a nonlinear doubling response, whereas X cells show excellent linear summation to all stimuli (for details, see Sherman & Spear, 1982; Shapley & Lennie, 1985; Sherman, 1985). With proper histological processing, the horseradish peroxidase provides a dense stain, allowing visualization of the entire somadendritic morphology. The dendritic arbor of the X cell has the tufted pattern, is elongated, and is oriented perpendicular to the plane of the layers, whereas the Y cell dendrites show a stellate distribution with an approximately spherical arbor. The X cell also has prominent clusters of dendritic appendages near proximal branch points. These are hard to see in the cell reconstructions, so three examples are shown at greater magnification, with dashed lines indicating their dendritic locations (the scale is 50 μm for the cell reconstructions and 10 μm for the dendritic appendage examples). Data from Friedlander et al. (1981).

2.A.3. The Possible Functional Significance of Cell Classifications in the Thalamus

There are two distinct ways of looking at the possible functional significance of differences between any two classes of relay cell in the thalamus. These two ways are generally implicit in past studies of relay cells, but they have rarely been made explicit or clearly distinguished from each other. One is that the different types of relay cell may have different integrative functions,[4] modifying receptive field properties or the nature of the message in characteristically distinct ways. The other is that all relay cells may do more or less the same thing in the transfer of information from afferents to cortex but differ either because different demands have to be met, in terms perhaps of impulse frequencies, conduction velocities, or cortical distribution patterns, or because of differing patterns of modulatory or gating actions that they can be exposed to. That is, on this second view, differences among relay cells represent either the nature of the traffic that is transmitted, or the cortical distribution of the message, or the characteristics of the modulation. They do not reflect differences in integrative functions.

This second view appears to receive experimental support in the lateral geniculate nucleus of the cat, because where functionally distinct afferent pathways can be defined in terms of the different receptive field properties that they transmit (the X and the Y pathways mentioned earlier [see figures 2.4 and 2.5] provide a good example), they use relay cells that can be distinguished from each other on the basis of many or all of the features just listed. However, they do not appear to be concerned to any great degree with modifying receptive field properties.

In the visual pathway, the receptive field properties change quite significantly at each relay from retinal receptor to the higher visual cortical areas *except* in the lateral geniculate nucleus. There is, to our knowledge, no clear evidence to suggest that the thalamus is concerned with the sorts of transforms that change receptive field properties in the other visual relays.[5] Nor is there any clear evidence that messages from two or more

---

4. We take integrative functions to be functions that sum different driver inputs to produce an output that differs *qualitatively* from that of any of the inputs.

5. A comparable absence of significant change in the transthalamic pathway also appears to characterize the somatosensory pathways, as well as the anterior dorsal thalamic nucleus (see chapter 10, section B.3).

inputs are combined in the thalamus.[6] It appears that the major definable function of thalamic relay cells is the transfer of a particular set of receptive field properties *without* significant modification of those properties. Instead, there are "gating" functions or "modulatory" functions that change the way in which the message is transmitted or that change features like receptive field size or contrast properties, without changing the essential content. We discuss these functions in chapters 5 and 6 and argue that they are characteristic for the thalamus in general, although evidence for most other thalamic relays is less clear-cut. At present there is no reason to think that any thalamic relay is concerned with the transformation of the message that it receives. If so, then it may prove to be a mistake to look for the "integrative" actions of the thalamus. One then has to ask what, on the second view, do differences in cell size, axon diameter, dendritic arbor, and so forth, of relay cells signify?

These differences may relate to the characteristics of the message transmitted, to the way in which the message is distributed, to the amount of convergence or divergence in the pathway, or to the way in which the message is modulated or gated. Thicker thalamocortical axons may transmit to more cortical areas or innervate more cells in any one cortical area, and may require larger cell bodies to sustain more axon terminals. Different cell sizes and dendritic architectures may relate to different patterns of modulator input. There may also be differences in the frequency with which the gating functions of the thalamus need to be employed. For any one transthalamic route, one of these functional properties may dominate over others, but on this view, the basic function of the thalamic relay, the transmittal of messages from its driving pathways to cortex with minimal modification of information content, would itself remain invariant. Whatever it is that the thalamus does, whether it is one gating function or several, each class of relay cell can then be thought to share this function or group of functions. An example

---

6. Merabet et al. (1998) have described some cells in the lateral posterior-pulvinar complex of the cat that respond selectively to the direction of moving targets and have suggested that this may reflect novel receptive field elaboration at the level of the thalamus from nonselective afferents. However, the authors acknowledge that it is also possible (and we think likely) that these receptive fields arise in the cortex or midbrain and are not generated in the thalamus. For the critical experiment to demonstrate the thalamic origin of these receptive field properties, it would be necessary to show that none of the afferents to the lateral posterior-pulvinar complex had these properties—a difficult experiment in view of the several afferents.

is given in chapter 5, section 5.C.1.a, where it is shown that one class of geniculate cell, the X cell (but not the Y cell), is subject to interneuronal actions that are likely to be concerned with mechanisms of gain control.

That is, it becomes important to look at differences among relay cells in order to define how the relay of information through the thalamus is modulated or gated in particular ways for particular thalamocortical pathways. One should regard the differences between relay cells as related, for example, to the different ways in which one pathway might be more readily brought into or out of an attentional focus. Further, the modulatory inputs that are needed by a relay concerned with rapid actions, such as a nociceptive pathway or one concerned with large, rapidly approaching objects, are likely to be distinct from the modulatory inputs required by pathways concerned with fine, detailed, discriminatory actions.

The main aim, then, of a classification of relay cells will be to establish features that characterize cells with functionally different properties. Although traditionally the most important feature of a thalamic relay cell concerns the type of information that it transmits to cortex, we have argued that this, strictly speaking, is not a property of the cell but of its input. That is, it is probable, indeed highly likely, that two thalamic relay cells that are indistinguishable on the basis of any of the features identified above, except perhaps for the cortical destination of their axons, will be responsible for relaying quite different messages. For example, a cell in the lateral geniculate nucleus may have precisely the same morphology, synaptic relationships, postsynaptic receptors, cable properties, voltage dependent membrane conductances, and so forth as one in the medial geniculate nucleus, and, if so, we would consider these cells to be of the same class, even though they relay different messages (i.e., visual versus auditory).

For any comparison of relay cells that one cares to make, whether the comparison be of cells within a nucleus or of cells in different nuclei, it is possible to assert that differences in structure and synaptic connectivity will relate to functionally significant differences. Conversely, where relay cells show the same features, no matter whether they are in one thalamic nucleus or another, dealing with auditory, visual, somatosensory, or other afferents, they will have similar relay functions. However, at present, we do not have sufficient evidence for a clear statement about exactly what the functionally relevant features are. Ideally one would like to be able to relate the intrinsic functional characteristics of cells, that is, their membrane properties, their receptors, transmitters, and so on (considered in chapters 4 and 5), to the morphological features that are the focus of this chapter. When we consider the detailed differences between X and Y cells illustrated in figures 2.4 and 2.5, we shall see that there are examples where the light and electron microscopic appearance of dendritic structures relates to the known synaptic connectivity patterns and thus to certain relay functions of some thalamic cells, but generally we cannot look at a cell, classify it on the basis of the structural details of its cell body, or dendrites, and arrive at functionally telling conclusions. This is an important task for the future, and one that is a challenge for many other parts of the brain, not just for the thalamus (see, e.g., Parra et al., 1998).

2.A.4. Classifications of Relay Cells Based on Dendritic Arbors and Perikaryal Sizes

Figures 2.4 and 2.5 illustrate some of the differences between the X cells and the Y cells of the lateral geniculate nucleus of the cat as seen with the light microscope. These two cell types are the best specified distinct relay cell classes for any thalamic nucleus and any species and are representative of three or more distinct cell classes demonstrable in the lateral geniculate relay of many different species. Summaries of these different cell classes, their possible functional characteristics, retinal inputs, and cortical axon terminals, have been provided by Sherman (1985) and Casagrande and Xu (2004; see also Kaplan, 2004). The major morphological differences between the X cells and the Y cells are summarized in the caption to figure 2.5, and their functional differences are considered further in chapter 5. The most striking structural difference relates to the pattern of branching of the dendrites, and to the clusters of dendritic appendages found close to the branch points of the dendrites of the X but not the Y cells.

The distinct branching patterns of dendrites seen in figure 2.5 is a commonly reported feature of thalamic relay cells. Kölliker already in 1896 described "bushy" and "radiate" cells in Golgi preparations of the thalamus of several different species, including *Homo sapiens*, and in several different nuclei (figure 2.6).

The radiate cells are larger, have a more angular cell body, are multipolar, and have dendrites that branch dichotomously, so that the number of dendritic branches increases gradually with increasing distance from the cell body. The bushy cells have somewhat smaller, rounded cell bodies, and their dendrites branch so as to resemble a paint-

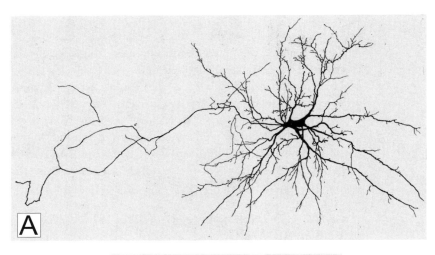

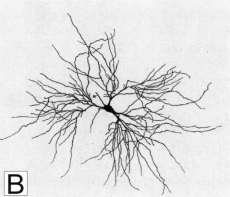

Figure 2.6
Thalamic cells illustrated by Kölliker (1896). *A* and *B* show individual radiate and bushy cells, respectively, *A* from a cat and *B* from a human thalamus. Golgi method.

brush. That is, these dendrites give off many branches close to each other, so that the number of dendritic branches increases rather suddenly with increasing distance from the cell body. These cells can be multipolar, triangular, or bipolar. Kölliker reported that the bushy cells often had a paler appearance in the Golgi preparations than the radiate cells.

Varying terminologies have been used in more recent accounts, but these two basic cell types are recognizable in Golgi preparations in several thalamic nuclei (Morest, 1964; Guillery, 1966; LeVay & Ferster, 1977; Winer & Morest, 1983; figure 2.7) although the pale appearance of the bushy cells is not mentioned. Where cells have been filled by intracellular markers such as horseradish peroxidase or biocytin (Friedlander et al., 1981; Stanford et al., 1983; Bartlett & Smith, 1999; see figure 2.7), one sees a more complete picture of the dendritic arbor, and the distinction between stellate cells and bushy cells is clear.

These distinctions among relay cells have not been identified in all thalamic nuclei and are sometimes blurred because there are intermediate types (Guillery, 1966; Pearson & Haines, 1980). Moreover, strict criteria for distinguishing between cells that represent two ends of a continuum have only rarely been applied. In addition, there is some confusion because observers have used different terminologies and seem to have used different criteria. In the visual and auditory pathways of the cat the bushy cells are smaller, have smaller cell bodies, and commonly have oriented, bipolar dendritic arbors, which the radiate type do not show, and this is in accord with Kölliker's description. The two cell types have been called "stellate" and "bushy" or "tufted," respectively, in the medial geniculate nucleus of the cat (Winer, 1985), and, confusingly, the cells that were described as class 1 (radiate) and class 2 (bushy), respectively, in the cat lateral geniculate nucleus (Guillery, 1966) were later called type 1 and type 2 by LeVay and Ferster (1977), and then type 2 and type 1 (respectively) in the cat ventral posterior nucleus by Yen et al. (1985b). However, Yen et al. claim that in the cat somatosensory pathways, tufted (bushy) cells are larger than the radiate type. Peschanski et al. (1984) and Ohara and Havton (1994; Havton & Ohara, 1994) found no distinctions among relay neurons in the ventral posterior nucleus of the rat, cat, or monkey, but a difference between bushy and radiate cells was described by Pearson and Haines (1980) for this nucleus in the bush baby (*Galago*). Possibly there is a species difference, or perhaps the cell types in the ventral posterior nucleus deserve further study.

We have pointed out that quantitative analyses of one or more parameters cannot prove that a cell population forms a single class. The

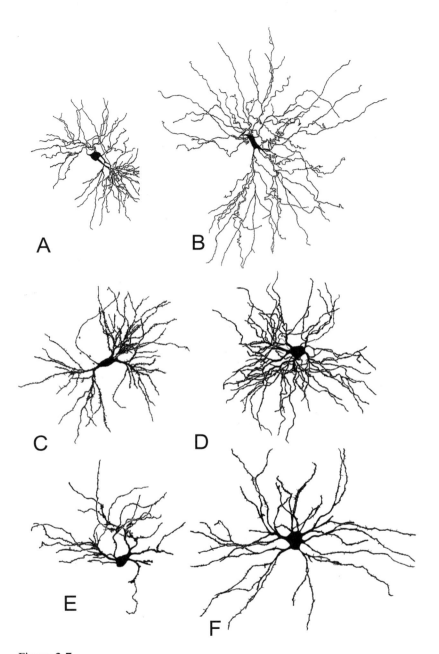

Figure 2.7
Three bushy (*A*, *C*, *E*) and three radiate (*B*, *D*, *F*) thalamic cells. *A* and *B* are cells from the medial geniculate nucleus of a rat that have been filled by intracellular injection of biocytin (Bartlett & Smith, 1999, with permission), *C* and *D* are from Golgi preparations of the medial geniculate nucleus of a cat (Winer & Morest, 1983, with permission), and *E* and *F* are from Golgi preparations of the lateral geniculate nucleus of a cat (Guillery, 1966, with permission). All magnifications are approximately × 200.

type of quantitative analysis used in the lateral geniculate nucleus of the cat by Sherman and colleagues (Friedlander et al., 1981; Stanford et al., 1983), who recorded dendritic intersections with spheres of increasing size centered around the perikaryon (the so-called Sholl circles), may provide a useful tool for identifying cell classes in other nuclei. Bartlett and Smith (1999) used this method in the medial geniculate nucleus of the rat and found that only bushy cells could be identified in the ventral division of the nucleus, but that the two cell types are distinguishable in the magnocellular division, suggesting that there may be an important difference between relay nuclei, with some containing only one type of relay cell and others having distinguishable stellate and bushy cells.

It is evident that defining distinct cell types on the basis of dendritic arbors has not been straightforward. However, there are enough hints in the literature for a reassessment of Kölliker's original account to be worthwhile. In the lateral geniculate nucleus of the cat, the more radiate type (class 1 of Guillery, 1966) has dendrites that appear to cross laminar boundaries relatively freely, whereas the bushy type (Guillery's class 2) has dendrites that tend to be confined to the lamina within which the cell body lies, suggesting that the two classes differ in the way that their peripheral dendritic segments relate to their afferents. Comparable relationships have been described for bushy cells in the ventral posterior nucleus of the rat, which have proximal dendrites confined within a single thalamic "barreloid," a well-defined cell group representing a single vibrissa, and have peripheral dendritic segments extending beyond their "home" barreloid (Deschênes et al., 2005). In the cat, the bushy cells are generally functionally identifiable as X cells, and the radiate cells are Y cells. Close to the site where the primary dendrites of the bushy cells characteristically give rise to several secondary branches, a number of prominent rounded dendritic appendages, described by Szentágothai (1963) as "grapelike appendages,"[7] tend to be grouped (Guillery, 1966; Friedlander et al., 1981; Stanford et al., 1983; see also figure 2.5). These are postsynaptic specializations that relate to the retinal afferents and to synapses formed by interneurons in complex synaptic arrangements called "triads" within "glomeruli" (Szentágothai, 1963; see chapter 3 for details), suggesting that the bushy cells establish complex synaptic connections with interneurons that the radiate cells lack. However, this

---

7. These appendages are not comparable, in their structure or their dendritic distribution, to dendritic spines such as are seen on pyramidal cells of the cerebral cortex or Purkinje cells in cerebellum.

difference, while it may apply to the cell classes found in the lateral geniculate nucleus of the cat and the ventral posterior nucleus of the bush baby (Pearson & Haines, 1980), is not likely to apply to the medial geniculate nucleus of the rat, where Bartlett and Smith (1999) have described bushy and radiate cells but where interneurons are absent or very rare (Winer & Larue, 1988; Arcelli et al., 1997), as also are the grapelike appendages.

The only conclusion one can reasonably come to at present is that relay cells differ in the patterns of their dendritic structures, that this difference relates to perikaryal size, and that some of the characteristic patterns seen in one thalamic nucleus can also be seen in others. A comparison of relay cells in the ventral posterior and pulvinar nuclei of monkey (Darian-Smith et al., 1999) did not focus on distinctions between relay cell types in either nucleus but did find that detailed quantitative comparisons showed no difference between these two nuclei. As a tool useful for distinguishing relay cell types, dendritic arbors and cell sizes have provided suggestive evidence for more than 100 years, but have so far not provided crucial evidence about a functionally significant classification. One reason for this is that classifying cells is more complex than is often recognized, which was our reason for starting this section with a discussion of classifications.

One might argue that the distinction between X and Y cells in the cat's lateral geniculate nucleus, which corresponds roughly to a distinction between bushy and radiate cells, provides the needed functional link to the morphological distinction. However, the major functional properties of the X and the Y pathways are established in the retina. These functional differences do not relate to the nature of the relay in the thalamus. The best clue to come out of a comparison of the cat's X and Y pathways is considered in chapter 3. The geniculate X cell dendrites relate to interneurons at "triadic" junctions, whereas the Y cell dendrites do not.[8] The possibility that the dendritic morphology relates to the way

---

8. Here and in subsequent sections we shall treat the cat's X pathway as postsynaptic to interneuronal dendritic processes and to triads, and regard the Y pathway as not having these synaptic relationships. This is based on several studies of the geniculate A layers (LeVay & Ferster, 1977; Friedlander et al., 1981; Wilson et al., 1984; Hamos et al., 1986). We recognize that two recent studies (Datskovskaia et al., 2001; Dankowski & Bickford, 2003) have provided evidence to show that some Y cell axons in the A layers are presynaptic to interneuronal dendritic processes (although actual triads appear to be rare). Dankowski et al. showed such postsynaptic interneuronal dendrites in the mag-

in which the dendrites contact interneurons is appealing and merits exploration in other thalamic nuclei. However, recent in vitro evidence from the lateral geniculate nucleus of rats and cats is discouraging in this context, because the presence of clustered appendages in the cat cells is indicative of a triadic input, whereas there seemed to be no correlation between appendages and triadic inputs for the rat cells (Lam et al., 2005). Further, as mentioned earlier, in the rat medial geniculate nucleus, where there are reputed to be no interneurons, and thus there can be no triads, there are distinct bushy and radiate cells (see Bartlett et al., 2000). The problem remains: which properties of thalamic cells relate to the nature of the message that is being transmitted and which relate to the ways in which the message is modulated on its way to the cortex? And how do these properties relate to the morphologically identifiable features?

---

nocellular C layer of the lateral geniculate nucleus, which is recognized as having Y relays but no X relays (reviewed in Sherman, 1985). Datskovskaia et al. showed some such postsynaptic interneuronal dendrites in the A layers. Their experiments involved large injections into the superior colliculus of biotynilated dextran amine (BDA). Since Y cells send axons that branch, going to the lateral geniculate nucleus and the superior colliculus, but X cells send branches to the pretectum but not the colliculus, the BDA injections were designed to label Y cell terminals in the lateral geniculate nucleus without also labeling X cell terminals. Because the precise uptake site of the BDA is difficult to define, there is a possibility that some pretectal X axons were also labeled, but we think it more likely that these studies revealed a second type of Y relay cell (see Colby, 1988, and section 2.A.6) found in the magnocellular C layers and at the borders of the A layers but not in the main part of the A layers. Thus, Datskovskaia et al. (2001), although they made relatively large injections into the tectum, which should have labeled all of the Y axons for a large part of the visual field representation, found only patchy labeling of terminal arbors in the lateral geniculate nucleus, with the patches distributed close to the laminar borders, and apparently largely absent in the main central part of the A layers. That is, it would appear that the retrograde labeling of axonal branches may be selective for a particular type of Y axon only (probably the thickest; see also Kelly et al. [2003], who report a failure of such labeling for corticothalamic axons that send a branch to the superior colliculus). We conclude that there are probably two, possibly more, types of Y cell in the cat's lateral geniculate nucleus, and that the main population of Y cell axon terminals in the A layers has very few postsynaptic interneuronal dendrites. Our discussion throughout the following will concern the main Y cell relay in the geniculate A layers and will stress the connectional difference between the two pathways. The possibility that there is another distinct Y cell pathway with a different connectional pattern, one that is also distinct from that of the X pathway, merits further study.

So far we have considered the two major classes of relay cell. A third, relatively small type of relay cell that is not readily identifiable as either bushy or radiate has also to be recognized, and will figure in the discussion that follows. In the lateral geniculate nucleus of the cat, Guillery (1966) described these cells as "class 4" cells, and in the following they correspond to the "W cells" of carnivores and to the "koniocellular" relay cells of primates. In terms of their dendritic morphology they have been described so far only in the cat (Stanford et al., 1983), and they can be more readily identified on the basis of their laminar position in the lateral geniculate nucleus or their cortical arborizations of their axons (Casagrande & Xu, 2004).

2.A.5. Laminar Segregations of Distinct Classes of Geniculocortical Relay Cells

Other criteria for distinguishing thalamic cells include the nature of the afferents they receive, the particular characteristics of their receptive field properties, and the sizes and patterns of distribution of their axons and axonal terminals in the cerebral cortex. For the mammalian lateral geniculate nucleus, all of these features are distinguishable, and the cells are segregated into distinct laminae on the basis of one or several of these features, almost as though they had been designed to illustrate discussions of thalamic cell classifications for a book such as this one (figure 2.8). The functional or developmental reasons for this laminar segregation are not clear, but different mammalian species show quite different patterns of laminar segregation, providing a useful approach to looking at ways of classifying thalamic relay cells.

We have briefly introduced the distinction between geniculate X cells, Y cells, and W cells of the cat to explore the possible significance of classifications that can be based on dendritic arbors and on the appearance and size of the cell body. In the lateral geniculate nucleus of carnivores and primates, three functionally distinct classes of relay cell have been recognized, and they may well contain subclasses (reviewed in Sherman & Spear, 1982; Sherman, 1985; Casagrande & Norton, 1991; Hendry & Calkins, 1998; Van Hooser et al., 2003; Casagrande & Xu, 2004; Kaplan, 2004). Each cell type receives afferents that have distinctive axon diameters (and conduction velocities), with the cat's Y cells having the thickest axons and the W cells having the thinnest. They come from functionally and structurally distinct classes of retinal ganglion cell. These retinal ganglion cell classes in the cat develop in a distinct sequence (X before Y before W; Walsh & Polley, 1985), and their axons occupy

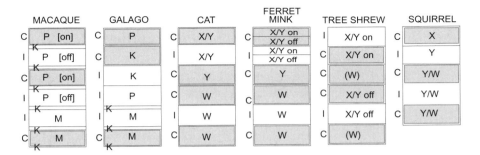

Figure 2.8
Schema to show the laminar distribution of cell types in the layers of the lateral geniculate nucleus of six different species (Kaas et al., 1972a; Sherman & Spear, 1982; Sherman, 1985; Casagrande & Norton, 1991; Hendry & Calkins, 1998; Van Hooser et al., 2003). The shaded boxes show layers innervated by a crossed pathway from the eye on the opposite side (C = contralateral), and the unshaded boxes show an uncrossed pathway from the eye on the same side (I = ipsilateral). The magnocellular (M), parvocellular (P), and koniocellular (K) pathways are shown for macaque and *Galago*; the X, Y, and W pathways are shown for cat, ferret, mink, and tree shrew. For the squirrel, the pathways were described as X-like, Y-like, etc., but are here labeled, X, Y, W. The on-center and off-center afferents are indicated by "on" and "off" for the ferret and mink and are shown as [on] and [off] for the macaque to indicate that there is some disagreement about this result in the monkey (see text). Note that there are often further subdivisions of the parvocellular layers in human and other primate brains, but their functional significance is not known (Hickey & Guillery, 1979; Malpeli et al., 1996). See text for further details.

correspondingly distinct positions in the optic tract (X deepest, Y and W most superficial). Each class of retinogeniculate axon has a distinct pattern of termination in the layers of the lateral geniculate nucleus (see figure 2.8), and each class of geniculate cell has axons with a distinct laminar distribution in the cortex. Further, in the cat, each ganglion cell class is characterized by the branches it sends to the midbrain (Fukuda & Stone, 1974; Wässle & Illing, 1980; Leventhal et al., 1985; Sur et al., 1987; Tamamaki et al., 1994). The X and Y relay cells in the cat also show distinctive types of synaptic relationships with retinal afferents and interneurons, which are discussed in chapter 3, section D.2.

The above summary shows that each class of geniculate relay cell provides an apparently independent channel for transmission from functionally distinctive retinal ganglion cells through to the visual cortex. These are the best-known examples of pathways that share a single thalamic nucleus or lamina and yet provide independent parallel relays with little or no interaction between the pathways apart from some modulatory interactions (for the cat: Sherman & Spear, 1982; Sherman, 1985). At this point, details of the known functional distinctions between the pathways are not relevant to the following consideration of the differences between the geniculate cells (for examples of such functional distinctions, however, see Lennie, 1980; Sherman, 1985; Van Hooser et al., 2003; Kaplan, 2004), because the distinctions depend primarily on the properties of the retinal ganglion cells that innervate the geniculate cells. This may seem strange at first sight; it is a measure of the difficulties we have in relating the structure and connections of thalamic cells to their function in the relay.

In primates, relay cells in descending order of cell body size and of axon diameter have been identified as magnocellular, parvocellular, and koniocellular. The first two lie in the correspondingly named geniculate layers (magnocellular layers 1 and 2, parvocellular layers 3–6 of Old World monkeys), and the koniocellular groups lie between these layers and, to a certain extent, scattered within them (see figure 2.8). In the bush baby, *Galago*, however, the koniocellular group forms distinct layers, and this provided a useful first experimental approach to these small cells in primates. In carnivores (cat, ferret, mink), the largest cells (Y cells) and the medium-sized cells (X cells) are almost entirely intermingled with each other in the major layers of the lateral geniculate nucleus (layers A and A1), whereas the smallest cells (W cells) are found in the small-celled C layers nearest the optic tract. Other parts of the nucleus show some segregation of Y and W cells from X cells. Again, cell body size relates to axon diameter. In the squirrel, the X-like cells are separated from the Y- and W-like cells, but the Y-like cells and the W-like cells share layers.

For each of these separate retinogeniculate pathways there is a so-called on-center system and an off-center system (for details of the two types of retinal ganglion cell that provide the afferents, see Rodieck, 1998), and these are also mingled in the A layers of cats. However, in ferrets (and mink), which have a geniculate relay basically similar to that of the cat, with the X and Y pathways mingled as in the cat, the on-center and off-center pathways lie in separate geniculate layers (LeVay & McConnell, 1982; Stryker & Zahs, 1983) and have separate cortical terminations. There is no evidence that the function of these pathways is significantly different in cat and ferret (or mink). In Old World monkeys, there is some evidence (Schiller & Malpeli, 1978; but see Derrington & Lennie, 1984) to suggest that the on-center parvocellular relay cells are partially separated from the off-center relay cells in distinct geniculate layers, but this is so only for central vision. For peripheral parts of the visual field the on- and off-center cells share geniculate layers, and here again there is no hint of a functional correlate. A comparison of carnivores and monkeys shows that the W pathway in carnivores has its cells in a separate layer, but that in the monkey (but not the bush baby) the koniocellular pathways have their cells scattered among the M and P cells. That is, although there is a definite tendency for functionally distinct cells to segregate within the nucleus, there is no general rule governing this segregation, and there is no reason to think that cell classes that share a layer are more likely to interact than those that occupy separate layers.

The lateral geniculate nucleus may be a useful example of how relay cells are segregated because there is one overriding rule for the visual pathways, which is the separation of left eye from right eye inputs. This separation of inputs is found in all mammals that have reasonably good vision, and the developmental mechanisms for producing this separation are likely to dominate other concurrent mechanisms that produce a separation of the functionally distinct cell classes. It has been proposed that the ocular separation of retinogeniculate inputs is influenced by distinct patterns of activity coming from each eye at the relevant stages of early development when the geniculate layers first start to separate (Wong et al., 1995; Shatz, 1996; Weliky & Katz, 1999; Crowley & Katz, 2002). The determinant of the further laminar segregation shown in figure 2.8 may well depend on how the developmental timing of the distinct retinal inputs relates to timing of the developmental processes that produce the ocular separation into distinct layers. Relatively small changes in the developmental maturation of any one cell class relative to another could thus lead to significant differences in the patterns of segregation found in the adult. The extent to which there may be a comparable segregation of functionally distinct relay cell classes in other thalamic nuclei is discussed further in chapter 8.

The possibility that the magno-, parvo-, and koniocellular pathways are homologous to the Y, X, and W pathways, respectively, has been raised in several of the studies cited above. However, at present there is insufficient information about the details of the connectional patterns and insufficient agreement as to which are the salient functional features for this to be readily accepted. One implication of such a homology across a wide span of mammalian species would be a common ancestor having the three classes of pathway, but this is not likely to be revealed by foreseeable research. The possibility that functionally similar specialized pathways developed independently, with significant structural and functional similarities but also with some important differences, should be taken as a serious possibility at present. For a fuller discussion of these issues see Van Hooser et al. (2005).

2.A.6. The Cortical Distribution of Synaptic Terminals from Relay Cell Axons

Thalamocortical relay cells differ in the nature of their terminal arbors and in the way in which they distribute their terminal arbors to different cortical layers and cortical areas, and these differences relate to the different classes of relay cell definable by other criteria, introduced for the visual pathways in the previous section.

2.A.6.a. The Laminar Distribution of Thalamocortical Axons

An early account of different patterns of termination of thalamocortical axons in the cortex was published more than 60 years ago and was based mainly on Golgi preparations. Lorento de Nó in 1938 showed two types of thalamocortical axon. He called one "specific," apparently having traced the fibers from medial or lateral geniculate nucleus or from the ventral posterior nucleus. These axons have dense terminals in cortical layer 4 and sparser extensions into layer 3. He traced other afferents, which he called "nonspecific," from the thalamus in the mouse, and found that these sent much less dense terminal branches to more than one cortical area. They ascend to layer 1 and give off a few branches to other cortical layers on the way, mainly to layer 6. This distinction between specific and nonspecific thalamocortical axons has had an important influence on subsequent studies of thalamocortical innervation patterns. Lorente de Nó's description has been widely cited and has been loosely and optimistically linked not only to important electrophysiological observations on cortical arousal, but also to more dubious speculations as to the distinctions and phylogenetic history of specific and nonspecific sensory pathways.

The nonspecific system was early linked to diffusely organized thalamocortical pathways going from the midline and intralaminar nuclei to the cerebral cortex (Jasper, 1960; reviewed in Macchi, 1993; Jones, 1998) and thought to be a widespread system concerned with mechanisms of arousal acting through the superficial layers of cortex. Further, an additional burden was placed on the distinction between the specific and the nonspecific pathways when an extension of older ideas concerning "protopathic" and "epicritic" sensory pathways (Bishop, 1959) was added to the conceptual structure. The protopathic pathways were considered to have generalized, nonlocalized, diffuse functions and to be made up of fine axons such as those in the spinothalamic pathways. The epicritic pathways were presented as having well-localized, "specific" functions and were made up of thicker axons, such as those in the lemniscal pathways (for details, see Head, 1905; Walshe, 1948). The argument was functional and phylogenetic. Fine axon pathways were thought to be phylogenetically old (Herrick, 1948) and thick axon pathways phylogenetically new; the former carried "more precise and specific" (Bishop, 1959) messages than the latter. This mixture of fact and speculation often still underlies contemporary views on the thalamocortical pathways. The relevant facts are sparse, and to a significant extent are yet to be defined. It is important to recognize that our knowledge about the evolution of central neural pathways is extremely limited; the evolutionary history of neural pathways is at best derived from comparative studies of extant forms, and one has to be dubious about the idea that axon diameter can serve as a marker that allows identification of distinct functional systems in species separated by enormous spans of evolutionary time. Further, distinguishing where thick axon systems are, indeed, specific, having local sign (as defined in chapter 1, section A.3) that fine axon systems lack, or defining the origin of the afferents that end in different layers of cortex, remain important but still unsolved questions for most thalamocortical pathways.

Although the difference between axons that distribute to cortical layer 1 and those that distribute to layers 3 or 4 is often treated as indicative of a functional difference between a system that is diffuse and "nonspecific" and one that is localized and "specific" (Jones, 2002a, 2002b), there is to our knowledge no clear evidence as to the nature of the message, driver or modulator (see chapter 7 for details), carried by the layer 1 component.

Recent studies have used several different techniques to define the laminar termination of thalamocortical axons. Small lesions or small injections of anterogradely transported tracer into the thalamus have shown the laminar distribution of the degenerating or labeled axons without showing the individual arborizations formed by the cortical terminals (Hubel & Wiesel, 1972; Harting et al., 1973; Abramson & Chalupa, 1985; Levitt et al., 1995; Ding & Casagrande, 1997). Small cortical injections of retrogradely transported tracers, limited to one or a few cortical layers (Carey et al., 1979; Penny et al., 1982; Niimi et al., 1984; Ding & Casagrande, 1998), have shown which thalamic cells have axons that reach any one layer or group of layers. The most informative experiments have involved the direct tracing of thalamocortical axons after injections of anterogradely transported markers into single thalamic cells or small groups of cells or axons (Ferster & LeVay, 1978; Humphrey et al., 1985a, 1985b; Ding & Casagrande, 1997; Aumann et al., 1998; Deschênes et al., 1998; Rockland et al., 1999).

In the visual and somatosensory cortex the densest thalamocortical terminals are in layer 4, with a sparser spillover from this plexus into layer 3; sparser projections go to layers 1 and 6, and there is evidence that the axons going to layer 6 are branches of axons going to more superficial layers (Ferster & LeVay, 1978; Blasdel & Lund, 1983; Humphrey et al., 1985a). In some other thalamocortical pathways the major afferent plexus is in layer 3 or 5 rather than layer 4 (Aumann et al., 1998; Deschênes et al., 1998). In the lateral geniculate nucleus and the ventral posterior nucleus of rats, cats, and monkeys, generally, the larger cells project mainly to layer 4, with a smaller projection to layer 6, while the smaller cells project mainly to layers 3 and 1, or just to layer 1 (Carey et al., 1979; Penny et al., 1982; Rausell & Jones, 1991; Rausell et al., 1992). Casagrande and Xu (2004) report that most geniculate cells, including some of the small koniocellular ones, innervate layer 4, but that other koniocellular projections go to layer 3 or to layer 1.

Patterns of projection from the medial geniculate nucleus are somewhat less clear, but in the monkey, some cells project mainly to middle layers and layer 6, whereas others terminate mainly in layers 3 and/or 1 (Hashikawa et al., 1991; Molinari et al., 1995; Niimi et al., 1984; Pandya & Rosene, 1993; Kimura et al., 2003). For the lateral posterior nucleus, Abramson and Chalupa (1985) found that in the cat, this higher order nucleus sends axons primarily to layers 1 and 4 of suprasylvian cortex, but only to layer 1 of areas 17 and 18. In relation to this finding are the observations of Tong and Spear (1986), who reported that after injections of distinct retrogradely transported tracers into area 17 and suprasylvian cortex, most of the nerve cells in the most densely labeled zone of the lateral posterior nucleus were double-labeled. This suggests that many of these individual thalamic cells have one type of terminal (to layer 1 only) in one cortical area and a different type of terminal (layers 1 and 4) in another cortical area. This is a relationship that merits further study. In the monkey, pathways from the pulvinar go to several extrastriate cortical areas, with varying patterns of laminar distribution, primarily to layer 3, but with some input to layer 1 and deeper layers (Rockland et al., 1999), a pattern similar to that described for axons that go from the medial dorsal nucleus of the rat to prefrontal cortex (Kuroda et al., 1998).

Whereas the results summarized above generally support Lorento de Nó's claim that there are two distinct patterns of thalamocortical axon distribution, they destroy the idea that they come from different nuclei, "specific" nuclei for layer 4 and other sources for layer 1, and they raise the possibility that both types of axon may be given off by a single thalamic cell.

The cortical distribution of thalamocortical axons coming from the intralaminar nuclei is of some interest, in view of the longstanding perception that they represent a "nonspecific" pathway to superficial layers of cortex, distinct from the "specific" pathways that come from first order nuclei. Evidence for the supposedly specific or nonspecific nature of this cortical projection varies considerably. Although there is a significant contribution from the intralaminar nuclei to layer 1 of cortex, there is also a contribution to the middle and deep layers of cortex (Kaufman & Rosenquist, 1985; Royce & Mourey, 1985; Towns et al., 1990). Further, whereas there is evidence that the projections from the intralaminar nuclei tend to be rather widespread, and in many experiments have shown no evidence of any local sign (Jones & Leavitt, 1974; Kaufman & Rosenquist, 1985), there are observations showing that different members of the intralaminar group of nuclei have distinct cortical projection areas (Ullan, 1985; Royce et al., 1989; Berendse & Groenewegen, 1991), and that not many of the individual intralaminar cells show evidence of axons that branch to innervate more than one cortical area (Bentivoglio et al., 1981). There is some evidence for distinct local sign in some of the cortical projection pathways (Royce & Mourey, 1985; Olausson et al., 1989). The problem was reviewed earlier by Macchi and Bentivoglio (1982), and more recently by Minciacchi et al. (1993) and Molinari et al. (1993).

It should be stressed that a major target of the intralaminar and midline nuclei, apart from the cerebral cortex, is the striatum (Jones & Leavitt, 1974; Macchi et al., 1984), but whereas in the past this striatal connection could be seen as a hallmark of the intralaminar nuclei, it now appears that striatal projections also arise from many other first and higher order thalamic nuclei (Harting et al., 2001; Cheatwood et al., 2003), and that in terms of their cortical connections, the intralaminar nuclei may prove to share many of the organizational features of other thalamic nuclei.

A survey of the laminar distribution of thalamocortical projections going to different cortical areas from individual thalamic nuclei would take us beyond the scope of the present inquiry, and would show that much of the relevant information for many thalamic nuclei and cortical areas is not yet available. The important point to be noted is that the pattern of projection from thalamus to cortex varies not merely from one nucleus to another but, perhaps more important, it varies from one cell type to another within any one nucleus. This aspect of the complexity of the thalamocortical pathways is well illustrated by the visual pathways, as shown in figure 2.9.

For the geniculocortical pathways to area 17 of primates, it has been shown that the parvocellular and magnocellular cells of the lateral geniculate nucleus project to layer 4, and most or all also branch to innervate layer 6, the magnocellular axons having richer and more widespread cortical arbors than the parvocellular axons (Hubel & Wiesel, 1972; Blasdel & Lund, 1983; Florence & Casagrande, 1987; Casagrande & Kaas, 1994). Within the cortex, the pathways initially remain distinct: the parvocellular and magnocellular projections go to different subdivisions of layer 4, the former deep to the latter. The parvocellular layers also send an additional component more superficially into layer 4, although this depends on the way in which the subdivisions of layers 3 and 4 are defined (Casagrande & Kaas, 1994). The koniocellular cells have a very different arborization pattern, terminating mostly in layers 3 and 1 (Diamond et al., 1985; Ding & Casagrande, 1997, 1998;

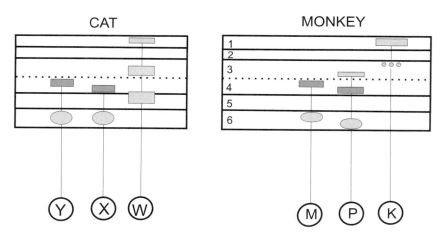

Figure 2.9
Schema to show the laminar distribution of geniculocortical afferents in the cat and the monkey. (Based on Casagrande & Kaas, 1994; Kawano, 1998; Casagrande & Xu, 2004.)

reviewed in Casagrande, 1994; Casagrande & Kaas, 1994; Hendry & Calkins, 1998; Hendry & Reid, 2000; Casagrande & Xu, 2004). The layer 3 terminals have a limited, patchy distribution, going specifically to specialized small regions of cortex, the so-called blobs, identified as having high cytochrome oxidase activity (Wong-Riley, 1979), and cells with color-opponent response properties (Livingstone & Hubel, 1984; Landisman & Ts'o, 2002a, 2002b). Most of the koniocellular axons branch to innervate both layers, but a minority seem to innervate only layer 3 or only layer 1 (Ding & Casagrande, 1997, 1998; Casagrande & Xu, 2004). Casagrande and Xu (2004) suggest distinct classes of koniocellular projections arising from distinct laminar positions in the lateral geniculate nucleus, but at present it is not clear that we have a complete classification of K cells.

A comparable pattern is seen in geniculocortical terminations of cats (Ferster & LeVay, 1978; Leventhal, 1979; Humphrey et al., 1985a; Kawano, 1998). The geniculate X and Y axons terminate mostly in layer 4, with branches innervating layer 6; X arbors terminate deep to Y arbors (Humphrey et al., 1985a, 1985b; Boyd & Matsubara, 1996); and the Y axons have richer and more extensive terminal arbors than do the X axons. W axons terminate mostly in layers 3 and 1. This general pattern has also been described for tree shrews, but in less detail, with one group of geniculate cells mainly innervating layer 4 and another innervating mainly layers 1 and 3 (Conley et al., 1984; Fitzpatrick & Raczkowski, 1990). The similarity in the gross pattern of geniculocortical terminations across such divergent mammalian representatives as primates, carnivores, and insectivores suggests that it is a general pattern for mammals, although as indicated earlier, we do not know whether this similarly represents a common evolutionary origin or whether it is imposed on the functionally distinct pathways by the functional specializations of particular cortical layers, about which we know all too little.

A revealing difference is seen when one compares the laminar arrangements in visual cortex, shown in figure 2.9, with those in the lateral geniculate nucleus, shown in figure 2.8. Whereas each eye has a termination in a distinct geniculate layer, in the cortex, for any one functional type, the two eyes share a layer. The cortical axons are distributed to alternating, side-by-side patches (not shown in figure 2.9), forming a part of the ocular dominance columns within one layer (Hubel & Wiesel, 1977). Further, where there is evidence for a separation of on-center from off-center pathways in distinct geniculate layers, there is also evidence that the two pathways terminate in alternating patches rather than in distinct laminae in the cortex (McConnell & LeVay, 1984; Zahs & Stryker, 1988). This difference suggests that cortical layers accommodate distinct functional systems, whereas, as we have seen, geniculate layers are not readily related to particular functional specializations and may rather represent an accident or epiphenomenon of developmental forces. The cortical processing required for left eye inputs is not likely to be different from that required for right eye processing, and comparably, the cortical processing for off-center and on-center pathways is likely to be very similar. In contrast to this, the functionally distinct X, Y, W or P, M, K systems are likely to be making quite distinct demands on cortical processing, and so we see their separation in cortex even where they are mingled in the geniculate. This arrangement stresses that each cortical layer, and even each subdivision of a layer, is likely to have a quite distinct intrinsic functional organization, whereas in the geniculate layers (and by implication, in subdivisions of thalamic nuclei more generally), there may or may not be a laminar separation of pathways that carry different messages, and there is no necessary spatial separation of the distinct types of intrinsic thalamic circuitry acting on the relay of the messages. The clearest example of this mingling of pathways in the thalamus is the shared laminar geniculate distribution of the X and Y pathways in cats, ferrets, and mink, each relating to distinct thalamic cell types and synaptic circuitry.

The difference between cortical and geniculate lamination not only throws an interesting light on the nature of the functional segregation related to the lamination, it also demonstrates that the ontogenetic or phylogenetic developmental mechanisms that lead to the production of thalamic and cortical segregation of functionally distinct pathways are likely to be fundamentally different. That is, in the cortex, the function of the cells appears to be determined primarily by their developmental history, that is, by their "birth dates," and through this by their laminar position. Each functionally distinct group of afferents from the thalamus distributes to particular cortical layers, and the comparative anatomy suggests that there is a general consistency across species in this laminar distribution, binding each type of functionally distinct afferent rather securely to a particular lamina, and, by implication, to the functional organization of that lamina. In contrast to this, in the lateral geniculate nucleus there is a laminar separation that is primarily a separation of functionally *identical* inputs (left eye, right eye) and that is secondarily a separation of functionally distinct inputs (X, Y, W). We have seen that this laminar separation is remarkably inconsistent across species but that it may well be related to the developmental period at which each pathway becomes active, or develops some other property that is relevant to establishing localized terminal connections.

2.A.6.b. The Distribution of Thalamocortical Axons to One or More Cortical Areas

Generally, a single axon or axon branch that goes to any one cortical area branches extensively to form multiple terminations within a localized part of that area. This pattern of branching is distinct from the branching pattern described in section 2.A.1 (see figure 2.2) that allows an axon access to two cytoarchitectonically and functionally distinct cortical areas. Where a dual innervation of two cortical areas relates to two identifiable maps of sensory surfaces, one expects both branches to innervate corresponding points on the map, and, where the evidence is available, they do (Bullier et al., 1984).

Whereas the classical approach, based on retrograde degeneration, assigned thalamic relay cells to particular nuclei and to particular cortical areas, it is now clear that this is only a first approximation. The highly sensitive methods currently available show that many cortical areas are innervated by more than one thalamic nucleus and that many thalamic nuclei have cells that send axons to more than one cortical area. In some instances, different cells within one nucleus send an axon to a different cortical area, but in other instances the axonal branches of single relay cells innervate more than one cortical area. That is, relay cells within one thalamic nucleus can also be distinguished on the basis of whether they innervate one cytoarchitectonically and functionally distinct cortical area or more than one. This has been demonstrated for the first order, visual geniculocortical pathways (Geisert, 1980; Kennedy & Bullier, 1985; Humphrey et al., 1985b; Birnbacher & Albus, 1987) and for somatosensory pathways (e.g., Spreafico et al., 1981; Cusick et al., 1985; but see Darian-Smith & Darian-Smith, 1993), and also for higher order pathways going through the pulvinar (Tong & Spear, 1986; Lysakowski et al., 1988; Miceli et al., 1991; Rockland et al., 1999). As methods become more sensitive and more widely used, one can expect to find more examples of multiple, complex interrelationships between thalamic nuclei and cortical areas. Here, again, we will not provide a survey of thalamocortical pathways in general but use the visual pathways to illustrate some of the relationships that have been established.

Looking specifically at the geniculocortical pathways in primates, the projection to the primary visual cortex (V1) is dominant, although there is evidence that some geniculate cells, scattered in the interlaminar zones and in the parvocellular laminae, also project outside V1 (Montero, 1986); some certainly go to area V2 (Fries, 1981; Yukie & Iwai, 1981) and some to area MT (Sincich et al., 2004), the latter from the koniocellular elements.

For the geniculocortical pathways of cats, X cells innervate area 17 only, whereas the largest, Y cells, which have more richly branching arbors in area 17 than do the X cells, also innervate area 18, with some of the geniculocortical axons sending branches to both cortical areas. The W cells, lying in the most ventral, small celled C layers, project to areas 17, 18, and 19, predominantly to areas 18 and 19 (Laemle, 1975; Holländer & Vanegas, 1977; Ferster & LeVay, 1978; Geisert, 1980; Kennedy & Bullier, 1985; Humphrey et al., 1985a, 1985b). However, the extent to which individual W cells innervate more than one area is not presently known.

The question as to what a particular system gains (or loses) by having cells that send axonal branches to more than one cortical area rather than having two separate cell populations, each going to a different cortical area, is not resolved, except for the relatively obvious probability that a branching axon will likely transfer a truer duplicate version of relay cell activity to the two cortical areas than two separate cells would. We do not know whether in the cat, the Y cells that innervate more than one cortical area differ in any other important respect from Y cells that apparently belong to the same morphological and functional class but innervate only one cortical area, nor do we know what the thalamocortical pathway gains by having some cells of each kind, and this seems to be true of branching axons in other thalamic relays such as the somatosensory pathways (Spreafico et al., 1981). Colby (1988) has provided evidence that two distinct types of geniculate Y cell can be recognized, one involved in a geniculocorticotectal pathway and the other not participating in the cortical innervation of the tectum, and it is possible that these two types of Y cells also differ in the branching pattern of their thalamocortical axons (see also footnote 8 on page 46). Alternatively, one could take a speculative, evolutionary view and suggest that the curiously mixed population of large cells in the cat's geniculo-cortical pathway represents an evolutionary stage, but one would be hard put to decide whether the branching cells are on their way in or on their way out. If there are rules that govern the distribution of such branching cells, they yet remain to be defined.

2.A.7. Perikaryal Size and Calcium-Binding Proteins

One generalization that emerges from the above description is that larger thalamic relay cells are most likely to innervate layers 4 and 6, while smaller ones tend to innervate layers 3 and 1. Recently, Jones and his colleagues (Hashikawa et al., 1991; Rausell & Jones, 1991; Rausell et al., 1992; Molinari et al., 1995; Jones, 1998, 2002a, 2002b, 2003) have shown that relay cells throughout the monkey's thalamus can be divided into two categories based on whether they are immunocytochemically reactive for parvalbumin or calbindin, two different Ca^{2+}-binding proteins. The smaller cells, which project mainly to superficial cortical layers, stained for calbindin, while the larger ones, which project mainly to middle layers, stain for parvalbumin (Hendry & Yoshioka, 1994; Munkle et al., 2000). This is a potentially useful distinction of cell types that are likely to have different functions. However, there are two problems. One is that we do not yet know the functional implications for a thalamic cell of having one or the other Ca^{2+}-binding protein. Further, since so far the distinction appears not to apply to many nonprimate forms (Ichida et al., 2000; Amadeo et al., 2001), the extent to which it can represent a basic distinction for thalamocortical systems is doubtful. Parvalbumin-positive cells dominate the main sensory relays of the thalamus, and calbindin-positive cells dominate the intralaminar nuclei in primates and raccoons (Herron et al., 1997), but both cell types are found in most thalamic nuclei (Diamond et al., 1993; De Biasi et al., 1994; Johnson & Casagrande, 1995; Goodchild & Martin, 1998).

Jones (1998) has recently used this correlation of immunocytochemistry and projection pattern in primates to suggest that for the thalamus in general, two distinct projection systems are recognizable. The smaller, calbindin-positive cells project mainly to superficial cortical layers, particularly to layer 1, in a diffuse pattern to form a "matrix" of thalamocortical input without local sign, whereas the larger parvalbumin-positive cells project mainly to middle cortical layers, primarily to layer 4, and do so in a specific, topographically organized fashion to form a thalamocortical "core" that has local sign. The proposal sees the core projections as bringing specific sensory information to cortex and the matrix projections as serving a role in recruitment of more widespread thalamocortical ensembles to reflect changes in behavioral state, or attention, and possibly to play a role in "binding" discharge patterns of cortical cells that represent different parts of a perceptual whole (Singer & Gray, 1995).

At present, it would appear that there is a functionally significant difference between the small cells and the large cells, a difference that is in part expressed by the calcium-binding proteins in primates and in part expressed by the more superficial distribution of the cortical terminals of the small cells. However, if one looks at the geniculocortical pathways as an exemplar of the proposed distinction of thalamocortical pathways, one finds that the small koniocellular cells in the monkey, which are calbindin-positive and thus should be part of the thalamocortical matrix, are not noticeably more diffuse than parvocellular and magnocellular cells. Their receptive fields, while somewhat larger, are nonetheless well focused and constrained to a small part of visual field, and the same is true for the cat if one compares the small W cells with the larger X or Y cells (Wilson et al., 1976; Sur & Sherman, 1982; Irvin et al., 1986, 1993; Norton et al., 1988). Further, as we saw earlier, although there is good evidence that the small W cells send axons to more than one cortical area (Kawano, 1998), the same has been shown for the larger Y cells (Geisert, 1980; Kennedy & Bullier, 1985). The small geniculocortical relay cells may well have some important functional characteristics in common, but they do not fit the description of a "diffusely organized" system, either in terms of the local sign of their cortical terminals or in terms of the number of different cortical areas that they innervate. Nor do the small cells all limit their terminals to layer 1 to form the nonspecific component of Lorente de Nó. A recent study of individual koniocellular axon arbors in cortex showed that most innervate only cortical layer 3 (a "middle" cortical layer), and most of those that innervate layer 1 do so via a branching axon that also innervates layer 3 (Ding & Casagrande, 1998; Casagrande & Xu, 2004). Thus, these koniocellular cells are, generally, neither diffuse nor targeted unerringly or dominantly to layer 1.

In summary, there are a number of differences among relay cells suggestive of distinct functional roles. The position of the cells in a particular nucleus, subdivision, or layer of a nucleus and in receipt of a particular set of afferents is perhaps the simplest and most obvious distinction, although we have seen that functionally distinct cells can share a lamina and be in receipt of functionally distinct inputs. The size of the cell and the structure and the branching pattern of the dendrites provide distinctions that may apply widely through the thalamus, but the precise functional significance of these features still remains to be defined. The distribution of the thalamocortical axons to a single functional cortical area or to more than one cortical area provides another distinction, as do the laminar distributions of the thalamocortical axons. The origin of the main driving afferents as coming either from ascending pathways to first order relays or from neocortex to higher order relays (see chapters 1 and 8) provides a way of classifying thalamic relay cells, and the Ca^{2+} binding proteins provide another variable that is likely to have functional significance, although the relationship of this classification to the others is not well defined. Perhaps the most important unknown about a classification of thalamic cells is whether the variable under consideration relates to the nature of the message that is being transmitted, to the nature of the modulatory influences that the message is exposed to in the thalamus, or to the way in which the message will be processed in the cortex and beyond.

2.B. Interneurons

Thalamic interneurons were described by Cajal (1911) on the basis of the Golgi method, which shows the local axons, but it was not until modifications of the Golgi methods based on aldehyde fixation, and suitable for adult tissues, were widely used that the complexity of these cells was recognized (Guillery, 1966; Tömböl, 1967, 1969; Ralston, 1971; figure 2.10). Intracellular fills (Friedlander et al., 1981; Sherman & Friedlander, 1988) subsequently showed that even the best Golgi pictures gave but a limited impression of the full richness that the dendritic arbors of some of these cells could attain (see figure 2.10; figure 2.11).

2.B.1. Interneuronal Cell Bodies and Dendrites

The interneurons have cell bodies that are among the smallest of the thalamus. They are recognizable by their size, by the fact that they cannot be retrogradely filled by tracers injected into the cortex, and because they are all GABAergic and thus immunoreactive to GABA and GAD. The proportion of cells in any one thalamic nucleus that are interneurons varies considerably, depending on the species and on the nucleus (Arcelli et al., 1997). In the lateral geniculate nucleus of the cat, the interneurons represent about 20%–25% of the total cell population (LeVay & Ferster, 1979), and a figure as high as 35% has been reported for the magnocellular layers of the monkey's lateral geniculate nucleus (Montero, 1986). Whereas in the rat, the lateral geniculate nucleus has 20%–30% interneurons, all other thalamic nuclei in the rat, including the ventral posterior nucleus, are reported as having less than 1%. Variation between these extremes, of 20%–30% for carnivores and primates and less than 1% for rats, has been reported for other species (Arcelli

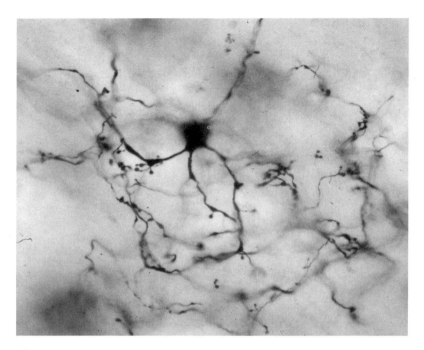

Figure 2.10
Interneuron from the ventral posterior nucleus of a cat. The Golgi method was used. (Figure courtesy of H. J. Ralston III.)

et al., 1997). However, there should be some caution about the reliability of some of the published figures. For example, Li et al. (2003b) illustrate a population of interneurons in the lateral geniculate and lateral posterior nuclei of the rat that suggests that the difference between these two nuclei is not as great as indicated by the earlier reports. Further, although 1% looks as though it represents a population that could easily be ignored, and sometimes is, it is important to recognize that a richly branched arbor of interneuronal processes can have several hundred (or even more) terminals, so even with only 1% of the cells being interneurons, there is a distinct possibility that all parts of the nucleus could be within reach of interneuronal processes and each relay cell could be interacting with the processes of several interneurons.

Figures 2.10 and 2.11 show that the terminal portions of the dendrites of interneurons differ strikingly from those of the relay cells. Whereas the dendrites of relay cells, like most dendrites in the vertebrate central nervous system generally, become thinner toward their ends and

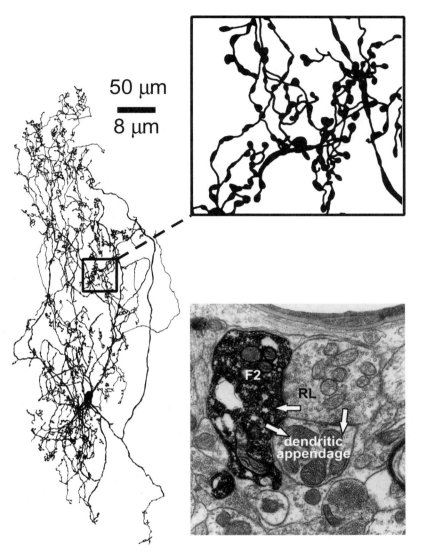

Figure 2.11
Interneuron from the lateral geniculate nucleus of a cat. Preparation by intra-cellular injection with horseradish peroxidase. (Redrawn from Hamos et al., 1985.) Inset at top shows an enlarged view of axoniform dendritic terminals. The electron micrograph shows a triad in one section, with the labeled (F2, see chapter 3) terminal from the interneuron indicated. Arrowheads point to the three synapses of the triad: from the F2 terminal to a dendritic appendage of an X relay cell, from the retinal terminal (RL) to the F2 terminal, and from the retinal terminal to the dendritic appendage.

have a simple branching pattern (see figures 2.5 and 2.6), the terminal parts of the interneuronal dendrites are more complex, have a relatively rich terminal branching pattern, and form enlarged en passage and terminal swellings of the sort more commonly seen on axons in most other parts of the brain. These dendrites have been described as "axoniform" for that reason. The term is further justified on the basis of electron microscopic studies which show that the terminals contain synaptic vesicles and make specialized synaptic contact on other cells, just as one would expect a classical axon to do (Ralston, 1971; Famiglietti & Peters, 1972; see also chapter 3). There is also recent pharmacological evidence to indicate that these dendritic terminals in fact do act to produce inhibitory postsynaptic potentials in relay cells (Cox et al., 1998; Cox & Sherman, 2000; Govindaiah & Cox, 2004). That is, although they are reasonably regarded as dendrites and serve as *postsynaptic* sites for the axons of incoming primary and other axons, many of their terminal processes and some of their en passage swellings also have the structure and function of axons and are *presynaptic*.

We show in chapter 3 that it has been possible to identify two distinct, parallel pathways through the cat's lateral geniculate nucleus to cortex, one, the X cell pathway, having extensive connections with dendritic and axonal outputs of interneurons, and the other, the main Y cell pathway through the A layers, having interneuronal inputs primarily from axons. The relative numbers of interneurons in any one relay nucleus may reflect the extent to which interneuronal activity is relevant to the relay as a whole, or they may reflect the extent to which one or another of two or more parallel pathways through a nucleus is dependent on interneuronal connections. For most thalamic nuclei we do not have information about either the proportion of nerve cells that are interneurons, the extent to which those cells do or do not have very rich terminal arbors, or the extent to which any one parallel pathway through the nucleus involves interneurons.

2.B.2. *On Distinguishing Interneuronal Axons and Dendrites*

2.B.2.a. The Nature of Presynaptic "Axoniform" Dendrites
At this point it is worth digressing briefly to consider a problem that is largely semantic and historic but that still often leads to puzzlement about processes such as these, which appear to be both dendrite and axon. The problem arises primarily because Cajal proposed two important conceptual tools for analyzing the nervous system. One was the neuron doctrine and the other was the "law of dynamic polarization"

(or the "law of functional polarity," in the 1995 translation of the 1911 book; see Guillery, 2005b, for more details). Each, the doctrine and the law, provided tremendously powerful tools for analyzing the nervous system, and they served well for half a century or more, but we now know that neither the doctrine nor the law is entirely correct in its original formulation, or indeed in any formulation that fails to recognize that each is merely a rough approximation that can serve as a guide for studying the brain. The names, the doctrine and the law, indicate the extent to which these concepts were used as propaganda. The fact that there has been confusion for most of the twentieth century reflects the success and the authority of these formulations. In the 1995 English translation of Cajal's 1911 book, the law is introduced and stated as follows:

Does this mean that incoming and outgoing impulses . . . pass indiscriminately from cell body to cell body, from one dendrite to another, from one axon to another, or from one of these three elements to any other? Or conversely, is there some well established and immutable rule that determines what parts of one neuron may contact another cell? Everything we know about the function of the nervous system points to the latter supposition as true, and indicates that there is in fact such a law. Our own observations have led us to define this law as follows: *A functional synapse or useful and effective contact between two neurons can only be formed between the collateral or terminal axonal ramifications of one neuron and the dendrites or cell body of another neuron.*

It is worth noting the "only" in the last, stressed phrase.

Although this law is a brilliant recipe for starting to analyze neuronal circuits in the vertebrate brain, it is also a quite extraordinarily limited and dogmatic statement. Cajal knew that most invertebrate neurons are unipolar, with processes that do not allow a ready distinction between axons and dendrites, and he clearly recognized that in vertebrates the granule cells of the olfactory bulb and the retinal amacrine cells lack axons, so that they were, according to the law, out of the business of influencing other neurons. The dogmatism of the law led to some interesting later discussions about various neuron types that did not fit readily into the law, such as the vertebrate dorsal root ganglion cell or the variety of neurons found in invertebrate brains (Bullock, 1959; Bodian, 1962), but there has never been any clear resolution of how to fit the law into the variety of known neuronal structures, and there is not likely to be. The variety of neurons is too great. Textbooks are generally less dogmatic about the functional distinction between axons and dendrites than they used to be, but this distinction is not one that should be lightly discarded.

For many nerve cells the distinction between axons and dendrites is useful. The former is a single slender process that almost invariably lacks ribosomes in the adult, conducts action potentials, is quite commonly myelinated, and terminates in presynaptic processes. The latter are generally represented by several processes for each cell. These processes are gently tapered, contain ribosomes, are commonly postsynaptic, and generally conduct decrementally, but, as we discuss in chapter 4, can perhaps also conduct spikes. More recent observations suggest that the orientation of the microtubules and the nature of the microtubule-associated proteins differ between axons and dendrites, and that several other groups of proteins are distributed differentially on the neuronal membrane (Black & Baas, 1989; Baas, 1999; Winckler & Mellman, 1999; Goldstein & Yang, 2000). However, there is no general law that relates axons or dendrites to their synaptic relationships. Axons can be postsynaptic and dendrites can be presynaptic (Guillery, 2003), and for any neural process, whatever we decide to call it, we need to know whether it contains and can release transmitter, how the release is controlled (e.g., by voltage and Ca^{2+} entry or by some other mechanism), whether it has receptors that can be influenced by transmitters released nearby, and what its membrane properties are that may or may not allow spike propagation. These issues are discussed in later chapters.

2.B.3. The Axons of the Interneurons

Whereas most thalamic interneurons have several characteristic axoniform dendrites, they have only a single axon that is recognizable on the basis of an axon hillock, a slim initial segment and, at least in some instances, myelin. This axon in turn leads into a long, branched process that does not taper significantly and that generally branches in the neighborhood of the dendritic arbor. On the basis of the axonal ramification, Tömböl (1969) has described two sorts of interneuron, one with a locally ramifying axon and one with an axon that goes beyond the dendritic arbor but generally stays in the same nucleus or nuclear group. In the lateral geniculate nucleus this type of axon may go into an adjacent lamina; in the medial geniculate nucleus, Tömböl described it going from one nuclear subdivision to another. She described such cells in the ventral posterior nucleus and the medial dorsal nucleus as well, but comparable accounts have not appeared subsequently, apart from the interneurons described by Winer and Morest (1983) in the medial geniculate nucleus of the cat, where they distinguished large and small interneurons and suggested that some of the interneuronal axons passed from one subdivision of the medial geniculate nucleus to another.

In Golgi preparations the distinction between the single axon and the axoniform dendrites is not always obvious, and it is not uncommon for a Golgi preparation to leave the axons unimpregnated or only partially impregnated. The possibility has been raised that interneurons may lack axons (Lieberman, 1973; Wilson, 1986), but in view of the difficulties of demonstrating the axons, this negative result needs to be interpreted cautiously. Electron microscopic studies may show the absence of a characteristic axonal initial segment arising from the cell body, but since axons can arise from dendrites, such evidence, which is based on a limited sample, leaves considerable room for doubt. Interneurons demonstrated by intracellular fills have shown axons, but this may be a highly selected sample, because in these experiments the neurons are usually identified on the basis of their action potentials, and, as shown in chapter 5, the dendrites of the interneurons, acting locally, can function without action potentials. That is, axonless interneurons may not have action potentials, and if so, then the method of filling interneurons by intracellular injections would favor neurons that have axons. Therefore, with the currently used methods of labeling by intracellular injection, one might expect to find no axonless interneurons, even if they exist. So, the question whether all thalamic interneurons have axons must be left open for the present. Given the available techniques, observations of interneurons that lack axons cannot be regarded as decisive evidence that such interneurons exist, and the demonstration that some interneurons have axons cannot be generalized to all interneurons.

The axonal terminals and the presynaptic dendrites of an interneuron are both GABAergic so that they may be thought of as having the same actions. However, the postsynaptic contacts made are different, and other differences in ultrastructure are noted in later chapters. Whereas the dendrites have terminals that are also postsynaptic, the axon terminals appear not to receive synaptic contacts from any other processes (Montero, 1987).

2.B.4. Classifications of Interneurons

We have seen that a classification has been proposed on the basis of the territory occupied by the axon relative to the dendrites. This feature stresses the possibility that the axon and the dendrites may be concerned with different aspects of the thalamic circuits. Other differences between interneurons may well depend on the extent to which individual cell processes have been revealed by the particular method used, so that the significant range of dendritic arbors that has been described for interneurons may not provide a categorization of interneurons that can be readily interpreted in functional terms. Montero and Zempel (1985) distinguished interneurons on the basis of cell body size (see also Winer & Morest, 1983), but on this criterion alone it is not clear whether one is dealing with a single class, represented by a continuum of cell sizes, or two distinct cell classes that differ in size and in some other measure that was not identified in the cited studies.

Recently Bickford et al. (1999) described two types of interneuron in the visual thalamus, both reacting positively to GAD immunostaining but one reacting positively and the other reacting negatively for nitric oxide synthase (see also Carden & Bickford, 2002). The former are somewhat larger than the latter and have a simpler dendritic form, resembling a cell type described earlier by Updyke (1979) as "class V" cells. These appear to be involved primarily in extraglomerular synapses, whereas the latter are seen more commonly in the glomeruli (see chapter 3).

Montero (1989) and Sanchez-Vives et al. (1996) described a somewhat special class of interneuron in the interlaminar regions of the lateral geniculate nucleus of the cat. These resemble the cells of the cat's reticular nucleus[9] (described below) rather than the other geniculate interneurons. These interlaminar interneurons are larger than other interneurons, show a somewhat distinctive orientation of their dendrites, and have some of the physiological properties of reticular cells (discussed in chapters 4 and 5).

The possibility that these cells may be displaced reticular cells has a clear functional implication. The interneurons of the lateral geniculate nucleus, and possibly of the thalamus in general, differ from the reticular neurons because the former receive synaptic contacts from primary, driving afferents (e.g., retinal axons for the lateral geniculate cells), whereas the latter do not (see chapter 3). Further, the reticular neurons send their axons to regions some distance from the cell body. In this they resemble the second of Tömböl's interneuronal classes, those having axons that extend beyond their dendritic arbors. These may, therefore, have included such interlaminar interneurons. Montero (1989) found no retinal input to the interlaminar interneurons, but he was not looking at labeled retinal axons, and his survey was limited to the cell body and the proximal parts of the dendrites. Because a significant part of the retinal

---

9. Strictly speaking, these are observations of the cat's perigeniculate nucleus (see chapter 9 for its identification as a part of the reticular nucleus).

input to geniculate interneurons contacts the distal, axoniform dendrites, the relationship of the interlaminar interneurons to the retinal input must remain an open question. Evidence obtained from intracellular filling of relay cells and their axons in slice preparations suggests that the interlaminar interneurons do receive afferents from collateral branches of the relay cell axons, which also branch within the perigeniculate nucleus (Sanchez-Vives et al., 1996). However, this may not represent a crucial distinction between the interlaminar interneurons and the type with axoniform dendrites in the major layers, since at least some geniculate relay cells filled with horseradish peroxidase have local collaterals (Friedlander et al., 1981; Stanford et al., 1983), and these contact the interneurons with axoniform dendrites (Cox et al., 2003). At present it is not known how common such local branches of relay cells are in the thalamus, or what proportion of the inputs to interneurons are formed by such axons.

The implication—that these interneurons actually represent migrated perigeniculate cells—would need developmental confirmation, which is currently not available. Such confirmation would be feasible if there were a specific marker of perigeniculate cells that is present at an early enough stage, and the result could prove of interest. Given the extent to which the segregation of functionally distinct cells in the lateral geniculate nucleus varies, so that X cells and Y cells, on-center and off-center cells can be either intermingled or not (see section 2.A.5) without apparently affecting their functional role, such displaced reticular cells may well be a further sign that the precise locus of a cell in the thalamus is not an important determinant of its functional connectivity. The developmental forces that might produce a migration of cells from ventral to dorsal thalamus are undefined. Possibly these cells should be included in the next section, on the reticular nucleus, rather than in this one, on interneurons, but at present that remains an open question.

2.C. The Cells of the Thalamic Reticular Nucleus

The thalamic reticular nucleus is made up of nerve cells that lie in a complex meshwork of intertwining thalamocortical and corticothalamic axons. The nucleus forms a slender shield around the dorsal and lateral aspects of the dorsal thalamus and is placed so that any axon passing between cortex and thalamus must go through the nucleus. Many of these traversing fibers (but see chapter 3) innervate the reticular cells, with glutamatergic afferents that are generally excitatory (see chapter 5 for exceptions). The reticular cells tend to have relatively large cell bodies and discoid dendritic arbors that lie in the plane of the nucleus (Scheibel & Scheibel, 1966; Lubke, 1993; figure 2.12). Like the thalamic interneurons, they are all GABAergic and provide an inhibitory innervation to the relay cells of the thalamus (Ohara & Lieberman, 1985; Jones, 1985; Sanchez-Vives & McCormick, 1997; Pinault & Deschênes, 1998b). There are some indications that the cells of the thalamic reticular nucleus are not a homogeneous group. The cells in the anterior part of the nucleus do not have the characteristic discoid shape seen in the main part of the nucleus, and there have been accounts that distinguish large from small cells on the basis of Golgi preparations (Spreafico et al., 1991).

Reticular cells and interneurons both send inhibitory axons back to thalamic relay cells. However, they have distinct developmental origins and lie in different parts of the diencephalon, the reticular cells in the ventral thalamus and the interneurons in the dorsal thalamus (see chapter 1). Further, there are other clear differences between the two cell groups. One is that the reticular cells do not show the striking axoniform terminal arbors on their dendrites like those seen on many thalamic interneurons (Scheibel & Scheibel, 1966; Ohara & Lieberman, 1985; Lubke, 1993; see, however, below). Another difference, mentioned earlier and treated more fully in the next chapter on afferents, concerns differences in the connectivity patterns of the two cell groups. Further, they also differ in the patterns of firing, particularly in the properties of burst firing, as discussed in chapters 4 and 5.

The axons of reticular cells terminate in the thalamus, where they generally form well-localized terminal arbors (Pinault et al., 1995a, 1995b; Deschênes et al., 2005). For the major sensory modalities the corticoreticular and reticulothalamic pathways show matching topographic maps, as do the pathways from the thalamus to the reticular nucleus (Montero et al., 1977; Crabtree & Killackey, 1989; Conley & Diamond, 1990; Crabtree, 1992a, 1992b; see chapter 8 for further details of these maps). That is, limited parts of any sensory surface produce activity within limited parts of the reticular nucleus since each small part receives afferents from thalamic and cortical regions innervated by axons representing the same parts of the sensory surface. The reticular cells in turn send their inhibitory axons back to the same parts of the thalamus.

The main part of the thalamic reticular nucleus can be divided into "sectors" on the basis of its afferent connections with groups of thalamic nuclei and groups of cytoarchitectonically and functionally

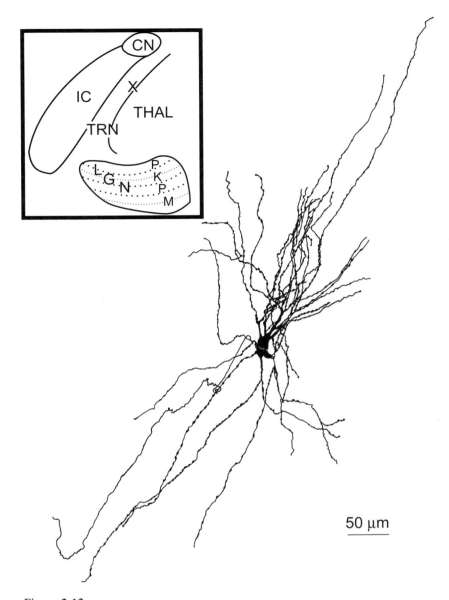

50 μm

Figure 2.12
Intracellularly filled neuron from the thalamic reticular nucleus of *Galago*. The cell was filled with neurobiotin and illustrates the pattern of orientation of the dendrites in the plane of the thalamic reticular nucleus. The inset shows the position of the cell from a coronal section through the lateral geniculate nucleus (LGN) and internal capsule (IC). CN, caudate nucleus; TRN, thalamic reticular nucleus; K, M, and P, layers of the lateral geniculate nucleus; X marks the position of the cell. (Drawing provided courtesy of by P. Smith, K. Manning, and D. Uhlrich.)

definable cortical areas (Jones, 1985; Guillery et al., 1998; Guillery & Harting, 2003; see also chapter 8), but there are no identifiable boundaries or architectonic distinctions between sectors in preparations that do not reveal the connections. Nor does it seem that the dendrites of cell bodies lying in any one sector respect the borders of the sectors. That is, the sectors of the reticular nucleus are not a morphologically distinct entity like the nuclei of the dorsal thalamus. Any one reticular sector, though generally limited in its connection to one modality or presumed functional group of pathways, can relate to more than one thalamic nucleus, and correspondingly, to more than one cortical area that is concerned with the same modality. In these connections and in the lack of clearly definable borders to the sectors there is an indication that the individual reticular cells may be less closely linked to any one functionally defined afferent pathway than are the cells of the dorsal thalamus. These topics are discussed in more detail in chapter 9.

The extent to which local interconnectivity patterns in the reticular nucleus might play a part in the control of rhythmic discharge patterns in the thalamocortical pathways has been important for theories of reticular function, particularly as they may relate to the synchronization of reticular activity that characterizes certain forms of sleep and epilepsy (Steriade et al., 1990; Destexhe & Sejnowski, 2002; Sohal & Huguenard, 2003; Sohal et al., 2003; Zhang & Jones, 2004). Although the complex axoniform dendritic appendages seen on thalamic interneurons have generally not been reported on reticular cells, they were shown by light microscopy in the rat by Pinault et al. (1995b). In addition, there is evidence that reticular cells have axons that can give off local branches within the nucleus itself in cat and rat (Yen et al., 1985a; Spreafico et al., 1988; Liu et al., 1995b). There is evidence for electrically coupled reticular cells (Landisman et al., 2002), and electron microscopic evidence for some local circuitry established by serial synaptic junctions in the nucleus, which will be considered in the next chapter.

When we look at the inhibitory afferents that thalamic cells receive from nearby neurons, we see that the inhibitory circuitry going to a thalamic relay neuron can come from interneuronal dendrites or axons or from thalamic reticular axons. Although the precise pattern of the inhibition in a nucleus may depend on the relative number of interneurons in that nucleus, we have seen that in a nucleus like the cat's lateral geniculate nucleus, which is rich in interneurons, there may be some cells, like the X cells, that have extensive connections with interneuronal presynaptic dendrites at triadic junctions, whereas other, adjacent cells, like the Y cells, lack such connections. The extent to which connections with interneuronal axons may play a comparable role is not known, although the connectivity patterns considered in the next chapter suggest that the interneuronal axons and dendrites have distinct functions. Further, it is not known whether the axons of reticular neurons may provide a functional replacement for interneuronal axons where interneurons are lacking. From this point of view the possibility that some geniculate interneurons should be seen as displaced reticular cells could either prove very interesting if the functions are clearly distinct or rather dull if they are not.

2.D. Summary

We have shown that there are morphological characteristics on the basis of which distinct types of thalamic relay neuron can be recognized, and that the same may prove to be true for interneurons and possibly also for the nerve cells of the reticular nucleus, although the functional heterogeneity of reticular cells does not currently have strong support. Relay neurons differ in several features, including perikaryal size, axon diameter, the pattern of dendritic arbors, thalamic position in a particular nucleus, nuclear subdivision or lamina, and site of cortical termination in a particular cortical area or lamina. However, it is difficult to interpret these features in functional terms. Perhaps the key issue is to define for each variable whether it relates to the nature of the message that is being passed through thalamus to cortex or to the nature of the thalamic control (modulation, gating) to which the message is exposed in its passage through the thalamus. Some of the morphological differences that have been described in this chapter, such as the difference between interneuronal dendrites and relay cell dendrites, clearly have direct and important functional implications, although it has to be recognized that exactly what it is that the presynaptic interneuronal dendrites are doing is still rather obscure. Other differences, such as those between bushy and radiate dendrites, or between axonal terminals in any one particular cortical layer, remain to be explored. The most important issues that have yet to be defined include the extent to which particular characteristics of thalamic cells that have been considered in this chapter are generalizable across all (or most) thalamic nuclei, and a resolution of exactly how each characteristic, whether generalizable or local, relates to the functional properties of the thalamic relay that are discussed in subsequent chapters.

2.E. Unresolved Questions

1. Are there structural features of thalamic relay cells that will lead to a functionally useful classification generally applicable across all of the thalamus?

2. How many functionally distinct types of relay cell can be identified in the major relay nuclei of the thalamus? Does the distribution of these cell types vary significantly across thalamic nuclei?

3. If the classes of relay cell reflect different functional gating properties (as opposed to integrative properties), how many distinct gating functions or classes can be defined in the mammalian thalamus?

4. What, if any, is the functional or developmental significance of regional segregations of cell classes across thalamic nuclei? Specifically, are there basic ground rules that govern the segregation of distinct functional cell types within the layers of the lateral geniculate nucleus?

5. Is there a basic difference between geniculate and cortical laminae such that distinct functional circuits are linked to particular cortical laminae and sublaminae, but can mingle in the thalamus?

6. Where a thalamic nucleus sends axons to more than one cortical area, are there functionally significant ground rules that govern whether the projection is established by branching axons or by two distinct populations of thalamic cells?

7. Are there several different types of thalamic interneuron? Do all interneurons have axons?

8. What is the functional significance of the different calcium-binding proteins found in thalamic relay cells?

3

The Afferent Axons to the Thalamus: Their Structure and Connections

3.A. A General View of the Afferents

The thalamus sends most of its outputs to the cerebral cortex, and the messages that are received by the cortex from the thalamus are the major focus of this book. To understand these messages it is necessary to look closely at the afferents to the thalamus. This chapter focuses on morphological features of the afferents, and chapter 5 focuses on their synaptic properties. We indicated in chapter 1 that the afferents can be classified as either drivers or modulators. It is the drivers that actually define the message carried to cortex, whereas the modulators produce changes in the way the message is transmitted or determine whether it is transmitted at all.

We shall see in this chapter that the drivers have a common terminal structure and pattern of synaptic connections in the thalamus (figures 3.1 through 3.3; compare with figures 3.4 and 3.5) even though they come from a variety of different sources, including the sensory pathways, the mamillothalamic tract, and the deep cerebellar nuclei for first order relays, and layer 5 of many different cortical areas for higher order relays. Many, possibly all, of the driver afferents have branches that innervate brainstem centers related to movement control. These branches, which do not end in the thalamus, provide an important clue about the nature of the messages that the drivers bring to the thalamus. They are considered in chapter 10.

Throughout the thalamus, the drivers contribute a minority of the synaptic junctions made onto relay cells. Where we have numbers, the proportion is less than 10% and may be as low as 2% (Van Horn et al., 2000; Wang et al., 2002a). That is, the modulators represent more than 90% of the synaptic junctions received by relay cells, and understanding the functional relationships of the modulators still represents one of the major challenges for understanding thalamic functions.

Figures 3.1 through 3.5 show two distinct types of afferent axons to first order (figures 3.1, 3.2, and 3.3) and higher order (figures 3.4 and 3.5) nuclei. Figures 3.1 through 3.3 show ascending driver afferents (type II axons) and figure 3.4 shows corticothalamic afferents (modulatory, type I axons) terminating in first order nuclei. Whereas the former have well-localized terminal arbors with relatively large en passant and terminal swellings and do not send branches to the reticular nucleus, the latter have more widespread terminal arbors, with small, scattered, terminal side branches and a few en passant swellings. They are often seen to send branches to the reticular nucleus (not shown in the figures). Figures 3.4 and 3.5 show the type I and type II axons that provide the same two sorts of afferent to higher order nuclei, both types here coming from the cortex but only the former having branches to the reticular nucleus (not shown in the figures).

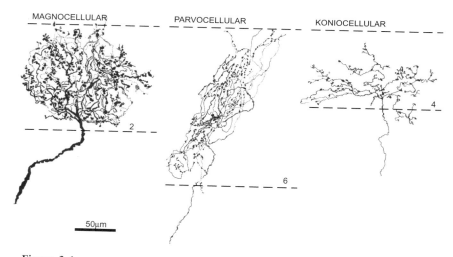

Figure 3.1
Three retinal afferent axons are shown terminating in different layers of the lateral geniculate nucleus in an adult *Galago* (from Lachica & Casagrande, 1988, with permission). Retinogeniculate axons were filled with horseradish peroxidase.

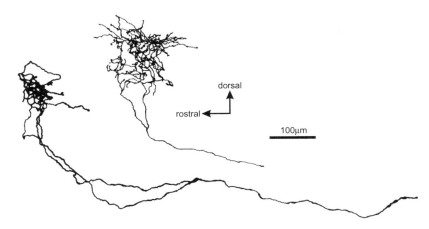

Figure 3.2
Two ascending driver afferents terminating in the medial geniculate nucleus of an adult ferret (from Pallas et al., 1994, with permission). Axons in the inferior colliculus were filled with horseradish peroxidase.

Modulators come from several different sources. The cerebral cortex sends excitatory, glutamatergic modulatory afferents, and these generally innervate the thalamic relays that supply the relevant area of cortex. They arise from pyramidal cells in layer 6. The brainstem sends cholinergic afferents, as well as serotonergic, noradrenergic, and histaminergic modulatory afferents. Inhibitory, GABAergic afferents come mainly from the thalamic reticular nucleus and from thalamic interneurons. Other examples of brainstem GABAergic or glutamatergic modulatory input to certain thalamic relays are considered separately in section 3.C.6.

Many of the afferent pathways to the thalamus, like the thalamocortical pathways themselves, have local sign. That is, there is an orderly map in the projection system, with different parts of the map representing differing functional loci. This mapping has been found for all of the driver afferents that have been studied from this point of view, and also for the modulatory afferents from layer 6 of cortex and for the local GABAergic inputs from the thalamic reticular nucleus and the interneurons, with the maps for the driver afferents and the modulatory afferents matching each other closely. Other pathways, particularly the cholinergic, histaminergic, noradrenergic, and serotonergic pathways, do not show a mapping that matches the thalamocortical projection, and current evidence suggests that they are not mapped. There is an

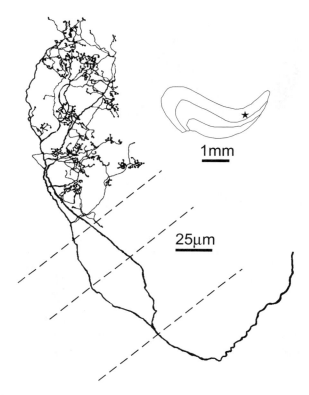

Figure 3.3
A retinogeniculate X axon terminating in layer A of the lateral geniculate nucleus
of a cat (from Sur et al., 1987, with permission). The axon was filled intracellularly with horseradish peroxidase and is shown in a coronal section. The star
in the small inset shows the location of the terminal arbor within the lateral
geniculate nucleus.

important functional distinction between a mapped modulatory projection, which can act on a small part of the functional system represented
by the thalamocortical pathway, and an unmapped one, which is likely
to affect all of any one system equally and may also act across several
distinct thalamocortical projection systems.

In this chapter we describe ways in which one can distinguish afferents on the basis of their light microscopic appearance, their fine structural, electron microscopic appearance, and their extrathalamic origins.
We show how these features may relate to the functions of the afferents
as drivers or modulators, and we look at the patterns of synaptic inter-

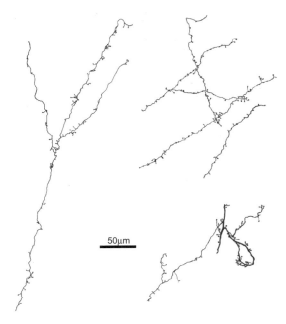

50μm

Figure 3.4
Corticogeniculate (type I) axons from the A layers of the lateral geniculate
nucleus of a cat; Golgi method (from Guillery, 1966, with permission).

connections established in the thalamus that help us to categorize each
of the major afferent groups.

3.B. The Drivers

3.B.1. Identifying the Drivers and Their Functions

We can use the morphological characteristics, synaptic relationships, and
functional properties of the drivers in well-studied thalamic nuclei, such
as the primary visual, auditory, or somatosensory relays, to identify the
drivers in other thalamic nuclei about which we currently have very
much less information. This idea forms an important part of this and
some of the later chapters. By identifying the drivers for any one thalamic nucleus, the origin of the main functionally significant input sent
by that nucleus to its cortical target can be defined. In this way it should
be possible to throw useful light on the function of those thalamic relays
and cortical areas that are currently not well understood. Each thalamic

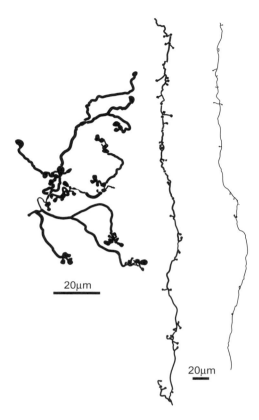

20μm

20μm

Figure 3.5
The terminal parts of three corticothalamic axons from a cat in the lateral posterior nucleus labeled by biotinylated dextran amine. A type II axon is shown
on the left, and two type I axons are shown on the right. *Note*: The drawing
shows the type I axons as thicker than they were in the section, in order to allow
adequate reproduction of the thinner parts of the axon. (From an unpublished
experiment by S. L. Feig and R. W. Guillery.)

nucleus may be capable of a variety of functional modes, but its essential function in awake behaving animals is to pass information received over its driving afferents on to its own cortical targets, and we regard this as a crucial feature of thalamic organization. The functional capacities of the receiving cortex depend critically on the nature of the messages that are carried to the thalamus by the driving afferents.

The primary visual cortex is regarded as visual because retinal messages reach it via the lateral geniculate nucleus and because of the closely related observations that its removal produces severe visual losses and its neurons respond to visual stimuli. For higher cortical areas, defining their functions rarely depends on defining the drivers of the thalamic relays to that area. Looking for functional losses after lesions can provide some clues, as can a study of the response properties of the cortical neurons. However, functional losses that are demonstrable depend on the observer's expectations, as do the response properties recorded from cortical neurons, and both can be elusive in higher cortical areas. Defining the role of the drivers to the relevant thalamic relay may not be much easier; it is an additional source of information that can strengthen our knowledge of a transthalamic pathway, but it is not one that is currently appreciated or used.

One can ask: what would be the consequence if drivers destined for one thalamic relay could be directed to another? The issue is not as purely theoretical as might appear at first. Sur and colleagues (Sur et al., 1988; Sharma et al., 2000; Von Melchner et al., 2000), working with young ferrets, redirected retinofugal axons into auditory thalamus after removing the visual cortex and superior colliculus. The auditory thalamus then received messages from the retina and sent them to the auditory cortex, where cells in the experimental adults responded to visual instead of auditory stimuli. That is, Sur and colleagues were able to show that nerve cells in the newly innervated cortex could be driven by visual stimuli and that the ferrets could respond to those visual stimuli.

This result illustrates not only the extent to which a cortical area depends on its thalamic input but also how important it is for investigators to know enough about the nature of the input to develop a better understanding of what it is that the cortex may be doing. Whereas when one is dealing with a sensory pathway, it seems fairly straightforward to define the functions of a cortical area on the basis of the driver inputs to its thalamic relay, the issue is more difficult for other pathways relayed through the thalamus. For example, there are a number of studies of neuronal activity in the cerebellar afferents to the thalamus in relation to activity in the recipient thalamic cells or the recipient motor cortical areas (Horne & Butler, 1995; Miall et al., 1998; Butler et al., 2000). These studies provide some clues as to the nature of the information that is transferred through the thalamus and how this information may relate to activity in the motor cortex. However, there is nothing comparable to the conceptual link between the inputs and outputs of the lateral geniculate nucleus, on the one hand, and activity in visual cortex on the other.

One thalamic link that illustrates the importance of understanding how inputs to a thalamic nucleus relate to the functions of the cortical recipient zone is the link going through the anterior dorsal thalamic nucleus. Cells in this, the smallest of the three anterior thalamic nuclei in rats, respond to specific head orientations in space (Taube, 1995). This nucleus sends thalamocortical axons to the retrosplenial cortex, where similar neurons can be recorded, as can neurons that respond when the animal is in a particular place in its environment. The driving afferents to the anterior dorsal nucleus come from the tiny lateral mamillary nucleus, which also has head orientation neurons, and these neurons in turn receive their innervation from neurons driven by inputs from the vestibular nuclei of the brainstem (Taube, 1995; Brown et al., 2002; Vann et al., 2003). There are many thalamic relays where this type of information, providing a comparable synthetic view of messages passed through thalamus to cortex, still remains to be defined. Such information is still lacking for some first order relays (e.g., the other two anterior thalamic nuclei) and is generally not available for any higher order thalamic relay. We can expect to learn more about relays in the medial dorsal, lateral dorsal, pulvinar, or intralaminar nuclei (see chapter 1) if we can define the origin and the functional nature of their driving afferents, a problem that is explored further in chapters 7 and 8.

We have stressed that not all afferents are equal. Drivers and modulators perform clearly distinct functions. Classifications of thalamic nuclei based on the origin or the total number of any one group of afferents are not likely to prove instructive unless the functional nature of the afferents has been taken into consideration (Macchi, 1983). It has been a general practice to classify thalamic nuclei in terms of the ascending afferents that they receive from lower centers, and to regard the inputs from cortex as categorically different, not contributing to this classification. We shall treat afferents in terms of their morphological relationships and the effects that they are likely to have on relay cells, no matter what their origin, and in the following account we recognize ascending drivers as well as drivers that come from the cerebral cortex. Similarly, modulators will be seen to have cortical as well as subcortical origins.

3.B.2. Identifying the Drivers on the Basis of Their Structure

The structure of the drivers, no matter what their origin, is readily recognizable and relates closely to their equally characteristic functional properties (discussed in chapter 7). The drivers resemble each other in their light microscopic and electron microscopic appearance, and they can be seen to establish similar synaptic relationships in the thalamus. On the basis of currently available evidence, driver afferents send branches to innervate nonthalamic brainstem centers and also innervate thalamic relay cells and interneurons, but they do not innervate the cells of the thalamic reticular nucleus. Modulators have a completely different light microscopic appearance, establish quite distinct patterns of synaptic relationships in the thalamus, and generally (perhaps always) innervate the thalamic reticular nucleus. The functional significance of the reticular connections is discussed in section 3.C.2 and in chapter 9.

At this point it is important to be clear about the basis of our identification of drivers in higher order relays. We argue that the drivers in the major sensory relays (the visual, auditory, and somatosensory afferents) are known on the basis of their receptive field properties in thalamus and cortex and on the basis of functional losses produced by damage to these afferents or to the relevant thalamic or cortical structures. When we see afferents that have the same structural, connectional, and physiological characteristics, we argue that they must therefore also have the same functions within the thalamic circuitry. That is, they must also be drivers. Even where the drivers do not have a readily demonstrable sensory function, and even where they may be carrying messages from cortical or other structures (cerebellum, mamillary bodies) with poorly defined or undefined functions, their function in the thalamus can reasonably be regarded as bringing to the thalamus the message that is passed to cortex, whatever that message may prove to be.

To illustrate this argument, it is useful to look at other well-characterized axonal terminal patterns, such as those in the cerebellum, where the morphology of the terminal arbor can be clearly related to the way in which a particular class of axon establishes its synaptic relationships (Eccles et al., 1967). The synaptic portions of basket cell axons are shaped to match the shape of the relevant receptive surface of the Purkinje cells, the climbing fibers match the branching pattern of their postsynaptic dendrites, and the parallel fibers show a distribution of synaptic swellings that relates closely to the contacts established as these fibers pass along the dendritic trees of the Purkinje cells. Above all, the mossy fibers, no matter what their origin from one of several different brainstem sources, show a common structure and connectivity pattern and are reasonably assumed to all perform the same basic functions in the cerebellar circuitry. Comparably, it is reasonable to assume that when one sees axons resembling those in figures 3.1 through 3.3, there is a shared pattern of connectivity, one that differs from that of the modulatory axons (e.g., figures 3.4 and 3.5), no matter where in the thalamus we are looking. We shall see that the structure, the synaptic connections, and the functional properties of the drivers show that the message is well localized to a relatively small part of the thalamus, and that the presynaptic axon terminal boutons are relatively large, allowing for a multiplicity of synaptic junctions that would correspond to the large postsynaptic potentials generally elicited by activity in a driver.

The drivers are readily recognizable in Golgi preparations or when displayed by injections of intracellular markers such as *Phaseolus* lectin, horseradish peroxidase, or biocytin (for an account of some of these methods, see Bolam, 1992), which reveal the structure of the terminals against a relatively clear background (see figures 3.1 through 3.5). They all show well-localized terminal zones that are characterized by relatively large, closely packed synaptic swellings (boutons) that may be en passant or terminal. Such structures have been described for ascending sensory pathways terminating in the ventral posterior nucleus, lateral geniculate nucleus, or medial geniculate nucleus (Cajal, 1911; Jones, 1983; Bowling & Michael, 1984; Sur et al., 1987; Pallas & Sur, 1994) and are sometimes generically referred to as lemniscal afferents. In earlier studies they were called type II terminals for the lateral geniculate nucleus (Guillery, 1966). Comparable terminals, called R-type terminals in the pulvinar (Rockland, 1996), have also been shown for corticothalamic drivers, which take their origin from cells in cortical layer 5 and terminate in higher order visual, auditory, and somatosensory thalamic relays (Deschênes et al., 1994; Ojima, 1994; Bourassa & Deschênes, 1995; Bourassa et al., 1995; Rockland, 1998; Darian-Smith et al., 1999; Kakei et al., 2001). The recent claim (Jones, 2001) that corticothalamic axons arising in layer 5 of cortex, that is, the driving corticothalamic axons (see below), form diffuse and widespread terminals in the thalamus is contrary to the many observations cited above showing well-localized terminal arbors comparable to those of ascending lemniscal afferents.

When the driver terminals are seen in electron micrographs, they form prominent, large terminal boutons that commonly establish complex synaptic relationships (figures 3.6 and 3.7). They were called

RL profiles because they contain round vesicles and are large. They have been identified in every thalamic nucleus that has been studied. They characteristically contain a dense group of mitochondria, suggestive of high metabolic capacities, and commonly, these mitochondria are significantly paler than the mitochondria in other nearby profiles, so that originally they were labeled RLP (P for pale) profiles (Colonnier & Guillery, 1964). The significance of this paler appearance is not known, and because the pale appearance is not always identifiable, we describe them as RL profiles and say no more about the mitochondria. The RL profiles are identifiable on the basis of several other features, particularly the multiple synaptic junctions that they make, which are indicated by arrows in figure 3.7 and considered in a later section.

Figures 3.6 and 3.7 show that the RL terminals commonly but not invariably lie close among a group of other profiles with which they establish synaptic junctions. These profiles lie packed adjacent to each other within a zone that is relatively free of glial cytoplasm and is called a glomerulus (Szentágothai, 1963) on the basis of its resemblance to the classical cerebellar glomerulus that surrounds the terminals of mossy fibers. A thalamic glomerulus can be defined as a specialized region where three or more, commonly more, synaptic profiles are closely related to each other, where several synaptic junctions are formed between these profiles, and where, characteristically, astrocytic cytoplasm (shaded in figure 3.7) is excluded from the regions close to the synaptic junctions and tends preferentially to collect as thin cytoplasmic sheets around the outer borders of the glomerulus.

Axon terminals having the characteristics of RL terminals have been identified as the driving afferents in the lateral geniculate nucleus (Szentágothai, 1963; Colonnier & Guillery, 1964; Peters & Palay, 1966; Guillery, 1969a), the medial geniculate nucleus (Jones & Rockel, 1971; Morest, 1975; Majorossy & Kiss, 1976), and the ventral posterior nucleus (Jones & Powell, 1969; Ralston, 1969; Ma et al., 1987a, 1987b; Ohara et al., 1989). The cerebellar axons that innervate the ventral lateral nucleus have also been identified as forming RL terminals (Harding, 1973; Rinvik & Grofova, 1974a, 1974b; Ilinsky & Kultas-Ilinsky, 1990; Kultas-Ilinsky & Ilinsky, 1991), as have the mamillothalamic afferents to the anterior nuclei (Somogyi et al., 1978). That is, the RL terminals are the drivers in every first order thalamic relay.

For higher order relays, more than 30 years ago Mathers (1972) showed that in the pulvinar of the monkey, corticothalamic axons having the characteristic RL (driver) structure degenerate after lesions are made

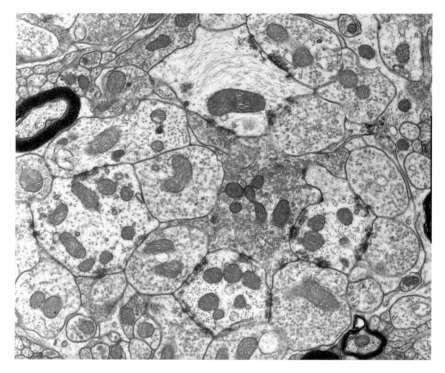

Figure 3.6
Electron micrograph of a glomerulus with a large central RL terminal from
lateral posterior nucleus of a cat. A schematic interpretation of the major profiles identifiable in this micrograph is shown in figure 3.7, where some of the
synaptic junctions are identified by arrows. F and RL identify the major types of
axon terminal (see text), and D identifies some of the dendritic profiles. This particular glomerulus shows very little evidence of the encapsulation by sheets of
astrocytic cytoplasm that is often regarded as a typical feature of thalamic
glomeruli. See text for details.

in visual cortex, and the cortical origin of these RL terminals was later
confirmed for the lateral posterior nucleus and pulvinar of the cat and
monkey, respectively (Ogren & Hendrickson, 1979; Feig & Harting,
1998), and the squirrel (Robson & Hall, 1977b). More recently Schwartz
et al. (1991) showed RL terminals in the medial dorsal nucleus that came
from frontal cortex. Kultas-Ilinsky et al. (1997) report that some RL
terminals in the ventral anterior nucleus of the monkey have a cortical
origin, and Hoogland et al. (1991), who traced axons marked by intracellular label from somatosensory cortex of the mouse to the (higher

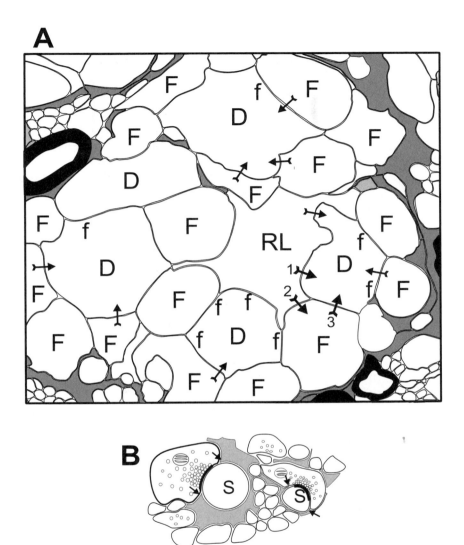

Figure 3.7
A. Interpretative schema to identify the major profiles in figure 3.6. The arrows indicate the positions of synaptic junctions, with the arrowheads pointing to the postsynaptic element. Astrocytic profiles are shown in gray, myelin in black. D, dendritic profiles; F, F-type profiles; f, filamentous contacts (desmosomes); RL, retinal terminal. Further details are given in the text. B. Comparable schematic representation at the same scale for the cerebellar molecular layer of synapses made onto Purkinje cell spines (S) to show the close relationship of the astrocytic cytoplasm to these synaptic junctions (*arrows*). (Based on figure 5.9 from Peters et al., 1991.)

order) posterior nucleus, have identified some of these as large, RL terminals within that thalamic nucleus. Comparable observations on cortical afferents to the (higher order) dorsal division of the medial geniculate nucleus have also been reported by Bartlett et al. (2000; see also Rouiller & Welker, 2000).

The common structural and connectional features of the thalamic afferents we have categorized as drivers argue strongly in favor of common functions. The functional properties are discussed further in chapter 7. Here it is important to stress the effect that can be seen when the cells giving rise to the drivers are silenced. In a first order sensory pathway such silencing produces a complete loss of the characteristic sensory receptive field. In a thalamic higher order relay that receives corticothalamic drivers from layer 5, as in the pulvinar of the monkey or the lateral posterior nucleus of the cat (Bender, 1983; Chalupa, 1991) or the posterior nucleus of the rat (Diamond et al., 1992), such silencing of the relevant cortical areas also produces a corresponding loss.

3.B.3. *The Origin of the Drivers and Their Heterogeneity*

We have indicated that the drivers for first order relays come from a variety of different sources, including the several sensory pathways, the mamillary bodies, and the deep cerebellar nuclei. The drivers for higher order relays come from the neocortex, specifically from pyramidal cells in layer 5. The precise relationships between the thalamocortical terminals and the layer 5 corticothalamic pathways for higher order relays still remain largely undefined. They are not likely to be reciprocal connections. Evidence for the cortical layer 5 origin of drivers comes from several different approaches. One approach entails the injection of label into single cells or of very small groups of cells that are identified in terms of their cortical locus and morphology and whose axons are traced into the thalamus (Deschênes et al., 1994; Bourassa & Deschênes, 1995; Bourassa et al., 1995). Another uses large injections of label made into one or another thalamic nucleus and the subsequent study of retrogradely labeled cortical cells. Such experiments (Gilbert & Kelly, 1975; Abramson & Chalupa, 1985) show that all thalamic nuclei receive afferents from cortical layer 6 but only some receive afferents from layer 5. Those that receive afferents from layer 6 only (e.g., the lateral geniculate nucleus) are the ones that receive ascending drivers but no corticothalamic drivers (see also Ojima, 1994). Those that receive afferents from layer 5 generally receive no, or only a few, ascending afferents. As indicated earlier and discussed further in chapter 8, there are nuclei that are likely to represent a mixture of first and higher order relays. Finally, focal electrical stimulation of corticothalamic axons from an in vitro slice preparation in the mouse shows that afferents from layers 5 and 6 have different properties, and that the former closely resemble other known driver afferents (e.g., retinogeniculate) in their properties (Reichova & Sherman, 2004; see chapters 5 and 7 for more details of these synaptic properties).

Although so far we have stressed the features that are shared by the driver afferents, it has to be recognized that not all drivers are the same. In chapter 2 we considered the differences among retinogeniculate pathways, distinguishing X, Y, and W pathways and parvocellular, magnocellular, and koniocellular pathways. These axons differ in their diameter and, correspondingly, in the size of the terminal structures they form in the lateral geniculate nucleus. The RL terminals formed by the W pathway are smaller than those formed by the X and Y pathways (Raczkowski et al., 1988, and figure 3.1). The X, Y, and W pathways also differ in the synaptic connections that they form onto relay cells (see below, section 3.D.2). Comparably, there is some variation in the structures of the corticothalamic driver afferents, although we know less about these. Guillery et al. (2001) showed that the light microscopic structure of the layer 5 corticothalamic terminals to the lateral posterior nucleus varied, with the most ventral and posterior terminals forming narrow, closely packed "cartridges" of terminal boutons and the more dorsal and anterior terminals forming a more open pattern. There was a striking similarity between the most ventral cartridges seen in the ventral parts of the lateral posterior nucleus and the terminal structures formed by retinogeniculate axons in the ventral C layers of the lateral geniculate nucleus (Guillery, 1966), where the W axons terminate.

3.B.4. The Relationship of Two Driver Inputs to a Single Thalamic Nucleus: Does the Thalamus Have an Integrative Function?

There is an important question about the driving afferents that has so far received limited attention for most thalamic nuclei. Where a cell group receives driving afferents from more than one source, one needs to know how the two groups of afferents relate to each other and to their postsynaptic neurons. The problem is again well illustrated in the lateral geniculate nucleus of the cat, where the X and the Y pathways have a common terminal site in one set of layers but show no significant interaction. With only rare examples of mixing, X cells have glomerular synapses, Y cells have mostly extraglomerular synapses, and any one geniculate cell serves as a relay for either the X or the Y pathways, not both (Cleland et al., 1971; Wilson et al., 1984; Hamos et al., 1987; Usrey et al., 1999). In general, there is little or no convergence among retino-geniculate inputs (see chapter 7), suggesting that at least for this driver input, there is no significant integrative function in thalamus. The question also arises in other nuclei, but has not been resolved in many. For example, in the ventral posterior nucleus of the rat, spinothalamic and lemniscal terminals overlap, and may share postsynaptic cells (Ma et al., 1987b). In the monkey, there is evidence that these two pathways terminate in adjacent but interdigitating parts of the nucleus (Krubitzer & Kaas, 1992), suggesting that they either do not share postsynaptic relay cells or do so only rarely.

For thalamic nuclei that may receive a mixture of first and higher order inputs (discussed further in chapter 8), there is no evidence about the possibility of shared postsynaptic sites. The nature of the relationships established by two (or more) driver pathways within a thalamic nucleus is likely to prove crucial to understanding the functional organization of that nucleus. If thalamic relays in general are like the lateral geniculate relay, and if functionally distinct relay pathways do not share cells in the transmittal of driver inputs, then one would expect to see no significant change in the nature of the message that is transmitted through the thalamic relay. That is, one could generalize from the lateral geniculate nucleus and say that the thalamic relay is concerned with the transmittal of a message, not with the integration of messages. Where one finds that two pathways share a relay, as possibly in the ventral posterior nucleus of the rat, one would need to look closely at how those two inputs interact functionally in the relay, in terms of the relay cell responses and also in terms of their synaptic arrangements on the relay cell dendrites and, where relevant, within the glomeruli.

3.C. The Modulators

3.C.1. Corticothalamic Axons from Layer 6 Cells

3.C.1.a. Structure, Origin, and Distribution
Numerically, one of the largest groups of modulators is made up of the axons of layer 6 cortical cells. These corticothalamic axons are generally

thinner than the layer 5 axons and have long, thin branches that run for considerable distances through the thalamus, with some en passage swellings and many short, stubby, terminal side branches, each of which ends in a tiny single swelling (see figures 3.4 and 3.5). These short side branches are an absolute hallmark of these corticothalamic axons and were aptly described as "drumstick-like" side branches by Szentágothai (1963) for the cat lateral geniculate nucleus. They were called type I axons by Guillery (1966) and type E axons by Rockland (1996). The terminals of the layer 6 axons are generally less tightly grouped and less well localized than are the terminals of the layer 5 axons (see figures 3.1 through 3.5).

Evidence that these modulatory axons come from layer 6 is comparable to the evidence summarized for the layer 5 projection above. That is, injections of retrograde tracers into first order nuclei such as the lateral geniculate nucleus have shown that all the corticothalamic axons come from layer 6 (Gilbert & Kelly, 1975) and that all the corticothalamic axons in these nuclei have the characteristic appearance described above (Guillery, 1967b; Robson, 1983). Most important, for first and for higher order nuclei, these axons can be traced from individual cortical cells or small groups of cells marked by anterograde tracers (Deschênes et al., 1994; Ojima, 1994; Bourassa & Deschênes, 1995; Bourassa et al., 1995; Murphy & Sillito, 1996; Ojima et al., 1996; Murphy et al., 2000).

The evidence for regarding these corticothalamic axons as modulators rather than drivers comes mainly from experiments in which the activity of thalamic cells is recorded in a nucleus such as the lateral geniculate nucleus, which receives only layer 6 inputs and no layer 5 inputs, while the cortical origin of the layer 6 input (area 17 or 18) is stimulated or silenced by cooling or destruction. A variety of modifications of receptive field properties have been reported in anesthetized preparations, but they are relatively mild and do not represent the total loss of receptive field that characterizes silencing of the drivers (Kalil & Chase, 1970; Richard et al., 1975; Baker & Malpeli, 1977; Schmielau & Singer, 1977; Singer, 1977; Sillito et al., 1994; Cudeiro & Sillito, 1996). Also, as noted above and described more fully in chapter 7, corticothalamic synapses from layer 6 behave differently from known driver synapses.

Although these axons vary considerably in thickness and in the density of their terminals, they are strikingly uniform in their basic structure, with the very short terminal side branches given off as shown in figures 3.4 and 3.5. This makes them readily distinguishable from other afferent types to the thalamus that have been described. The axons are remarkably similar in appearance, not only from nucleus to nucleus but also from species to species. It should be recognized that it is the shape of the terminal arbor more than the thickness of the axons or the size of the terminals that represents the crucial distinguishing feature between layer 5 and layer 6 axons. In many nuclei, as, for example, the lateral geniculate nucleus of the cat, the drivers (retinogeniculate axons) invariably have larger terminal boutons than do the layer 6 modulators, but in other regions the sizes can be more evenly matched. Thus, we have seen some relatively small layer 5 terminal boutons in the cat's lateral posterior nucleus, and in rats we have seen several examples of layer 5 axons with terminal boutons in a size range overlapping the larger layer 6 boutons (R. W. Guillery and S. L. Feig, unpublished light microscopic observations).

In electron micrographs, the terminals of the modulatory layer 6 corticothalamic axons have a characteristic appearance. They contain round synaptic vesicles and are relatively small. With rare exceptions, they make single synaptic contacts with adjacent dendritic processes. Such RS profiles are relatively common in all thalamic nuclei, but not all of the profiles that can be identified as RS profiles represent the corticothalamic modulators. In the lateral geniculate nucleus about half of these profiles come from the brainstem and represent cholinergic afferents (Erişir et al., 1997b). They are considered in more detail below. Most of the RS profiles lie outside the glomeruli (see above), and those that are in the glomeruli can generally be identified as belonging to the cholinergic brainstem component. A similar arrangement has been described for the cat's pulvinar (Patel & Bickford, 1997), where most of the cholinergic terminals are in glomeruli, but the cat's lateral posterior nucleus may be somewhat different, since most of the cholinergic terminals there seem to target distal dendritic shafts rather than glomeruli (Patel et al., 1999).

It should be noted that the two types of cortical cell (layer 6 and layer 5) contributing afferents to any one thalamic nucleus are not necessarily found in the same areas of cortex. For example, in the cat, area 17 contributes a layer 5 input to the lateral posterior nucleus but essentially no layer 6 input, and sends a layer 6 input but no layer 5 input to the lateral geniculate nucleus (Gilbert & Kelly, 1975; Abramson & Chalupa, 1985). Both of these nuclei, the lateral geniculate nucleus and the lateral posterior nucleus, receive layer 6 inputs from several other visual cortical areas, some of which also send layer 5 inputs to some of the same extrageniculate regions of the thalamus (Updyke, 1977, 1981; Abramson & Chalupa, 1985).[1]

We indicated earlier that drivers differ from modulators in that drivers do not innervate the thalamic reticular nucleus, whereas modulators commonly, possibly always, do (Uhlrich et al., 1993; Deschênes et al., 1994; Bourassa & Deschênes, 1995; Bourassa et al., 1995; Murphy & Sillito, 1996; Murphy et al., 2000; Uhlrich et al., 2003). This is potentially an important functional distinction, but there are many thalamic nuclei; for most, the corticothalamic inputs have not received any study from this point of view, and relatively few individual axons have been traced. It is not known whether every layer 6 corticothalamic axon has such a branch, or whether only some of them do. A preparation that reveals a group of corticothalamic axons passing through the reticular nucleus and continuing on to the thalamus shows that the plexus in the reticular nucleus is well localized and relatively dense, but in its total extent it is modest compared to that developed in the thalamus (Murphy & Sillito, 1996; Murphy et al., 2000). An intuitive, nonquantified view would suggest that either each reticular branch is rather modest, or that only some of the corticothalamic axons passing through the nucleus have reticular branches. Further, whereas axons arising from cortical areas 17, 18, or 19 show such branches (Murphy & Sillito, 1996; Murphy et al., 2000; Guillery et al., 2001), unpublished observations (R.W.G.) of several robust layer 6 corticothalamic axons arising in the lateral suprasylvian cortex and with numerous well-stained terminals in the thalamus have shown either short and extremely fine branches in the reticular nucleus with very few terminals, or (12 axons) with no identifiable branches in the reticular nucleus at all. That is, while the failure to stain fine branches does not demonstrate their absence, the varied appearance of reticular branches from different cortical areas indicates that the degree to which any one cortical area does or does not innervate the reticular nucleus may vary and merits further attention.

---

1. An observation (Feig & Guillery, 2000) that both types of corticothalamic axon appear to innervate small blood vessels in the regions close to their terminal thalamic arbors raises two interesting possibilities that warrant further study. One is that these axons may play a role in controlling the blood supply to the regions that they innervate, and the other is that they may alter the permeability of vessels in those regions, producing modulatory actions quite distinct from those produced by transmitter release from the axon terminals.

3.C.1.b. Topographic Organization of Corticothalamic Afferents

Evidence from early fiber degeneration studies and from more recent labeling studies (Guillery, 1967b; Bourassa & Deschênes, 1995; Bourassa et al., 1995; Murphy & Sillito, 1996; Murphy et al., 2000) indicates that the layer 6 corticothalamic axons that go to the first order nuclei all show a topographic organization that matches the thalamocortical projection relatively closely (figure 3.8; compare this figure with figure 2.1). However, when single axons are traced, individual layer 6 axons show more scatter in the relevant part of a thalamic nucleus than do the individual driver axons described above. This has been demonstrated in a comparison of corticogeniculate and retinogeniculate axons for the visual pathways by Murphy and Sillito (1996; Murphy et al., 2000) in the cat's lateral geniculate nucleus. It has also been shown for the two types of cortical afferent, one coming from layer 6 and one from layer 5, for the somatosensory pathways in rat and monkey (Bourassa & Deschênes, 1995; Bourassa et al., 1995; Darian-Smith et al., 1999), for the motor cortex of the cat (Kakei et al., 2001), and for the visual pulvinar (Rockland, 1998). This relationship may to some extent reflect the

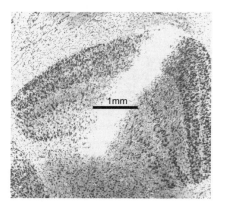

1mm

Figure 3.8

A coronal section through the lateral geniculate nucleus of an owl monkey showing a "pencil" of autoradiographic label passing through all of the geniculate layers. Radioactive proline had been injected into a small zone of the primary visual cortex (area 17) on the same side. The proline was incorporated into proteins or polypeptides in the cortical cells and transported along the corticothalamic axons to the lateral geniculate nucleus. The radioactivity in the terminals of the labeled corticothalamic terminals shows up on the photographic emulsion with which the section was coated, and in this dark-field micrograph appears as a bright streak. (From a photograph by Jon Kaas, with permission.)

fact that the layer 6 axons distribute to the peripheral segments of relay cell dendrites (see below), whereas the layer 5 axons distribute to proximal dendritic segments.

Murphy et al. (2000) found that there is not a strict reciprocity between the thalamocortical and the corticothalamic pathways in the corticogeniculate projections of the cat. Their study showed that the pathway tends to favor reciprocal connections, with cortical areas 17 and 18 each showing a preference for the geniculate layers from which they receive afferents, extending Updyke's (1977) demonstration that the geniculate C layers, which project to area 19, also receive a major input from that cortical area. In terms of more detailed connections, Murphy et al. (2000) showed that individual corticogeniculate axons terminate most densely in a zone corresponding to the region where geniculate receptive fields matched those of the corticofugal axons. However, even when allowance is made for the fact that these corticothalamic axons relate to the peripheral dendrites of the geniculate cells, the corticogeniculate axons also extended well beyond that, but as a less dense zone. Further, in the geniculate relay one finds that where retinal afferents are limited to a single set of monocularly innervated layers, most cortical afferents distribute to adjacent layers, one receiving from each eye. That is, some scatter of the corticothalamic modulators around the relevant geniculocortical cells beyond strict reciprocity is demonstrable. For most other parts of the thalamus, evidence about the reciprocity of the thalamocortical and the layer 6 corticothalamic pathways is not yet defined. Darian-Smith et al. (1999) showed examples of layer 6 terminals that scattered well beyond the region of retrogradely labeled cells in the ventral posterior nucleus of monkeys, suggesting that strict reciprocity of the pathways is not a general rule, although there may be a tendency for the densest layer 6 input to relate reciprocally to thalamocortical cells (Van Horn & Sherman, 2004).

For most higher order relays we lack specific information about the mapping of the layer 6 inputs. The majority of studies show that the corticothalamic projections are mapped (Updyke, 1977, 1981; Groenewegen, 1988; Shipp, 2001, 2003). However, these studies used methods that do not allow a distinction to be made between the layer 5 driver input and the layer 6 modulatory input. In experiments that allow a distinction between the two cortical inputs from a single small cortical injection site (see above; see also Bourassa & Deschênes, 1995; Bourassa et al., 1995; Rockland, 1998; Darian-Smith et al., 1999), the layer 6 inputs extend well beyond the layer 5 inputs, and in some instances (Guillery et al., 2001) also tend to surround the layer 5 input but not occupy the zone of the layer 5 terminals itself. Here we are seeing the distribution of the cortical modulators in relation to the corticothalamic drivers that define the receptive field of the relevant thalamic cells, not in relation to the relevant thalamocortical pathway that might define the reciprocity of the modulatory corticothalamic pathway. That is, assuming that cells in layers 5 and 6 of a single cortical column have a common receptive field, the modulators here are not going back to the thalamic relay cells whose receptive fields they share, as they do to a great extent in the lateral geniculate nucleus (Murphy et al., 2000).

3.C.1.c. The Heterogeneity of the Corticothalamic Axons from Layer 6

Although we have indicated that the thalamic terminal structures of the layer 6 axons are essentially similar in all thalamic nuclei, there is reason to think that there are differences in the cortical cells that give rise to these axons. In chapter 2 we discussed the dangers of creating distinct classes on the basis of a few criteria that have not been shown to have a clear bimodal or multimodal distribution. However, the opposite danger must also be recognized, namely, of looking for a single function where several functions contribute to a system. Tsumoto and Suda (1980) described three types of cortical cell projecting to the lateral geniculate nucleus of cats, basing these types on axonal conduction velocities and receptive field properties. They found that one type, having intermediate values for conduction velocity, is absent from the monocular segment of the nucleus, which led them to suggest that this particular type of corticothalamic cell may be specifically concerned with binocular interactions, a function that was earlier proposed by Schmielau and Singer (1977) for corticogeniculate axons and that would fit well with the observation that many corticogeniculate axons pass through the layers in the direction of the lines of projection and can have terminals in adjacent layers that receive retinal innervation from different eyes (Guillery, 1967b; Robson, 1983; Murphy & Sillito, 1996; Murphy et al., 2000).

Katz (1987) described two types of cell in cortical layer 6 of area 17 projecting to the lateral geniculate nucleus in cats. These cell types differed in the richness of their dendritic arbors and local cortical collaterals. In primates, distinct populations of cortical cells project to different layers of the lateral geniculate nucleus (Fitzpatrick et al., 1994; Casagrande & Kaas, 1994), and Bourassa and Deschênes (1995) showed that cells in the upper parts of cortical layer 6 of area 17 in the rat project to the lateral geniculate nucleus, whereas cells in the lower parts send axons to the lateral posterior nucleus and the lateral geniculate nucleus, with some single axons innervating both nuclei.

We have said that the small "drumstick-like" side branches of the layer 6 corticothalamic afferents are an absolute hallmark of the corticothalamic modulators, and we have indicated that the density of the distribution of corticothalamic terminals varies considerably for any one corticothalamic pathway. The right part of figure 3.5 shows two layer 6 corticothalamic afferents, one at a significantly lower magnification than the other, showing that the side branches can be distributed relatively densely or sparsely along the course of one of these axons. One might anticipate that where the cortical input is sparse the side branches would be widely spaced, and where it is dense they would be closely spaced along any one axon. However, the relationship is more complex, so that one can see closely spaced side branches occurring far from the focus, and widely spaced branches at the densest focus. Whether the density of the side branches relates to distinct cortical cell types or to distinct types of terminal relationships (or both) remains to be determined. The illustrations of single axons shown by Murphy and Sillito (1996) suggest considerable variability in the density of side branches on single axons, so that for these axons this feature appears to be related to the character of the terminal distribution, not to the cortical origin of the axon.

Apart from the heterogeneity of the cells that provide the corticothalamic modulators for any one cortical area, there is also the heterogeneity of the cortical areas within which the cells lie. The precise origin, in terms of particular cortical cytoarchitectonic areas, of layer 6 corticothalamic afferents has only been defined to a limited extent for some thalamic nuclei. There is a need for more information for each thalamic nucleus about precisely which cortical areas send layer 6 afferents to that nucleus and how these several inputs relate to each other. It will be important to define where two thalamic nuclei share a cortical afferent, as do the first and higher order visual relays in the study of Bourassa and Deschênes (1995), and it will be equally important to know where several distinct corticothalamic afferents relate to a single thalamic relay cell or group of relay cells. That is, this is a system that shows both divergence and convergence. For example, we know that the lateral geniculate nucleus of the cat receives layer 6 afferents from cortical areas 17, 18, and 19. There is significant overlap of these three inputs, but the extent to which inputs from two different cortical areas impinge on the same geniculate cell or the same parts of any one geniculate cell is unknown. Areas 17 and 18 distribute to all geniculate layers, with the layer 18 afferents being somewhat more focused on intralaminar regions, whereas area 19 sends its axons to the geniculate C layers and also sends a significant layer 6 component to the lateral posterior nucleus and pulvinar (Updyke, 1977; Murphy et al., 2000; Guillery et al., 2001). There are additional afferents to parts of the lateral geniculate nucleus from other visual cortical areas (Updyke, 1981), but we know nothing about how these several afferents interact in modulating geniculate activity.

Other examples of the complexity of these modulatory inputs are represented by the anterior thalamic nuclei, which receive RS afferents not only from the cingulate cortex, which is the area of cortex to which the relay cells project, but also from the hippocampus (Somogyi et al., 1978). The cortical projection to the medial dorsal nucleus as described by Négyessy et al. (1998) is of interest because there is a bilateral corticothalamic pathway. The uncrossed pathway is relatively large and includes axons that have RS terminals as well as some axons that have RL terminals. The smaller crossed projection possibly also includes both types of terminal (see Kaitz & Robertson, 1981; Preuss & Goldman-Rakic, 1987; Carretta et al., 1996; Négyessy et al., 1998; Shibata, 1998). For the center median nucleus it has been reported that injections of retrograde tracers into the nucleus label cortical pyramidal cells in layer 5 but not in layer 6 of the motor cortex (Catsman-Berrevoets & Kuypers, 1978; Royce, 1983). This pattern of labeling suggests that there should be a significant RL or type II input to the center median nucleus from motor cortex, with no significant type I or RS input. However, fine structural studies of this pathway (Harding, 1973; Balercia et al., 1996) show a predominant RS input. Possibly the layer 6 cells in motor cortex are resistant to the retrograde marker used, perhaps most of the RS terminals that come from the motor cortex come from layer 5 cells, or possibly the RS terminals that were described were mainly parts of larger RL terminals and would have been identified as such had the studies used serial sections. The issue remains unresolved.

Experiments designed to test the action of corticothalamic afferents coming from visual cortex have generally focused on one or two cortical areas (17, 18) in anesthetized animals (Kalil & Chase, 1970; Richard et al., 1975; Baker & Malpeli, 1977; Schmielau & Singer, 1977; Singer, 1977; Sillito et al., 1994; Cudeiro & Sillito, 1996) and have demonstrated generally subtle effects of cortical cooling, destruction, or stimu-

lation. We argue in chapters 6 and 7 that the effects produced by manipulations of these modulatory pathways may well be elusive and more
likely to be relevant to the responses of an awake, behaving animal than
an anesthetized one. The nature of the modulatory influence that the
layer 6 cells exert in the thalamus is discussed in chapter 7, but if one is
to understand the circumstances under which this modulatory influence
acts, then one needs to know about the activity patterns of the relevant
layer 6 cells. There is relatively little information available on this score,
and generally it is recorded in terms of receptive field properties of the
layer 6 cells in anesthetized animals. An important point is that the functional significance of at least some of the corticothalamic axons may be
entirely lost in an anesthetized animal. They are likely to be functional
in a conscious animal that is maintaining attention on one particular part
of its sensory environment or is in the process of switching attention
from one part of the environment to another. For instance, Tsumoto and
Suda (1980) reported corticothalamic cells that were silent in their anesthetized preparations and that could only be identified on the basis of
antidromic stimulation from the thalamus. To address the function of
such silent cells requires detailed study of the firing patterns of these layer
6 cells under different conditions of visual stimulation and behavioral
state, and the firing patterns seen under these conditions may well be
quite different from those observed in the classical receptive field studies.

Since there is evidence for precise reciprocal mapping for at least
some of the components of this modulatory pathway, it may prove
important to look for functions that are highly specific in terms of topography, and this may be another reason why global manipulations of
cortex have failed to produce dramatic changes in thalamic relays. The
details of the precise cell-to-cell connections that are established are also
important and are discussed later in this chapter, in section 3.G. It is reasonable in the first instance to search for the action of corticothalamic
afferents that come from primary receiving areas, such as area 17, but
in the long run we will need to know how each of the several areas giving
rise to a layer 6 innervation acts, and what happens when several cortical areas send concurrent afferents to a thalamic relay.

3.C.2. Afferents from the Thalamic Reticular Nucleus to First and Higher Order Nuclei

Axons from the reticular nucleus to the thalamus have been demonstrated
by electrophysiological methods in vivo (Sefton & Burke, 1966; Ahlsén

et al., 1984) or in slice preparations (Von Krosigk et al., 1993; Lam & Sherman, 2005), and have also been shown on the basis of anterograde labeling of single reticulothalamic axons (Yen et al., 1985a; Uhlrich et al., 1991, 2003; Pinault et al., 1995a, 1995b; Cox et al., 1996). The reticulothalamic pathway is GABAergic (Houser et al., 1980; Ohara & Lieberman, 1985), and, so far as is known, all thalamic nuclei receive these GABAergic afferents from the thalamic reticular nucleus. Although many of the illustrations of these reticulothalamic axons do not show the details of the terminal morphology, the most common picture shows beaded axons with few side branches (Uhlrich et al., 1991; Cox et al., 1996; figures 3.9 and 3.10), and in this they are readily distinguishable from the

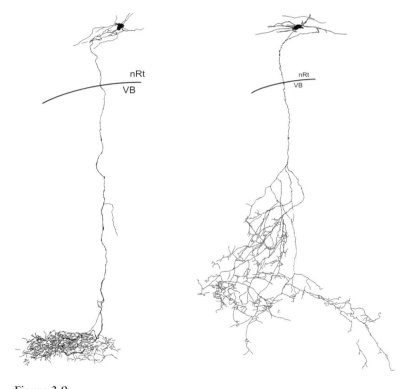

Figure 3.9
A. Reticulothalamic axon with a closely clustered terminal arborization in the ventral posterior nucleus of a rat. (Modified from Cox et al., 1996, with permission). *B.* Reticulothalamic axon with a relatively diffuse terminal arborization in the ventral posterior nucleus of a rat. (Modified from Cox et al., 1996, with permission.)

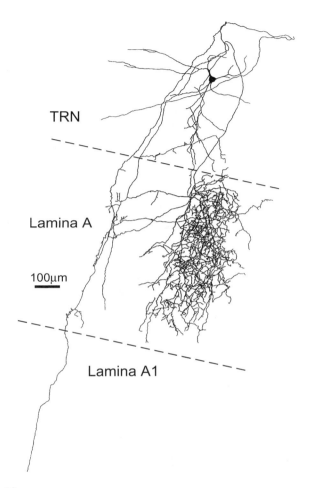

Figure 3.10
An afferent axon from the perigeniculate nucleus of the cat passing to the A layers of the lateral geniculate nucleus, showing a medial (to the left) slender branch and a lateral branch with a broader distribution. The axon was filled with horseradish peroxidase and is shown in a section cut in the coronal plane. (Modified from Uhlrich et al., 1991, with permission.)

driver afferents and from the layer 6 corticothalamic afferents considered above. However, reticulothalamic axons may not have a uniform structure. They differ in the degree to which their terminals are tightly localized or widespread, and they may also differ in the detailed structure of their terminals. Cox et al. (1996) described a range of terminal patterns in the ventral posterior nucleus of the rat, with some showing a very small, well-localized terminal plexus and others showing a more widespread but still localized arbor. The latter produce a weaker inhibitory action on the thalamic relay cells of the ventral posterior nucleus than do the former (Cox et al., 1997; see also figure 3.9A and B); these may represent extremes of a continuum rather than distinct cell classes. Whereas Yen et al. (1985a) and Uhlrich et al. (1991) described relatively fine-beaded axons in first order thalamic nuclei in the cat, Pinault et al. (1995a) described a more complex pattern of terminal branches in the rat, not unlike that of driver afferents described above, also suggesting that there may be a range of reticulothalamic axon terminal patterns that vary in their terminal localization and their terminal structure.

In electron microscopic sections, the terminals of the reticulothalamic axons have the appearance that is now widely associated with GABAergic, inhibitory terminals. That is, they contain synaptic vesicles that have a flattened or irregular ("pleomorphic") shape, and they make "symmetrical" synaptic contacts primarily with relay cell dendrites. The significance of vesicle shape and synaptic symmetry is discussed further in section 3.D.1. These profiles have been called F1 profiles (F for the flattened vesicles, and 1 to distinguish them from the terminals formed by the dendrites of interneurons, which are F2 profiles, described below). F1 profiles are most commonly not in the glomeruli, although they can be found in the outer parts of glomeruli. Apart from the reticulothalamic axons, there are other inhibitory axon terminals in the thalamus that also have the appearance of F1 terminals. These terminals are probably predominantly the terminals of interneuronal axons, although other inhibitory inputs considered later in this chapter also have the characteristic appearance of the F1 profiles.

Earlier methods seemed to show a rather widespread and diffuse projection for the reticulothalamic axons (Scheibel & Scheibel, 1966; Yen et al., 1985a), but there is now good evidence for a topographically organized pathway going from the reticular nucleus to the major first order nuclei. Locally limited injections of retrograde tracers into some of these thalamic nuclei have produced localized zones of labeled cells in the reticular nucleus (Crabtree & Killackey, 1989; Crabtree, 1992a, 1992b; Lozsádi, 1995), and small fills of one or a few reticular cells with an anterograde tracer can reveal individual axons with locally ramifying branches within one thalamic nucleus, which can be either first or higher order (Uhlrich et al., 1991; Pinault et al., 1995a, 1995b; Cox et al., 1996; Pinault & Deschênes, 1998a). Using photostimulation of caged glutamate in an in vitro preparation from the rat, Wan and Sherman (2005) were able to show functionally that a high degree of topography exists in the projection from the thalamic reticular nucleus to the ventral posterior nucleus. There is some evidence that the topographic map of sensory surfaces is less clearly preserved in the reticulothalamic and thalamoreticular pathways of higher order thalamic nuclei than for first order nuclei (Conley & Diamond, 1990; Conley et al., 1991; Crabtree, 1996; see also chapter 9).

In some instances the innervation of a higher order nucleus is formed by a branch of an axon that is also innervating a first order nucleus (Pinault et al., 1995b; Crabtree, 1996, 1998; Crabtree et al., 1998; Pinault & Deschênes, 1998a, 1998b; Crabtree & Isaac, 2002). Pinault and Deschênes (1998b) found in rats that, of 22 single-cell injections of reticular cells, 16 showed an axon localized in the ventral posterior (first order) nucleus, four showed an axon in the posterior (higher order) nucleus, and two showed an axon that branched to innervate both nuclei. Crabtree (1998) reported reticular cells that were double-labeled after injections of retrograde tracers into distinct auditory nuclei of the thalamus. His results, though not quantified, suggest a more common occurrence of the branched reticular axons innervating two thalamic nuclei.

Uhlrich et al. (1991) described axons that pass from the cat's perigeniculate nucleus (which is usually considered to be part of the thalamic reticular nucleus; see chapter 1) to the A layers of the lateral geniculate nucleus (see figure 3.10). They showed that these axons generally have two branches, a medial one distributing to a very narrow column of geniculate cells that must correspond to a tiny part of the visual field, and a lateral branch with a broader but still rather limited distribution. This branch shows two types of local sign. In the first place, it distributes to geniculate layers receiving from left or right eye in accordance with the dominant ocular input to the parent perigeniculate cell, and second, it distributes to a column of geniculate cells that corresponds roughly to the position of the receptive field of that perigeniculate cell.

3.C.3. Connections from Interneurons to Relay Cells

Interneurons provide a numerically major source of inhibitory afferents to relay cells in some but not in all thalamic nuclei. For example, in cats

evidence for the globus pallidus and substantia nigra leaves some room for doubt. The pallidal and nigral cells do send GABAergic afferents to the thalamic reticular nucleus (Cornwall et al., 1990; Paré et al., 1990; Gandia et al., 1993; Asanuma, 1994). However, Asanuma's study showed that the projection to the reticular nucleus arose in the external segment of the globus pallidus, and her account showed no component to the motor thalamus coming from this segment. In contrast to this, Sidibe et al. (1997), who demonstrated the projection from the internal segment of the globus pallidus to the thalamus, showed no projection to the thalamic reticular nucleus, although there was a projection to the zona incerta, adjacent to the reticular nucleus. Functionally, such an incertal connection cannot be treated as a reticular component, so it would appear that the pallidal cells that send axons to the reticular nucleus do not innervate thalamus, and conversely, that the pallidal cells that innervate the thalamus do not innervate the reticular nucleus. Comparable evidence is not available for the nigral afferents to the thalamus, but there is no evidence currently available to show that the cells that provide the thalamic afferents themselves have branches innervating the reticular nucleus. Finally, GABAergic axons from the basal forebrain innervate the thalamic reticular nucleus but not the dorsal thalamus (Bickford et al., 1994).

Electron microscopic studies (Balercia et al., 1996; Kultas-Ilinsky et al., 1997) show that the pallidal axons can form the presynaptic components to F2 terminals and relay cell dendrites in triadic junctions (see section 3.D.2 and section 2.C), and that at least some relate to primary branch points of dendrites. That is, they show some resemblance to the RL axons, although they have flattened vesicles and make asymmetrical junctions, both characteristic of inhibitory junctions (see below). Their position in a triad might be taken as evidence for thinking of these as drivers, but, since the cholinergic afferents that come from the brainstem and that are not likely to be drivers also show a similar relationship, we cannot regard this as a useful criterion in itself for determining the function, driver or modulator, of these axons. We have included these axons in the section on modulators for reasons discussed in chapter 7, where we suggest that it is unlikely that inhibitory afferents can act as drivers.

3.C.5. Cholinergic Afferents from the Brainstem

Other afferents include cholinergic axons coming from the brainstem (figure 3.11), which represent a significant proportion of the total number of synapses, up to perhaps 30% or more (Erişir et al., 1997b).

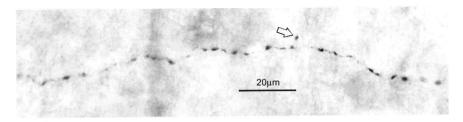

Figure 3.11
Photomicrograph of part of terminal arbor of axon labeled from the parabrachial region. This view is from the A layers of the cat's lateral geniculate nucleus, and the anterograde label placed into the parabrachial region is the lectin, *Phaseolus vulgaris* leucoagglutinin. The synaptic boutons are evident mostly as en passant swellings, with an occasional terminal found at the end of a short side branch (arrow). (From Uhlrich et al., 1988, with permission.)

Cholinergic axons from the brainstem have been described in rats, cats, and monkeys (Hallanger et al., 1987; Cucchiaro et al., 1988; Raczkowski & Fitzpatrick, 1989; Bickford et al., 1993; Erişir et al., 1997a). The density of the distribution of these axons varies both among thalamic nuclei and among species (Hallanger et al., 1987; Cucchiaro et al., 1988; Raczkowski & Fitzpatrick, 1989; Bickford et al., 1993; Erişir et al., 1997a). Cholinergic axons coming from the parabrachial region[3] of cats have been described as fine, branching, beaded terminal axons, some of which have a relatively localized zone of termination within one or two functionally related thalamic nuclei. In the lateral geniculate nucleus they go mainly to the A layers, whereas in other parts of the thalamus they show a less localized and more widely distributed terminal arbor (Uhlrich et al., 1988). Another cholinergic projection to parts of the lateral geniculate nucleus comes from the parabigeminal nucleus (Hashikawa et al., 1986; Fitzpatrick et al., 1988). The cholinergic axons from the parabrachial region colocalize nitric oxide, a presumed neurotransmitter,

---

3. The terminology for these brainstem cholinergic afferents to thalamus has been confusing. Among other terms commonly used for these cells are "pedunculopontine tegmental nucleus" and "laterodorsal tegmental nucleus." The problem is that in many species, such as the cat and the monkey, the cholinergic cells are intermixed with noradrenergic and possibly other afferents to thalamus, whereas in other species, such as rodents, the pedunculopontine tegmental nucleus effectively includes only cholinergic afferents and the noradrenergic afferents are gathered in the locus caeruleus. For the cat, we prefer the term "parabrachial region" because it does not imply a homogeneous, well-demarcated cell group.

whereas those from the parabigeminal nucleus do not (Bickford et al., 1993).

In the lateral geniculate nucleus of the cat, the cholinergic brainstem afferents form RS terminals similar to those described for the layer 6 corticothalamic terminals above, but slightly larger on average than the cortical terminals, although there is considerable overlap in the size distribution (Erişir et al., 1997a). Whereas the cortical RS terminals contact relatively small, peripheral dendritic profiles of relay cells and the dendritic shafts of interneurons (Wilson et al., 1984; Weber et al., 1989; Montero, 1991; Erişir et al., 1997a) outside glomeruli, the brainstem cholinergic terminals make their contacts closer to the relay cell body (Wilson et al., 1984; Erişir et al, 1997a) commonly within glomeruli (see below).

3.C.6. Other Afferents to Thalamic Nuclei

Other afferents from the brainstem include serotonergic axons from the dorsal raphé nucleus (de Lima & Singer, 1987b; Kayama et al., 1989; Gonzalo-Ruiz et al., 1995), histaminergic axons from the hypothalamus (Uhlrich et al., 1993), and noradrenergic axons from the parabrachial region (Morrison & Foote, 1986; de Lima & Singer, 1987a). The cells that give rise to the latter are mixed with the cholinergic afferents in some species and separated into a well-defined locus coeruleus in others (Morrison & Foote, 1986; de Lima & Singer, 1987a). There are also certain ascending pathways from the brainstem that appear to be specific to particular thalamic nuclei, such as inputs from the superior colliculus to the C layers of the cat or the K layers of primates (Harting et al., 1986, 1991).

The vast majority of terminals in the thalamus form conventional, symmetrical or asymmetrical synaptic contacts. The structure of the thickenings and the postsynaptic processes associated with each contact provides important identifying criteria for each major terminal type, discussed further in the next section. However, a few terminals appear not to form such conventional morphologically recognizable synaptic contacts, instead releasing neurotransmitter at nonspecialized sites to act on any nearby processes that have the appropriate receptors and are within the range of the transmitter's action. It appears that both noradrenergic inputs from the parabrachial region (Jones, 2002a) and histaminergic inputs from the tuberomamillary nucleus of the hypothalamus have such nonspecialized release sites (Wilson et al., 1999).

3.D. The Arrangement of Synaptic Connections in the Thalamus

3.D.1. *The Four Terminal Types*

We noted in chapter 2 that in most thalamic nuclei there are relay cells and interneurons and that there may be more than one type of each. In this chapter we have described several different types of afferent, each with a characteristic terminal structure as seen by light or electron microscopic study. We now have to examine how these several structures relate to each other, first in terms of the synaptic relationships that are established and then (in the next section) in terms of the connectivity patterns that may be formed. The functional relationships are discussed in more detail in later chapters.

Electron micrographs show a "generic" structure that is present in essentially all thalamic nuclei. At a relatively low magnification, a section of a thalamic nucleus shows primarily dense bundles of myelinated axons that represent the many afferent and efferent axons, blood vessels, glial cells, neuronal cell bodies with relatively few synaptic contacts on their surface, many dendritic profiles that receive a few more, but still not many, synaptic contacts, and then patchy areas of closely grouped synaptic profiles, the "glomeruli" (figures 3.6 and 3.7A), where several different sorts of structure appear to be making specialized synaptic contacts with each other.

The synaptic terminals of afferent axons are primarily one of four types described above, two containing round synaptic vesicles (RL and RS, above), and two containing flattened or irregular ("pleotropic" in some accounts) vesicles (F1 and F2). The shape of the vesicles is determined by the vesicular contents and the osmolarity of the solutions used in the early processing of the tissue (Valdivia, 1971). That is, high osmolar solutions tend to produce a flattening of all synaptic vesicles, whereas with low osmolarities the vesicles are all round. At intermediate osmolarities some vesicles, specifically those that contain inhibitory transmitters, are flattened, whereas others remain rounded (Uchizono, 1965). It appears from immunohistochemical studies that in the thalamus, as in many other parts of the mammalian brain, the F profiles are all GABAergic, whereas many of the profiles containing round vesicles are glutamatergic.

We have seen that the RL profiles represent the driver afferents; they are characteristically seen within the glomeruli, although they can also be found in extraglomerular regions. The RS afferents represent a mixed population, including modulator afferents from cortex and from the brainstem. Virtually all of the cortical RS terminals are extraglomerular, and all of the RS terminals within glomeruli are of brainstem origin, although brainstem terminals are also found outside of glomeruli. The F1 profiles represent terminals from the thalamic reticular nucleus and from the axons of local interneurons. For some thalamic nuclei, they also represent other extrinsic GABAergic afferents. However, all seem to be from axons, whereas the F2 profiles represent the axoniform dendritic processes of interneurons (see chapter 2). F1 and F2 profiles are not distinguishable on the basis of size, but the former are never postsynaptic to another process, whereas the latter commonly are.

Before considering the synaptic contacts established by these various profile types it is useful to look more closely at the basis of their classification and naming. Problems concerning classifications in general were discussed in the last chapter, and the same issues apply whether one is classifying nerve cell bodies, synaptic terminals, or synaptic vesicles. Given that most successful and functionally significant classifications will depend on several variables, an obvious but not widely recognized problem of naming arises. The traditional approach to the naming problem as applied to axons and their terminals was to identify the origin and the termination of a particular group and then name them accordingly as spinothalamic, retinogeniculate, and so on. However, in an electron microscopic study one is initially faced with the problem of identifying axons on the basis of their fine structure and synaptic relationships. There may be good experimental evidence that a particular terminal type defined in this way comes from a particular source, and then it would seem sensible to name those terminals in accordance with that knowledge. Currently we are close to being able to name all RL terminals as driving afferents for their particular nucleus, so that such a terminal in the lateral geniculate nucleus is reasonably treated as a retinal terminal. But it could be coming from the tectum or possibly, on the basis of the light microscopic evidence discussed above, there may yet be a few having a different origin. So we continue with the more neutral term, RL. In general, whenever a particular morphological class is likely to include afferents from more than one source, as is the case for the RS terminals, which have at least two distinct origins, in cortex and brainstem, it is best, in accounts that do not identify the origin, to work with a neutral terminology.

It should be stressed that a number of characteristics other than vesicle shape (roundness) and terminal size (largeness) contribute to our recognition of the RL terminals, and this is also true for all of the other terminal types. We stress that the terminology should be regarded as neutral and interim. The R and F, the L and S should be treated as labels for terminals that combine several distinct morphological features, some of which are not part of the name. These features are dealt with more fully later and include synaptic relationships, mitochondrial appearance and distribution, types of contact made, and others. Terminal size alone, vesicle shape alone, or even the combination of the two would provide a very limited basis for classification. Some RL terminals are smaller than others, and in single sections some RS terminal profiles can be as large as some of the smaller RL terminal profiles. However, as a population, RL terminals are significantly larger than RS terminals, and in at least some regions, such as the A layers of the cat lateral geniculate nucleus, there appears to be no overlap in their size distributions when measured from serial reconstructions (Van Horn et al., 2000).

3.D.1.a. The RL Terminals

RL profiles make asymmetrical synaptic junctions on stem dendrites, which are among the largest dendritic profiles in the region and therefore are near the cell body of a relay cell. They also contact grapelike dendritic appendages (see chapter 2) and, very rarely, a cell body. They also synapse on F2 terminals (see figure 3.6). In figure 3.6, some of the dendritic profiles (labeled D in figure 3.7) that are postsynaptic to the central RL terminal are likely to be grapelike appendages and have swirls of filaments, and others, which have microtubules and filaments running a relatively straight course (left side of figure), are likely to be dendritic stems. The two types of dendritic profile have not been separately identified in this figure because their certain identification would require analysis of serial sections.

The asymmetry of the synaptic junctions made by the RL terminals wherever they establish synaptic contacts relates to their excitatory action. Gray (1959) characterized synaptic junctions as symmetrical or asymmetrical on the basis of the relative thickening of the postsynaptic specialization, which probably relates to the nature of the receptor at the junction (Cowan et al., 2002). The presynaptic thickening is roughly the same across all synapses in the brain. "Asymmetrical" means that the postsynaptic thickening is much more pronounced than the presynaptic, and "symmetrical" means that the pre- and postsynaptic thickenings are about equal. Colonnier (1968) showed that asymmetrical junctions are generally associated with round vesicles in the presynaptic process and that symmetrical junctions are associated with flat vesicles.

There is some variation in the part of the relay cell to which the RL terminals relate: not only is there variation within any one nucleus of the thalamus, but there is also a systematic difference between nuclei and even between geniculate layers (Kultas-Ilinsky & Ilinsky, 1991; Feig & Harting, 1994). For example, in the magnocellular and parvocellular layers of primates, the RL terminals are often found close to the cell body, whereas they are further from the cell body in the koniocellular layers (Guillery & Colonnier, 1970; Feig & Harting, 1994).

RL terminals are never postsynaptic to any other process. In addition to these synaptic junctions, the RL terminals, and occasionally the F terminals, establish some desmosome-like contacts with adjacent dendrites. These contacts are not associated with synaptic vesicles and so are regarded as nonsynaptic. They are associated with groups of intermediate filaments that accumulate on either side of the junction (f in figure 3.7) and for this reason have been called filamentous junctions (Guillery, 1967a; Lieberman & Spacek, 1997). They may represent an unusual adhesive junction (Peters et al., 1991). Their functional role has not been explored, but they provide a useful clue for distinguishing RL from RS terminals.

The RL terminals establish triadic junctions (see section 3.C.3) in glomeruli. A triad is formed where an RL terminal is presynaptic to two adjacent profiles, one a dendrite of a relay cell and the other an F2 terminal. The F2 terminal in turn is then presynaptic to the same dendrite (see figure 2.11 and the three numbered arrows to the lower right of the RL profile in figure 3.7). This is the classical form of the triad and, in most of the examples that have been documented for the thalamus, involves an RL terminal as the common presynaptic element. Triads that involve RS profiles as the common presynaptic element are considered in the next section. Because the RL terminals contact F2 terminals, which are the axoniform dendritic processes of interneurons, and also contact the dendrites of the relay neurons, they are presynaptic to both types of thalamic cell. However, whereas interneurons receive the retinal driver contacts primarily on the (presynaptic, axoniform) distal dendritic appendages, the relay cells receive their afferents on the proximal dendrites. RL terminals do form some contacts on the stem dendrites of interneurons (Hamos et al., 1985; Weber et al., 1989; Montero, 1991;

Wilson et al., 1996; Van Horn et al., 2000), and functionally these two types of contact are likely to have quite distinct actions (Cox et al., 1998; Cox & Sherman, 2000; see also chapter 5). The synaptic contacts on the presynaptic dendrites may well act locally on individual dendritic processes, whereas the contacts on stem dendrites nearer the cell body are more likely to produce action potentials capable of discharging the axon and invading at least parts of the dendritic arbors of the interneurons.

3.D.1.b. The RS Terminals

The RS terminals are smaller than the RL terminals in single sections and in reconstructions. Figures 3.12A and B show that in the A layers of the cat's lateral geniculate nucleus there is no overlap between RS and RL terminal sizes (Van Horn et al., 2000) when measured from serial reconstructions. The vesicles are generally more closely packed in the RS than in the RL terminals. The RL terminals make multiple junctions in single sections (see figure 3.6), whereas the RS terminals do not. The RS terminals do not show filamentous junctions, and where the differential appearance of the mitochondria is evident, the RS terminals have dark mitochondria, the RL terminals pale ones. RS terminals are somewhat more likely to be found outside the glomeruli than in them, and where they occur in the glomeruli they contribute fewer synapses than do the RL terminals. In terms of the overall visual impression and of the volume occupied, the RL profiles dominate in the glomeruli, where RS profiles are seen more rarely. However, since the RS terminals are significantly smaller than the RL terminals, they are less likely to be cut, and the visual impression cannot be taken to represent the numerical relationships, which are considered separately below.

We have seen that there are two major sources of the RS terminals, the cortex and the brainstem. In the lateral geniculate nucleus of the cat the cortical RS terminals contact relatively small, peripheral dendritic profiles of relay cells and the dendritic shafts of interneurons (Wilson et al., 1984; Weber et al., 1989; Montero, 1991; Erişir et al., 1997a; see also section 3.C.7). The brainstem cholinergic RS terminals make their contacts closer to the relay cell body (Wilson et al., 1984; Erişir et al., 1997a). Both types of RS terminal (from cortex and brainstem) contact the dendritic shafts of interneurons, but those from the brainstem are the major and perhaps only type of RS terminal contacting the distal axoniform processes (F2 terminals) of the interneuronal dendrites, with few if any cortical RS terminals contacting these (Vidnyánszky & Hámori, 1994; Erişir et al., 1997a).

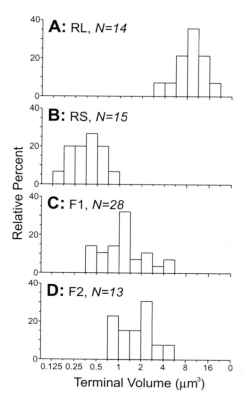

Figure 3.12
Histograms showing the volumes of representative populations of terminal types from the A-laminae of the cat's lateral geniculate nucleus. (Redrawn from Van Horn et al., 2000.)

When RS profiles that come from the brainstem are selectively labeled in the lateral geniculate nucleus of cats, it is possible to see that they often form a type of triad. This involves two different RS terminals, from two branches of a common brainstem axon, making contacts, which are comparable to the contacts made by the single RL in the classical triad (Wilson et al., 1984; Weber et al., 1989; Montero, 1991; Erişir et al., 1997a). We shall refer to this as a pseudotriad. RS terminals of cortical origin do not show this pattern of synaptic contacts.

The terminology that was used in the past to describe RS terminals and our own usage need brief consideration (Ide, 1982; Erişir et al., 1997a, 1997b). As mentioned earlier, in many preparations the RS profiles have dark mitochondria whereas the RL profiles have pale mitochondria, so they were called RSD and RLP terminals (Colonnier & Guillery, 1964). Later, however, some observations led to the introduction of further distinctions between RSD and RLD profiles (the "D" referring to dark mitochondria), and the latter were recognized as clearly distinct from the RLP profiles, which are generally even larger than the largest RLD profiles and which also differ in the other respects considered above. However, because mitochondrial appearance is somewhat variable, and because it has been shown that in the lateral geniculate nucleus the RSD and RLD profiles form a continuum and cannot be distinguished from each other without specifically labeling one or the other (Ide, 1982; Erişir et al., 1997b), it continues to be useful to refer to all of these as RS. Further, there are terminals in the reticular nucleus that are thought to come from the thalamus (Ide, 1982; Ohara & Lieberman, 1985; Williamson et al., 1993; Liu & Jones, 1999; see section 3.E); these terminals are larger than most of the RS terminals in the thalamus, and in the past were also called RLD (Ide, 1982). We will use the simple term RS throughout for the terminals in the dorsal thalamus, identifying axon terminals by other criteria where this is possible and useful.

3.D.1.c. The F terminals: F1 and F2

We have presented the F1 terminals as axons of reticulothalamic cells and interneurons. In addition, where GABAergic afferents come to the thalamus from other sources, these appear as F1 terminals (see section 3.C.4). F2 terminals are the axoniform terminals of interneuronal dendrites and, more rarely, the stems of interneuronal dendrites. Reticulothalamic axons form medium-sized F1 terminals. In the lateral geniculate nucleus of the cat, F1 and F2 terminals are comparable in size (see figures 3.12C and D) but differ in other respects, chiefly in that F2 terminals are both presynaptic and postsynaptic, whereas F1 terminals are strictly presynaptic. In the lateral geniculate nucleus of the rat, F1 terminals from the thalamic reticular nucleus form symmetrical, extraglomerular, axodendritic synapses (Montero & Scott, 1981). Similarly, in the cat, where they mainly contact relay cells, they terminate predominantly outside the glomeruli: about 90% are on the peripheral dendritic segments that receive the cortical RS terminals, and only about 10% are on the more proximal dendritic segments receiving the retinal RL afferents (Cucchiaro et al., 1991; Wang et al., 2001). The significance of the difference in dendritic location is considered in chapters 4 and 5.

Other sources for F1 terminals in the lateral geniculate nucleus include the axons of interneurons and the GABAergic axons that innervate the lateral geniculate nucleus from the pretectum (Montero, 1987; Cucchiaro et al., 1993). In general, morphological distinctions among F1 terminals from different sources are elusive (but see Montero, 1987). Because the vast majority of reticular F1 terminals are onto peripheral dendrites, by a process of elimination, it seems likely that most of the proximally located F1 terminals, including those within glomeruli, are from interneuronal axons, which represent the only other major source of F1 terminals.

3.D.1.d. Other Terminal Types

There are also rare terminals that are noradrenergic from the parabrachial region, serotonergic from the dorsal raphe nucleus, and his-taminergic from the tuberomamillary nucleus of the hypothalamus. These have the general appearance of the RS terminals described above. While at least some of these modulatory terminals may end in conventional synapses, others, as indicated earlier, may not (de Lima & Singer, 1987a; Wilson et al., 1999), instead releasing neurotransmitter into the extracellular space to act on any appropriate nearby receptors.

3.D.2. The Glomeruli and Triads

Glomeruli represent a specialized region where three or more, commonly more, synaptic profiles are closely related to each other, where several synaptic junctions are formed between these profiles, and where, characteristically, astrocytic cytoplasm is excluded from the regions close to the synaptic junctions and tends preferentially to collect as thin cytoplasmic sheets around the outer borders of the glomerulus. The complexity of a glomerulus can vary greatly. In the cat's lateral geniculate nucleus, where several serial reconstructions are available (Wilson et al., 1984; Hamos et al., 1986; Van Horn et al., 2000), glomeruli always include at least one triad, and therefore at least one F2 and one RL terminal. It is not known whether this applies to all other thalamic nuclei, and one would expect the rule not to apply in nuclei that lack interneurons (i.e., the thalamus of the mouse and rat other than the lateral geniculate nucleus; Arcelli et al., 1997). Glomeruli generally contain one, occasionally more than one, RL profile, and so one can treat the RL profiles, together with the F2 profiles that tend to be grouped around the RL profile, as characteristic of glomeruli. However, we know of no systematic study to demonstrate whether every glomerulus contains at least one RL profile. In the A layers of the cat's lateral geniculate nucleus, a nonsystematic survey carried out in Sherman's laboratory showed that every glomerulus did have an RL terminal. To some extent the complexity of glomeruli relates to the presence of interneurons, since interneuronal processes provide all of the F2 profiles and possibly some of the F1 profiles in a glomerulus. However, this may not be a general rule. Kultas-Ilinsky and Ilinsky (1991) claim that in the ventral lateral nucleus of the monkey about 25% of the nerve cells are interneurons, but that glomerular formations and triads are unusually rare in this nucleus. A detailed comparison of this nucleus with one like the lateral geniculate nucleus of the same species could prove rewarding in showing exactly what are the critical features of the interneuronal structure, the distribution of interneuronal dendrites or the synaptic connectivity of the relevant processes that produce the reported difference.

We have noted that a common feature of the primary afferents is their synaptic involvement in three closely associated synapses that form a triad. These triads relate to the grapelike dendritic appendages of relay cells described in chapter 2, but are not an essential part of all thalamic relays. Thus, when one compares the retinogeniculate X and the Y pathways that were introduced in chapter 2, the innervation of X relay cells commonly involves such triads and glomeruli, but the innervation of Y relay cells does not (Wilson et al., 1984; Hamos et al., 1987; but see Datskovskaia et al., 2001, and footnote 2.8). This relates to the observation that the X relay cells are more likely to have grapelike appendages at their primary branch points than the Y relay cells. In the ventral posterior nucleus of the rat, axons that come from the dorsal column nuclei relate to triads, thus resembling the X pathway, but spinothalamic axons do not, and may be more like the Y pathway (Ma et al., 1987b) . The functional significance of this difference is not clear. It is discussed further in chapter 5, which deals with the properties of synaptic inputs.

We have seen that within the glomeruli, the RL terminals often lie centrally (see figure 3.6) among many other synaptic profiles of the glomerulus. Although they vary considerably from one thalamic nucleus to another in their complexity, the glomeruli are a characteristic feature of many thalamic nuclei,[4] and it is reasonable to ask about the possible

---

4. Kelly et al. (2003) describe "tubular clusters" of synaptic terminals around proximal dendrites of relay cells. From their illustrations, which show very little astrocytic cytoplasm within these tubular clusters, we would regard them as glomerular structures in terms of the definition provided earlier.

functional significance of these quite striking synaptic arrangements. That is, given that the glomeruli are such a visually impressive and characteristic feature of thalamic synaptic arrangements, we need to ask what it is about the glomerular structures that differentiates them from other synaptic groupings and that may be relevant to the way in which these particular synaptic arrangements function.

The glomeruli are generally described as regions of many closely grouped synaptic processes with slender sheets of astrocytic cytoplasm wrapped around the whole glomerulus. The implication of this description focuses on the possible function of the astrocytic sheets that appear to be wrapping the glomeruli and leads one to look at the sheets as though they may provide a barrier that prevents transport into or out of the glomeruli. However, an effective diffusion barrier requires a quite significant wrapping, some significant reduction of the extracellular space, the strategic placement of tight junctions, or a specialization of extracellular material. There is no evidence for any of these in the regions surrounding the glomeruli. And the astrocytic ensheathment is often incomplete. It may be more instructive to regard the glomeruli as regions that are essentially free of any astrocytic processes (see figures 3.6 and 3.7A). It is as though there had been a developmental process that cleared the astrocytic cytoplasm from within glomeruli and removed it to the glomerular periphery, where the appearance of a wrapping is produced. This alternative view of the glomerulus, as a zone free of glia, has two important consequences. One is to help counter the idea that the astrocytic sheets that wrap around glomeruli may actually serve as diffusion barriers, preventing the passive diffusion of materials out of (or into) the glomeruli. The second consequence arises from a comparison with nonglomerular synapses, such as are seen in many other parts of the brain, for example in the cerebral cortex, the molecular layer of the cerebellar cortex, or the nonglomerular parts of the thalamus. The relationships are shown schematically in figure 3.7B and can be contrasted with figure 3.7A. In the nonglomerular synapses there is almost invariably a tongue of astrocytic cytoplasm on each side of the synaptic cleft, whereas in the thalamic glomeruli, and also in the cerebellar glomeruli where mossy fibers contact granule cells, the synaptic clefts are all at some distance from the astrocytic cytoplasm.

In view of the known functions of astrocytes, which include ion transport and transmitter uptake at synaptic junctions (Pfrieger & Barres, 1996; Bacci et al., 1999), the absence of astrocytic processes from the glomeruli may reflect functional properties not shared by extraglomeru-

terior nucleus in rats, Gentet and Ulrich (2003) provided evidence based on synaptic properties (see also chapters 5 and 7) that the afferents to reticular cells from relay cells were drivers. This identification of thalamo-reticular axons as drivers does not rule out the possibility that other inputs may also function as drivers, nor does it necessarily imply that this pattern exists throughout the reticular nucleus, but it is reasonable to consider that it represents a general plan, that relay cells provide the driving input to reticular cells and that the other inputs are modulatory. This evidence concerning thalamoreticular axons can be viewed in relation to the observations, summarized earlier, that modulators for the thalamic relays send branches to the reticular nucleus, whereas drivers for the thalamic relays do not. The thalamocortical axons, which are drivers for cortex, are an exception in that they have reticular branches. We recognize that an axon could be a driver with one branch and a modulator with another (see chapter 7), but the presence of a reticular branch on the one recognizable driver pathway that is also a candidate to be the driver for the reticular nucleus suggests an important relationship that is special to the thalamocortical axons. This relationship, as well as the broader issue of how drivers and modulators to thalamic relay cells in general relate to drivers and modulators of thalamic reticular cells, merits more detailed study. A recent report by the same authors showed that the layer 6 cortical inputs to these same reticular cells act as modulators (Gentet & Ulrich, 2004).

3.F. Afferents to Interneurons

Although there are several types of interneuron (see chapter 2), only one type is known to receive inputs from drivers (the RL terminals). These interneurons, which are common to first order relays such as the lateral geniculate and the ventral posterior nuclei, receive, apart from the drivers, inputs from F terminals and from RS terminals. They do not contain brain nitric oxide synthase (BNOS, an enzyme involved in the formation of nitric oxide and generally thought to indicate the presence of that neuroactive substance within neurons), and in the lateral geniculate nucleus are found in the main layers. (Quantitative relationships are considered in section 3.H.) The drivers relate particularly to the vesicle containing axoniform dendritic terminals (F2 terminals), and to a lesser extent to the dendritic stems of the interneurons. The F1 terminals represent afferents mostly from the local axons of interneurons and from the other GABAergic afferents summarized in section 3.D.1.c; few

F1 terminals from reticular cells contact these interneurons (Cucchiaro et al., 1991; Wang et al., 2001). At present it is not clear exactly how these afferents are distributed to the various parts of the interneuron except that F1 profiles, many presumably from axons of other interneurons, are presynaptic to vesicle-containing F2 profiles in glomeruli and also contact dendrites of the interneurons outside of glomeruli. The RS profiles represent corticothalamic axons and cholinergic axons from the brainstem, as well as local axon branches from relay cells.

Two types of interneuron mentioned in chapter 2—one found in the pulvinar of the cat, which contains BNOS, and one in the interlaminar regions of the lateral geniculate nucleus, which may represent a displaced cell of the perigeniculate nucleus—both differ from the above in lacking a clear driver input. The other inputs to these cells remain to be defined.

Another source of inputs to these interneurons has recently been described. It has been found that stimulation of relay cells produces EPSPs in local interneurons but not in nearby relay cells, and that axons of relay cells can be seen to give off collaterals not only in the thalamic reticular nucleus but also within the main layers of the lateral geniculate nucleus itself. It appears that these collaterals innervate relatively proximal dendrites of interneurons (Cox et al., 2003). Not every relay cell shows such a local collateral, but the collaterals are extremely thin (see also Guillery et al., 2001) and might very well be difficult to label, or be missed if labeled. A very limited electron microscopic survey of one of these collaterals showed that they form RS terminals (Van Horn et al., 1986). Because the targets of these local collaterals of relay cells are interneurons, one might not expect to see such collaterals in regions of thalamus lacking interneurons, as in rat or mouse thalamus outside the lateral geniculate nucleus (Arcelli et al., 1997).

3.G. Some Problems of Synaptic Connectivity Patterns

A number of problems arise when one considers the details of connectivity patterns. We raise these problems here to illustrate the extent to which we still need details of exactly how the patterns of synaptic connections described in the preceding sections relate to the details one will eventually need in order to understand the circuitry at the level of individual cells. The fact that the corticothalamic pathway from layer 6 innervates relay cells directly and also indirectly via the thalamic reticular nucleus means that the pathway can excite relay cells via the direct connection and inhibit them via the reticular connection. The actual effect on relay cells of activating these cortical afferents depends critically on the details of connectivity at the single-cell level. This dependence is illustrated in figure 3.13A and B for two variants among the many more that are possible. In the version schematically shown in figure 3.13A, a single corticothalamic axon branches to innervate a reticular cell (cell 2) and relay cell (cell b), and the reticular cell contacts the same relay cell. This is an example of feedforward inhibition, and the result would be that strong activity in the corticothalamic axon would produce monosynaptic excitation of the relay cell and disynaptic inhibition via the reticular cell. Whereas at first one might view this as an arrangement with little purpose, it could serve as a gain control mechanism (see

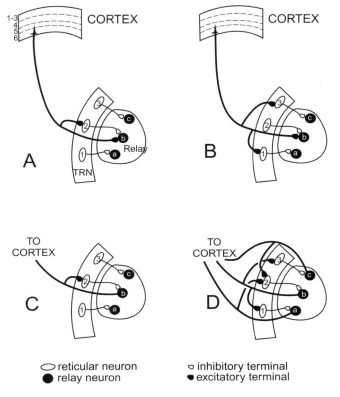

Figure 3.13
Schematic representation of possible patterns of interconnections of thalamic relay cells with reticular cells and corticothalamic type I axons. See text for details.

chapters 6 and 7). The schema in figure 3.13*B* is radically different. Here, the corticothalamic axon branches to innervate reticular cells 1 and 3 and relay cell b. However, reticular cells 1 and 3 do not contact relay cell b, but instead contact its neighbors (cells a and c). This arrangement would not produce feedforward inhibition; rather, it would tend to excite a central relay cell, or a small group of cells, and inhibit neighboring cells. This can also be regarded as a form of lateral inhibition. The schema of figure 3.13*B* would thus produce zones of quite strong excitation and inhibition that are topographically organized, and these zones would tend to form center/surround patterns.

The schemas of figure 3.13*A* and *B* could produce distinct outcomes only if corticothalamic activity were modulated with a very fine grain. For instance, thalamic cells would respond to large-scale inactivation or activation of cortex in much the same way with either schema. The one relevant study, which suggests that figure 3.13*B* is present, was published by Tsumoto et al. (1978). They excited a small cluster of cells in layer 6 of area 17 in cats with iontophoretic application of glutamate while recording from relay cells of the lateral geniculate nucleus. They found that if the receptive fields of the relay cells overlapped or were within about 1° of those of the excited layer 6 cell cluster, the geniculate relay cell response was increased; if the receptive fields of the geniculate cells were offset by about 1°–2° from those of the cortical site, the geniculate cell responses were reduced; if the receptive field offset was more than about 2°, there was no effect of cortical glutamate application on geniculate cell responses. Whether this observation can be generalized to favor the circuitry of figure 3.13*B* for all corticoreticulothalamic examples remains to be determined, and a combination of the schemas shown in figure 3.13*A* and *B* may also exist.

Currently there is much of the same ambiguity for the reticulothalamic connections as described above for the corticoreticulothalamic connections. Some of these connections are illustrated in figure 3.13*C* and *D*. In figure 3.13*C*, the relay cell b contacts reticular cell 2, which projects back to innervate cell b. This is a classic example of feedback inhibition and means that strong activity in a relay cell will be somewhat suppressed after two synaptic delays. The scheme drawn in figure 3.13*D* is more complex and more interesting. Here, relay cell b contacts reticular cells 1 and 3, but not reticular cell 2. However, cells 1 and 3 do not contact cell b, but rather contact its neighbors (cells a and c), and reticular cell 2, which does innervate cell b, is in turn innervated by cells a and c. Consider what this means when a relay cell becomes highly active: activity in cell b would produce disynaptic inhibition (via reticular cells 1 and 3) of its neighbors, cells a and c; the reduced activity in the neighboring relay cells means that reticular cell 2 would be less activated, and thus its inhibitory contribution to cell b would be reduced. This scheme would thus yield feedback disinhibition, precisely the opposite of the scheme illustrated in figure 3.13C. Clearly, we cannot understand how the thalamoreticulothalamic circuit functions until we know whether figure 3.13C, figure 3.13D, or some combination best represents the functional connectivity.

On the evidence that the reticulothalamic pathway shows local sign, it appears to be in a topographically reciprocal relationship with the thalamoreticular pathway. That is, the part of a thalamic nucleus receiving local afferents from the reticular nucleus sends branches of its thalamocortical axon back to roughly the same part of the reticular nucleus. Pinault and Deschênes (1998a) labeled cells in the thalamic reticular nucleus of the rat so that they could trace the axons of these cells into the thalamus, and at the same site they labeled the axon branches that thalamocortical relay cells sent to the same region of the reticular nucleus. The thalamic relay cells in the lateral dorsal, lateral posterior, and ventral lateral nuclei themselves were labeled retrogradely in these preparations. The results showed that these retrogradely labeled thalamic relay cells lay outside, but close to, the limited volume of the relevant thalamic relay nucleus within which the terminal arbor of the labeled reticular cell ramified. This is an elegant, and so far as we know unique, morphological demonstration of the sorts of relationship that are schematically represented in figure 3.13. However, there is some evidence from intracellular recording from geniculate relay cells of rats, cats, and ferrets that action potentials in a relay cell are sometimes followed disynaptically by an IPSP (Lo & Sherman, 1994; Kim & McCormick, 1998; Gentet & Ulrich, 2003), implying a direct feedback (as in figure 3.13C). However, while such a feedback does occur, it is not clear how strong it is, nor does this preclude the circuit described in figure 3.13D.

3.H. Quantitative and More Detailed Relationships

Quantitative studies have addressed a number of different issues. At first they were used to counter the classical view of the driver afferents as the major or even the sole source of synaptic inputs to a thalamic nucleus. For the lateral geniculate nucleus, Glees and Le Gros Clark (1941), on the basis of light microscopic observations, expressed the view that there is a 1:1 relationship between retinogeniculate synapses and geniculate cells in the macaque monkey. Early counts from electron microscopic sections, carried out with no correction for the sampling error that over-estimates large and underestimates small structures, showed only about 20% of all of the synapses in the A layers of the cat's lateral geniculate nucleus as coming from the retina (Guillery, 1969b). More recently, counts have been undertaken in order to obtain quantitative distributions of inputs to thalamic neurons. Most importantly, such information will ultimately prove an essential link between morphology and synaptic integration in the postsynaptic neuron. That is, as we learn more about the integrative properties of the dendrites of these cells (see chapter 4), knowledge of how the various inputs distribute to different parts of the dendritic arbor, along with specific synaptic properties of the various inputs, will be a necessary prerequisite to understanding how relay cells respond to their various inputs. Also, such details will provide information about the extent of variability or constancy in circuitry among thalamic relays and species.

Whereas earlier counts did not correct for sampling errors mentioned above (Weber et al., 1989; Montero, 1991; Erişir et al., 1998), more recent counts (Van Horn et al., 2000) have made the corrections. These studies have shown that for synapses on relay cells, the retinal afferents represent only about 7% of the total synapses in the lateral geniculate nucleus. These counts have also shown the relative distribution of synapses on the different parts (cell body and proximal or distal dendrites) of a neuron (summarized by figure 3.14). We have argued that the number of synapses is not in itself a good estimate of the relative importance of an afferent system, and the small number of drivers seen in the lateral geniculate nucleus and visual cortex (Ahmed et al., 1994; Latawiec et al., 2000) supports such a view. Relative numbers are hard to interpret in functional terms because a numerically large input may be modulatory, with a relatively subtle or finely graded effect, whereas a powerful driver input, if it is critically located, can have a dominant effect, even though numerically it forms only a small proportion of the terminals. (We return to this point in chapter 7). Relative numbers for the lateral geniculate nucleus of the cat provide a general guide, but there may be considerable variation among nuclei and species. Figure 3.14, based on results from Wilson et al. (1984) and Van Horn et al. (2000), schematically shows the numerical distribution of synapses onto different parts of the surface of different classes of relay cells in the lateral

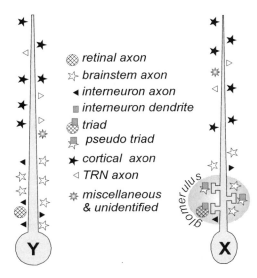

Figure 3.14
Schematic view of synaptic inputs onto an X cell and a Y cell of the cat's lateral geniculate nucleus. For simplicity, only one, unbranched dendrite is shown. Synaptic types are shown in relative numbers. Note that for both cell types, cortical synapses occur on distal dendrites and brainstem and retinal synapses are found on proximal dendrites; there is no overlap of these two zones. Also, for the most part, reticular inputs end distally and interneuronal inputs end proximally. The main difference between the X and the Y cell is that the X cell has numerous triadic inputs in glomeruli involving F2 terminals and either retinal or brainstem terminals. These inputs typically occur on dendritic appendages. The Y cell is essentially devoid of such triadic inputs and glomeruli.

geniculate nucleus of the cat. (As noted below, the distribution on interneurons is different.)

Numbers for the ventral posterior nucleus (Liu et al., 1995a) are comparable to those cited above for the lateral geniculate nucleus, but the presumed resemblance is based on estimates of various terminal distributions being similar before correction for oversampling of the larger RL terminals (Van Horn et al., 2000). In contrast to these results for first order relays, a recent study of the cat's pulvinar has shown that the RL synapses represent only about 2% of all the synapses there, as compared to 7% for the lateral geniculate nucleus (Wang et al., 2002a). Preliminary evidence has extended this observation to the somatosensory relays (ventral posterior as first order and posterior medial as higher order) in cats, with the same result, the first order relay having relatively more driver inputs to relay cells than the higher order relay (Wang et al., 2003). The implication that higher order relays may have relatively more modulatory inputs than first order relays is of interest and worth exploring in other first and higher order relays and in species other than the cat.

Van Horn et al. (2000) in their counts also used GABA immuno-histochemistry in the lateral geniculate nucleus of the cat to distinguish postsynaptic profiles of relay cells (i.e., GABA–) from those that were interneurons (i.e., GABA+). They found that, for relay cells, 7% of the synaptic contacts are from RL terminals, 31% are from F terminals, and 62% are from RS terminals. For interneurons, the values are 47%, 24%, and 29% from RL, F, and RS terminals, respectively. These numbers can be further broken down by the estimate that roughly half of these RS terminals are from corticogeniculate axons, and nearly all the rest are from parabrachial cholinergic afferents (Erişir et al., 1997b). Thus, provided that the distribution of these terminals is evenly shared by relay cells and interneurons, corticogeniculate and parabrachial afferents each provide roughly 30% of the synapses on relay cells and roughly 15% on interneurons. The uncorrected data for interneurons and relay cells on which these figures are based (Erişir et al., 1998) are similar to those reported by Montero (1991), but the corrections increase the numbers for the smaller RS profiles and reduce the numbers for the larger RL profiles.

Overall, the results summarized above show that the interneurons receive a relatively much larger share of their inputs from the retina than do the relay cells. Correspondingly, the interneurons receive a smaller share of F and RS inputs. For the RS terminals, it is not clear what subset is from cortex or brainstem. Two classes of interneuron not included in the above and likely to have a different pattern of inputs are the interneurons found in pulvinar that contain BNOS, and the interneurons described in the interlaminar zones of the ferret (Montero, 1989; Sanchez-Vives et al., 1996; see chapter 2). Both lack direct clear driver inputs.

One further point about these figures is that they represent ratios of numbers of synapses as identified in terms of electron microscopic specializations. They do not represent terminals, since, in the cat's lateral geniculate nucleus, a single RL terminal commonly makes about nine distinct synaptic contacts, F terminals make about three, and RS terminals make only one (Van Horn et al., 2000).

The point that synaptic junctions can only be recognized as such when they are cut in a suitable plane roughly perpendicular to the cleft has been discussed by Guillery and August (2002). When cut parallel to the cleft, a synapse is no longer identifiable as such and becomes essentially invisible. One can expect that the proportion of any one synaptic type that is invisible in serial sections will depend on the size of the specialization and on its curvature, large, curved junctions having a smaller chance of being missed in a count. We do not at present know how this feature affects the counts summarized above but stress that whereas the invisibility of a proportion of all synapses will introduce significant errors into absolute counts, the ratios presented above will be less seriously affected. A further point about counts of synaptic junctions is that some afferents function without synaptic specializations, as noted above.

3.I. Summary

The most important distinction among afferents to the thalamus is likely to be that between drivers and modulators. For some of the afferents to first order nuclei, the functional distinction is clear: the axons that have RL terminals (type II or R type light microscopically) are drivers, whereas the axons with RS terminals (type I or E type light microscopically) are modulators. The former are represented by ascending afferents to first order relays and by corticothalamic afferents from layer 5 to higher order relays. The latter are corticothalamic afferents from layer 6, as well as the RS terminals from the brainstem. We have proposed that this functional distinction applies to all thalamic nuclei, and have explored differences in the distribution and the synaptic connectivity patterns with relay cells and with interneurons formed by the several different major afferent types. The generality of this proposed distinction for the thalamus remains to be tested, and in chapter 7 functional tests for distinguishing drivers from modulators are proposed. The possibility that there are several types of modulator with distinct functions remains largely unexplored. Apart from these two major afferent types, an appreciation of thalamic circuitry must include the patterns of connectivity of several other axonal groups, which include candidate modulatory axons from brainstem and basal forebrain, as well as the important afferents that come from the thalamic reticular neurons and from the interneurons. The presynaptic dendrites of the interneurons provide yet another source of input to many but not all thalamic relay cells.

A survey of thalamic afferents and of the major synaptic connections that they establish in the thalamus shows, in the first place, that the details of the synaptic connections, and the possibilities for interactions between drivers and modulators, are extremely complex. In the second place, such a survey shows us how little we really understand about what the circuitry of the thalamus is like. If we focus on the way in which afferents from different cortical areas, different cortical layers, or different cortical cell types relate to each other, to other afferents, and to particular thalamic relays, we find that most of the facts that are critical for a functional appreciation of these pathways are not yet available. The same is true if we look for the details of synaptic interconnections in any one thalamic nucleus. The introduction of the electron microscope and, more recently, the development of a variety of techniques for tracing axons individually or in bundles have provided a great deal of new information about the thalamus, but perhaps the most important conclusion that can come out of this chapter is the literally abysmal degree to which we still lack key information about details of thalamic organization, information that is technically obtainable but that will require a clear sense of what the important questions are and a significant amount of painstaking work.

3.J. Unresolved Questions

1. What are critical structural features by which one can unmistakably recognize a driver, and, more importantly, how do these structural features relate to the functional features? (These questions are explored further in chapter 7.)

2. Is it possible to define for each thalamic nucleus, and consequently for each corresponding neocortical area, one or more sets of driving afferents, and can this information be used to clarify the functional role of each thalamocortical pathway?

3. Is the pattern of several functionally distinct parallel (driver) pathways seen in the lateral geniculate nucleus common to all first order relays?

4. Is this pattern also seen in higher order relays? That is, are the layer 5 cells that send their axons to any one higher order nucleus functionally all of the same class? (This question is considered further in chapter 8.)

5. Are there thalamic cells that receive inputs from two functionally distinct drivers and that thus serve as thalamic integrators?

6. Can driver afferents be generally characterized as not having a reticular branch? Does the reticular branch of the thalamocortical axons (drivers of cortical cells) relate to the fact that such afferents may be the drivers for the reticular cells?

7. Can the heterogeneity of the layer 6 corticothalamic modulators be defined in terms of the functional properties of the layer 6 cells and in terms of the terminal, thalamic distribution of their axons? How are these two features related to each other and to the morphology of the layer 6 cells?

8. Do all corticothalamic axons from layer 6 innervate relay cells and thalamic reticular cells and interneurons, or do some innervate just one or two of these cell classes?

9. What are the functional consequences of having groups of synaptic processes arranged within glomeruli, and how important are the glial relationships in producing these consequences?

10. To what extent are glomerular synapses in the thalamus functionally comparable to glomerular synapses in the cerebellum?

11. What are the possible functions of the triads? (This question is considered further in chapter 5.)

12. What are the detailed connections, at the single-cell level, established between relay cells, reticular cells, and layer 6 corticothalamic axons?

13. How common throughout the thalamus are the detailed circuit properties that have been defined best for first order relays such as the lateral geniculate nucleus?

4 Intrinsic Cell Properties

4.A. Cable Properties

One of the key questions that needs to be answered is how thalamic circuitry affects the relay of information to cortex. There are likely to be several different ways in which thalamic circuitry can act on the relay, and each of these ways will involve many interrelated properties of the relay, including the nature of the various driver and modulator inputs, the properties of synaptic transmission from these afferents to the thalamic neurons, and finally the intrinsic properties of these neurons, since these properties dictate how synaptic inputs will be integrated to control the cell's firing properties. We begin with a consideration of these intrinsic neural properties. In chapter 5 we consider the nature of synaptic inputs to these cells.

In the general case of a classical neuron, with an output limited to an axon, the only signal that can be relayed for the sort of distances (i.e., several millimeters to centimeters) required by thalamocortical axons requires the generation of conventional Na^+/K^+ action potentials. Such axonal signaling is used by thalamic relay cells, reticular cells, and probably most interneurons. We need to understand how synaptic potentials generated in the dendrites, where the vast majority of synaptic inputs are found, affect the soma or axon hillock, the site where action potentials are usually generated.[1]

A few decades ago, our view of a neuron was that it more or less linearly summed excitatory and inhibitory postsynaptic potentials (EPSPs

---

1. In some neurons in other parts of the brain, there is evidence that action potentials can be initiated in the dendrites, but this issue has not been addressed for thalamic cells. Also, some neurons have axons that emanate from proximal dendrites rather than the soma, but in thalamic relay cells and interneurons, axons generally arise from the soma.

and IPSPs, respectively) to create a net voltage change at the axon hillock, where firing of action potentials is initiated. This was thought to be all that was needed to predict the output of the neuron. That is, when post-synaptic potentials were summed to depolarize the cell past its firing threshold, an action potential would be initiated, or, if the cell were already firing, the further depolarization would increase its firing rate. Conversely, if the summed postsynaptic potentials produced a net hyper-polarization, the cell's firing rate would drop or cease altogether. We now know that this concept of a linearly summing postsynaptic potential is an oversimplification, because membrane properties show highly non-linear, voltage dependent properties. Nonetheless, it is a first step to understanding how inputs to a cell can be integrated to control the cell's output.

Even with the simplifying assumption that postsynaptic potentials sum linearly, the problem of how this can be analyzed by the investiga-tor is not trivial. Imagine that a synaptic input at some specified den-dritic site locally changes an ionic conductance in the postsynaptic membrane, allowing current in the form of charged ions to flow into (or out of) the cell at that site. How does this event change the membrane potential at the soma or axon hillock? This will depend on the flow of current that is initiated and on how it spreads through the cell. The actual pattern of current flow is mostly related to the complex three-dimensional architecture of dendritic arbors. Not all the current will flow directly to the soma, because some will flow in the opposite direction, toward more distal dendrites. As each dendritic branch point is passed in either direction, the current flow will divide from the active branch into adjacent branches. Thus, if we start with the current flowing toward the soma, once a branch point is reached, the current will divide, part heading down the parent branch toward the soma and part heading down the other daughter branch(es) away from the soma. This process is repeated as other branch points are reached, regardless of the direc-tion of current flow, toward or away from the soma, until either the soma or a dendritic ending is reached. Finally, because the membrane enclos-ing the dendrites and soma is itself somewhat permeable to electric current, some of the current will flow out of all parts of the dendrites and the cell into the extracellular spaces.

A hydraulic analogue often helps to explain this phenomenon. We can think of the dendritic tree as an intricately branched rubber hose with tiny holes all along the surface. These holes make the hose slightly leaky, and thus water will leak in much the same way current leaks across the neuronal membranes. If water is injected at some specific "dendritic" site, that will increase the water pressure, which is the hydraulic analogue of increasing the voltage difference across the membrane of the neuron. This leads to water flow in all directions throughout the branched hose, with some of it leaking out through the surface holes. A more formal term for electrical "leakiness" as applied to cell membranes is "conductance": the greater the conductance, the more current (or water) will flow across the membrane. The amount of leakiness or conductance matters: the less the conductance (i.e., with fewer or smaller holes), the larger the amount of injected current that will reach the soma and axon hillock. Now, to further complicate the determination, let us imagine that the amount of membrane conductance (to electric current) or leakiness (to water) varies in a complicated fashion with time. To make matters even worse (but not quite hopeless), we can imagine finally that multiple sites along the dendritic tree (or hose) can have current (or water) injected with variable temporal interrelationships. This is the analogue of different synapses becoming active with a variety of temporal interrelationships. The problem is to determine the amount of extra electric current (or water) that will appear at the soma, because this is the ultimate determinant of the pattern of action potentials that will ensue.

To begin solving this difficult problem, neurons may be modeled as passive cables (Jack et al., 1975; Rall, 1977), and the postsynaptic potentials can be thought of as being conducted electrotonically through the dendritic arbor, and particularly from synaptic sites, to the soma or axon hillock. Such modeling remains the chief hypothesis linking cell shape, the distribution of synaptic inputs, and the efficacy of synapses in the production of postsynaptic action potentials. It has thus proved to be a useful first step in assessing the impact of synapses at different dendritic locations. One must be mindful of the many assumptions and simplifications typically used in cable modeling, because these limit the validity of the model. For one example, various parameters that are often impractical to measure in neurons, such as electrical resistance of the cytoplasm and electrical resistance and capacitance of the membrane, can be estimated from measurements made in other cell types (Jack et al., 1975). Although these values have not been explicitly tested for neurons, the cable values computed with these parameters seem to be within reasonable bounds. For another, these parameters are typically, but not always, assumed to be uniform spatially and temporally, but there is evidence to the contrary that is based on, among other factors, nonuniform distribution of voltage-sensitive ion channels, the opening or closing of which alters membrane conductance. However, membrane conductance can be viewed as just another cable parameter, and these dynamic alterations can be taken into account in cable modeling. Finally, most cable models assess only the effects of an isolated synaptic event and do not attempt to compute the various spatial and temporal combinations of multiple synaptic activations. For a real neuron, the electrical properties of the membranes or cytoplasm may not be distributed uniformly throughout, these values almost certainly change with time (see below), and complex spatiotemporal combinations of synaptic activation are common. Here the effect of active synapses is to change membrane conductance locally, and this can be accounted for in cable modeling.

4.A.1. Cable Properties of Relay Cells

Several experiments have described the cable properties of thalamic relay cells from in vitro slice preparations, but properties measured from in vitro preparations tend to differ from the more physiological properties of the in vivo preparation, for two reasons (Holmes & Woody, 1989; Bernander et al., 1991; Destexhe et al., 1996; Destexhe et al., 1998a). First, slices often tend to cut off significant portions of the dendritic arbors of relay cells, leaving a cell with only a partial arbor. Although the cut ends of dendrites appear to close, thus repairing major leaks caused by the cuts, this partial arbor has less surface membrane area and thus less overall leakage or membrane conductance than does the intact cell. Second, and probably more significant, compared with the in vivo condition, there is much less spontaneous activity in most in vitro slice preparations, and thus much less synaptic activation of a recorded cell. Less synaptic activation means much less membrane conductance, because most active synapses result in opening ion channels, thus making the postsynaptic cell more leaky. Both of these differences make cells appear less leaky to electric current in vitro, and this affects the final estimation of cable properties. It is probably more physiologically appropriate to consider the cable properties of thalamic cells as determined from in vivo experiments. However, while it is true that in vivo experiments in principle offer a more physiological estimate of cable properties, the fact that recordings are generally of higher quality and easier to control in vitro somewhat negates these arguments.

The only thalamic relay cells that have been formally tested for cable modeling during in vivo recording are those of the lateral geniculate nucleus in cats (Bloomfield et al., 1987). Two of the major factors that determine cable properties of neurons are dendritic geometry and the electrical properties of the cytoplasm and membranes of the cell. Since the morphological variation among relay cells is quite similar across a wide range of thalamic nuclei and species, and since passive, intrinsic electrical properties are generally assumed to be quite similar for neurons throughout the brain, it seems a good guess that the passive cable properties seen for geniculate relay cells generally apply to other thalamic relay cells. This is, nonetheless, a point that has not been experimentally verified.

When modeled as passive cables, relay cells of the lateral geniculate nucleus in cats appear to be electrotonically compact, suggesting that steady-state (i.e., DC) voltage changes applied even at the most distally located synaptic sites will attenuate by less than half en route to the soma. In the water analogy developed above, this would be like a hose with relatively little leakage, because the holes are either few or small. Also, current injected into one point in the dendritic arbor by an active synapse will have significant effects throughout the dendritic arbor, as well as at the soma. This is illustrated in figure 4.1A and B for two typical relay cells. Here the cable parameters have been modeled based on morphological features, electrophysiological measures of input resistance and membrane time constant, and assumed values for membrane resistance and capacitance, cytoplasmic resistance, and so forth (Bloomfield et al., 1987). Steady-state current was then injected into a distal dendritic locus of each model to roughly mimic a synaptic activation there, and this effect was determined on the membrane voltage at various dendritic loci and at the soma (and axon hillock).

It should be noted that this example and further considerations of figure 4.1 below show the effect of the spread of *steady-state* current injections or those that vary slowly with time. This is because the resistive-capacitative properties of the membrane act like a low-pass temporal filter with a time constant of roughly 10–50 msec, sometimes longer, meaning that steady-state or slow voltage changes are electrotonically conducted with less attenuation than are fast ones, and thus faster postsynaptic potentials would be more attenuated in peak amplitude and more spread out in time during electrotonic conduction. As noted in chapter 5, postsynaptic potentials result from activation of two different classes of postsynaptic receptor, *ionotropic* or *metabotropic*. Activation of the former leads to postsynaptic potentials sufficiently fast that they will be significantly attenuated by the resistive-capacitative properties of

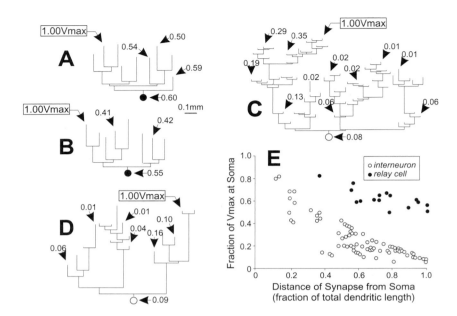

Figure 4.1

A–D. Cable modeling of the voltage attenuation that occurs within the dendritic arbors of two relay cells (*A* and *B*) and two interneurons (*C* and *D*) following the activation of a single synapse (i.e., of a single voltage injection). The cells from the cat's lateral geniculate nucleus were labeled by intracellular injection of a dye in vivo, and the stick figures represent a schematic view of one primary dendrite from each cell with all of its progeny branches. Each branch length is proportional to its calculated electrotonic length. The site of voltage injection is indicated by the boxed value labeled 1.00 V_{max} (maximum voltage). Voltage attenuation at various dendritic endings within the arbor and soma is indicated by arrows and given as fractions of V_{max}. *E.* Attenuation at the soma of a single voltage injection placed at different dendritic endings within the dendritic arbor as a function of the anatomical distance of the voltage injection from the soma. Each voltage injection mimics the activation of a single synapse. The abscissa represents relative anatomical distances normalized to the greatest extent of each arbor, and the plotted points represent values from the four cells shown in *A–D*. (Redrawn from Bloomfield & Sherman, 1989.)

the membrane, whereas activation of the latter produces such slow post-synaptic potentials that they will be minimally attenuated by these membrane properties.

A major reason why these relay cells are electrotonically compact is that their dendrites are relatively thick through most of their extent. The cross-sectional area of a dendrite is proportional to the square of its diameter, but the surface membrane area is only linearly proportional to the diameter. Thus the ratio of its cross-sectional area to its membrane area for a dendrite increases with increasing thickness. Since the relative resistance of the cytoplasm is related to its cross-sectional area and that of the membrane to its total area, the larger the ratio of cytoplasmic cross-sectional area to membrane area, the lower the resistance of the cytoplasm relative to that of the membrane. As a result, a thicker dendrite allows more current from synaptic activation to flow down the path of least resistance through the cytoplasm to the soma, and less of this current will leak out through the membrane.

4.A.2. Cable Properties of Interneurons and Reticular Cells

The interneurons of the cat's lateral geniculate nucleus appear to be much larger electrotonically than the relay cells, which means that, if the dendrites act as passive cables, voltage changes created at distal dendrites are likely to be much more attenuated at the soma. Two examples based on modeling from morphological and electrophysiological data are shown in figure 4.1C and D, with the same methodology as applied to the relay cells used to compute measures of membrane voltage expected at the soma and various dendritic loci when a current is injected at one distal dendritic locus (Bloomfield & Sherman, 1989). A major reason for the electrotonically extensive dendritic arbor of interneurons appears again to be related to dendritic diameter: whereas the dendrites of interneurons are roughly as long as the dendrites of relay cells, those of interneurons are much thinner, which would result in more current from synaptic activation leaking across the membrane en route to the soma.

As is the case for relay cells, to date the only formal cable modeling of interneurons recorded in vivo has come from the lateral geniculate nucleus of the cat (Bloomfield & Sherman, 1989). The interneurons illustrated in figure 4.1C and D are of the type represented by figure 2.11. Given evidence of other classes of thalamic interneuron (see chapter 2), it is possible that other patterns of cable properties are present in other interneurons. More information is needed about the general properties of interneurons and their variation across thalamic nuclei and species.

Cable modeling of neurons of the thalamic reticular nucleus in rats suggests that they are electrotonically extensive (Destexhe et al., 1996). If the only output of a reticular cell is the axon, as is the case with relay cells, one might conclude from teleological arguments either that such cells must be relatively compact electrotonically or that their dendrites are not passive and may actively conduct postsynaptic potentials toward the soma (and evidence for this latter argument clearly exists, as described below). Otherwise, synaptic inputs located peripherally in the dendritic arbor would be ineffective in influencing the neuronal output, and the creation of such inputs would seem pointless. If, however, a neuron has dendritic outputs (with or without axonal ones), it might make sense for its dendritic arbor to be relatively extensive, since inputs that can influence dendritic outputs nearby need not influence the soma or axon hillock to affect the cell's output. Indeed, as we argue in the following paragraphs for interneurons, it makes sense for cells with dendritic outputs to be electrotonically extensive. Thus one might predict that reticular cells in the rat would have dendritic outputs, with reticular cells forming dendrodendritic contacts with each other, and evidence for such dendrodendritic contacts in this species exists (Pinault et al., 1997), although it has also been questioned (Ohara & Lieberman, 1985). Furthermore, evidence for such dendrodendritic contacts has been found among reticular cells of the cat (Ide, 1982; Deschênes et al., 1985), but not the monkey (Williamson et al., 1994). Unfortunately, no published evidence of cable properties of reticular cells for species other than the rat exists. In light of claims of interspecies differences in dendrodendritic connections among these cells, their cable properties might prove particularly interesting.

4.A.3. Implications of Cable Properties for the Function of Relay Cells and Interneurons

In view of their cable properties, it is interesting to compare and contrast how relay cells and interneurons integrate synaptic inputs. Because relay cells have a single axonal output, it is sufficient to consider synaptic integration in terms of how inputs affect membrane voltage at the soma or axon hillock. The dendritic architecture and branching pattern of these cells suggest rather efficient current flow throughout the dendritic arbor, meaning that postsynaptic potentials will attenuate relatively little from the dendritic site of origin to the soma. As indicated earlier and shown in figure 4.1, the maximum voltage attenuation for steady-state voltage changes from the most distally located synapse to the soma is estimated to be less than one half (Bloomfield et al., 1987; Bloomfield & Sherman, 1989). In relay cells, it thus seems likely that all active synapses, regardless of their location in the dendritic arbor, may significantly influence the axon hillock and that synaptic integration in relay cells involves large-scale summation of all such active synapses.

Interneurons appear to function quite differently. Many, perhaps all, interneurons have axons (Hamos et al., 1985; Montero, 1987; see chapter 2 for more detailed discussion). However, in addition to the synaptic outputs of these axons, interneurons also have synaptic terminals emanating from peripheral dendrites. These are the F2 terminals described in chapter 3, and they form inhibitory synapses onto relay cells. Most, perhaps all, are postsynaptic as well as presynaptic. They receive synaptic input from various terminals, mostly retinal, but also some from brainstem or from GABAergic axons forming RS or F1 terminals, respectively (see chapter 3). Typically, they engage in the triadic synaptic arrangements in which the F2 terminal is postsynaptic to a retinal terminal and both the F2 and retinal terminals are presynaptic to the same relay cell dendrite.

The typical interneuron thus has two distinct types of output pathway, which are summarized schematically in figure 4.2 (Sherman, 2004). The outputs of the axon are effectively controlled only by the inputs to the soma or proximal dendrites, because the inputs to more distal dendrites and especially onto the F2 terminals are electronically too distant to have much effect on membrane potential at the axon hillock. Evidence to support this comes from pharmacological studies (summarized in the next chapter) in which drugs thought to depolarize the F2 terminals directly have no recordable effects in the soma (Cox et al., 1998; Cox & Sherman, 2000; reviewed in Sherman, 2004). In turn, events at or close to the soma are too distant electrotonically to have much effect on the F2 terminals. The F2 terminal outputs are controlled by their local inputs, so that there is multiplexing in the interneuron: this cell can permit both synaptic input/output routes to operate simultaneously. It also seems likely that clusters of F2 terminals are themselves effectively isolated from each other, so that the dendritic arbor of the interneuron contains many local circuits performing independent input/output operations. As indicated in chapter 2, all geniculate interneurons so far studied with intracellular dye injection after

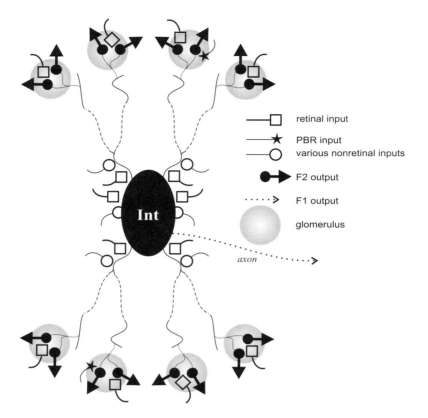

Figure 4.2
Schematic view of hypothesized functioning of interneurons in the cat's lateral geniculate nucleus. Retinal and nonretinal inputs are shown both to the glomeruli and to the proximal dendrites and soma. The inputs to the glomeruli lead to F2 (dendritic) outputs, whereas the inputs to the proximal dendrites and soma lead to F1 outputs from the axon, both outputs acting on relay cells. The dashed lines indicate the electrotonic isolation between glomeruli and the proximal dendrites plus soma. This isolation suggests that the two sets of synaptic computations, peripheral for the glomerular F2 outputs and proximal for the axonal F1 outputs, occur in parallel and independently of one another. Most glomeruli are also functionally isolated from one another.

electrophysiological recording have axons, although the number studied this way is small (Friedlander et al., 1981; Hamos et al., 1985; Sherman & Friedlander, 1988). The methods used to sample these interneurons before filling require that they fire action potentials, otherwise they would be missed, and thus any existing axonless interneurons, which might not generate action potentials, would not have been detected in these experiments (see also chapter 2). An interneuron without an axon would still provide outputs via the dendritic F2 terminals and thus may not require action potentials to function.

4.B. Membrane Conductances

It used to be thought that cable modeling alone provided a reasonably complete and accurate picture of how neurons integrate their synaptic inputs to produce specific firing patterns. However, starting about two decades ago, it became clear that neurons and their dendritic arbors do not act in the manner of simple cables. Instead, they display numerous nonlinear membrane properties that further complicate the job of understanding neuronal input/output relationships.

These membrane nonlinearities are due to various membrane conductances that can be switched on or off, thereby affecting the flow of electric current in the form of charged ions into or out of the cell. In addition to affecting membrane potential, these conductance changes also affect membrane resistance, and thus the cell's passive cable properties. We can consider as an example the interneuron. Cable modeling based on one specific membrane resistance leads to one value of electrotonic length, and, as noted earlier, typical values for this length suggest that these cells are electrotonically extensive. If membrane resistance can vary based on variable conductances (described more fully below), then so can electrotonic extent. Perhaps in some functional modes when the membrane is relatively leaky because a conductance is active (e.g., a K^+ conductance; see below), the interneuron is so extensive electrotonically that effects at dendritic F2 terminals are isolated from the soma, as argued above; but if the conductance can be switched off, then the membrane resistance increases, leading to a more electrotonically compact cell with a possible breakdown of the isolation between soma and F2 terminals. Evidence for precisely this sort of dynamic change in cable properties exists for interneurons of the rat lateral geniculate nucleus (Zhu & Heggelund, 2001).

Synaptic inputs create changes in ionic conductances (see chapter 5), which underlie changes in membrane potential or postsynaptic potential. Many of the variable membrane conductances seen in cells can also be affected by membrane voltage, being regulated simply by changing membrane potential, so synaptic inputs can have other effects on certain conductances through postsynaptic potentials. Still other conductances are controlled by the changing intracellular concentration of specific ions (e.g., Ca^{2+}), which, as shown by examples provided below, can be controlled by certain synaptic events. Thalamic cells are fairly typical of neurons throughout the brain in having a rich array of these membrane conductances. Because the discovery of these conductances is still ongoing, it is likely that their full array has yet to be defined. Because these conductances ultimately change membrane potential, and many also have complicated temporal properties, they represent a complex influence on the axon hillock that is not a part of the cable model but must now be taken into account. Thus, cable modeling, although useful, is severely limited. We now look at these nonlinear membrane conductances and at the quite dramatic effects they have on how a cell responds to its synaptic inputs. Chapter 5 adds to this account.

4.B.1. Voltage Independent Membrane Conductances in Relay Cells

The transmembrane voltages that are the signature of neurons and other electroresponsive cells, such as muscle cells, are created initially by specific ionic pumps that create differential concentrations of various ions across the membranes. However, the membranes are not completely impermeable to ions, and they constantly leak across the membrane. The ionic conductances underlying these leaks generally do not depend on membrane voltage. The result of the leaks and pumps is a stable equilibrium concentration gradient for each ion, and this leads to the typical resting membrane potential. For a typical neuron, the resting potential is usually between -65 and $-75\,mV$. Of the ions that dominate this process, namely K^+, Na^+, and Cl^-, passive leakage is greatest for K^+. This is the so-called K^+ "leak" conductance. However, if only K^+ leaked across the membrane, the resting potential would be at the reversal potential for K^+, or about $-100\,mV$. The smaller leakages of Na^+ and Cl^-, which are driven by more positive reversal potentials, combine with the K^+ "leak" conductance to create the resting membrane potentials observed, typically between -65 and $-75\,mV$. As we shall see in chapter 5, one important effect of certain synaptic actions is a change in the K^+ "leak" conductance.

4.B.2. *Voltage Dependent Membrane Conductances in Relay Cells*

There is a large class of membrane conductances that are generally known as voltage dependent but that also have a time dependency, so that their behavior is typically a complex function of voltage and time. That is, changes in membrane potential will often alter a conductance, but there is typically a delay in the alteration, and this delay may vary. Often, for instance, a small change in membrane potential may alter a membrane conductance relatively slowly, while a larger voltage change will produce a faster change.

4.B.2.a. Action Potentials

Voltage dependent conductances should not seem mysterious, because the action potential as classically defined for the squid giant axon by Hodgkin and Huxley (1952) is itself the result of voltage (and time) dependent Na^+ and K^+ conductances and is thus an excellent example of these nonlinear membrane properties. For this reason, it is useful to review these properties for the action potential of the squid giant axon, which are summarized in figures 4.3 and 4.4. Many readers are likely to be familiar with this material and are encouraged to move ahead to the next section. Others, however, will find it a useful introduction to the sections that follow. Whereas the details of kinetics and voltage dependency and also the nature of the various K^+ conductances differ somewhat across cell types, and the actual conductances for thalamic cells probably differ quantitatively from this illustration, the action potential of the squid giant axon nonetheless serves as an excellent model for many other voltage dependent conductances described for thalamic neurons. As shown in figure 4.3A, the action potential has a very rapid rise or upstroke from rest and a somewhat slower fall or downstroke that slightly overshoots rest to create a period of relative hyperpolarization, known as the afterhyperpolarization.

First, we can consider the Na^+ channels. These have two voltage activated gates (see figure 4.4): an *activation gate* that opens at depolarized levels and closes at hyperpolarized ones, and an *inactivation gate* that shows the opposite voltage dependency. For Na^+ to flow into the cell, which leads to an inward Na^+ current (I_{Na}), both gates must be open, and the channel and I_{Na} are now said to be *activated*. Because of the close

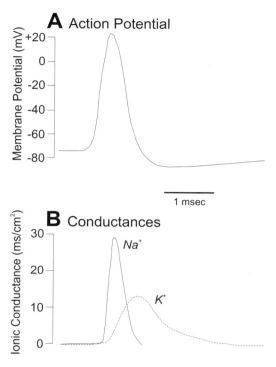

Figure 4.3
Typical action potential. *A*. Voltage trace. Note that just following the action potential there is a period of modest hyperpolarization, known as the *afterhy-perpolarization*. *B*. Voltage dependent Na⁺ and K⁺ conductances underlying the voltage changes of the action potential.

relationship between channel conductance and transmembrane current, the phrases and concepts are often interchanged; for instance, an increase in the conductance of the Na⁺ channel leads to an increase in I_{Na}, and we can refer to both the channel and the current as being activated, inactivated, and so on. The channel and I_{Na} are *inactivated* when the inactivation gate is closed, and they are *deactivated* when the activation gate is closed.

Figures 4.3*B* and 4.4*E* show the time course of changes for Na⁺ channel conductance and I_{Na} during a typical action potential. At rest, Na⁺ channels and I_{Na} are de-inactivated and also deactivated (figure 4.4*A*). However, sufficient depolarization from rest opens the activation gate, and I_{Na} is activated, so Na⁺ flows into the cell to depolarize it further

The Action Potential

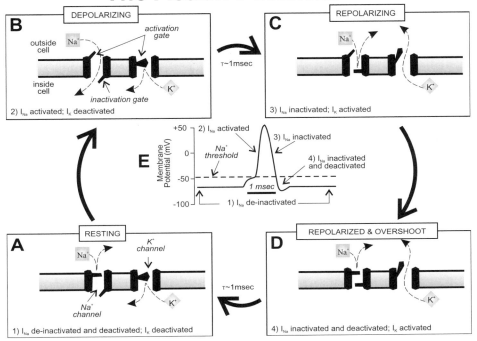

Figure 4.4

Schematic representation of voltage dependent Na^+ and K^+ conductances underlying the action potential. *A–D* show the channel events, and *E* shows the effects
on membrane potential. The Na^+ channel has two voltage activated gates: an
activation gate that opens at depolarized levels and closes at hyperpolarized
levels, and an *inactivation gate*, with the opposite voltage dependency. Both must
be open for the inward, depolarizing Na^+ current (I_{Na}) to flow. The K^+ channel
(really an imaginary amalgam of several different K^+ channels) has a single activation gate, and when it opens at depolarized levels, the outward, hyperpolarizing K^+ current (I_K) is activated. *A.* At a resting membrane potential (roughly −60
to −65 mV), the activation gate of the Na^+ channel is closed, and so it is deactivated, but the inactivation gate is open, and so it is de-inactivated. The single
gate for the K^+ channel is closed. *B.* With sufficient depolarization to reach its
threshold, the activation gate of the Na^+ channel opens, allowing Na^+ to flow
into the cell. This depolarizes the cell, providing the upswing of the action potential. *C.* The inactivation gate of the Na^+ channel closes after roughly 1 msec
(roughly, because closing of the channel is a complex function of time and
voltage), and the slower K^+ channel also opens. These combined actions lead to
the repolarization of the cell. While the inactivation gate of the Na^+ channel is
closed, the channel is said to be inactivated. *D.* Even though the initial resting
potential is reached, the Na^+ channel remains inactivated, because it takes
roughly 1 msec (roughly having the same meaning as above) of hyperpolarization to de-inactivate it; it also takes a bit of time for the various K^+ channels to
close, leading to an overshoot or afterhyperpolarization.

(figure 4.4*B*). Typically the voltage threshold for this effect occurs at around −50 mV when the membrane is depolarized from more hyperpolarized levels, such as a resting potential of about −70 mV. This is the upswing of the action potential. The resulting depolarization serves to inactivate the Na$^+$ channels and I_{Na} rapidly, after about a millisecond or so (figure 4.4*C*). Such inactivation means that, no matter what the membrane voltage, the channels will not open. (Thus, whereas we normally think of depolarization as an excitatory event because it promotes cell firing, depolarization that is sufficiently strong and prolonged will actually prevent action potentials, because it inactivates the Na$^+$ channels.) With I_{Na} now shut down, the cell begins to repolarize to its previously hyperpolarized level, and the opening of various slower voltage dependent K$^+$ channels[2] speeds this process of repolarization by activating an outward K$^+$ current (I_K). The voltage gated K$^+$ channels are simpler than the Na$^+$ channels, because they lack an inactivation gate: they and their related I_K are thus either activated or deactivated, but do not inactivate. Also, just as the K$^+$ channels are slower to activate than the Na$^+$ channels, they are also slower to deactivate, and this leads in most neurons to the above-mentioned afterhyperpolarization (figure 4.4*D*). Eventually, the repolarization and afterhyperpolarization remove the inactivation of the Na$^+$ channel, but this takes about 1 msec. It is this slight delay before I_{Na} is de-inactivated that creates the refractory period during which another action potential cannot occur, thereby limiting the firing rates of most neurons to roughly 1,000 spikes/sec. Actually, there are two refractory periods: an absolute one, during which I_{Na} remains inactivated, and a relative one caused by the afterhyperpolarization.

It should be noted here that the Na$^+$ channels actually exist in four quite different states, as outlined in figure 4.4: (1) At rest, when de-inactivated and deactivated, the channels are closed, but they can be rapidly opened by activation via a suprathreshold depolarization (figure 4.4*A*). (2) When activated by a suprathreshold depolarization, they are open (figure 4.4*B*). (3) Further depolarization inactivates the channels and closes them, leaving them temporarily unopenable (figure 4.4*C*). (4) When hyperpolarized from a depolarized level, the channels will remain closed until the inactivation is relieved (figure 4.4*C*). There are thus three

2. As detailed later in this chapter, a number of different K$^+$ conductances may contribute to this process.

closed channel states, inactivated and deactivated, or both, and one open state, activated.

Finally, while activation seems to be very fast, the switch between de-inactivation to inactivation and back is slower, at about a millisecond, and this switch between inactivation states is a complex function of time and voltage so that the larger the polarization change, the faster the switch.

The voltage-sensitive ion channels involved in the Na^+ and K^+ conductances of the action potential are located in the soma and axon hillock (and also often in dendrites; see below), where they are concerned with the initiation of action potentials, and all along the axon, where they produce the conduction of the nerve impulse. As a result, a sufficient depolarization in the soma or axon hillock that triggers the Na^+ and K^+ conductances will propagate down the axon as a wave, since the depolarization due to Na^+ entry depolarizes nearby voltage sensitive Na^+ channels. The refractory period dominates the wake of the action potential as it sweeps down the axon and prevents a backward-propagating spike. A special case occurs for myelinated axons, where the voltage sensitive Na^+ and K^+ channels are concentrated at the nodes of Ranvier, so that instead of a smooth, wave-like propagation, the action potential jumps from node of Ranvier to node of Ranvier down the axon in a saltatory fashion. In general, myelinated or not, thicker axons conduct action potentials to their targets with a faster conduction velocity. However, this saltatory conduction in myelinated axons produces a much faster conduction velocity than would be expected to occur in unmyelinated axons of the same diameter. In any case, whatever the speed of thalamocortical transmission, the transmission itself depends critically on the presence of the Na^+ and K^+ channels in the axons.

While the presence and role of the Na^+ and K^+ channels along the axon are quite clear, their possible dendritic location and role are less certain. In fact, this has not yet been adequately addressed for thalamic cells. However, the possibility is interesting, because studies of hippocampal and neocortical pyramidal cells indicate the presence of Na^+, K^+, and Ca^{2+} channels in the dendrites (Kim & Connors, 1993; Johnston et al., 1996; Hoffman & Johnston, 1998; Magee et al., 1998) that may affect the transmission of EPSPs generated in dendrites. They may serve to promote transmission of EPSPs toward the soma and also play a role in "back propagation" of the action potential from the soma (Schiller et al., 1997; Stuart et al., 1997a, 1997b), which means that an action potential generated in the soma or initial segment may propagate throughout the dendritic arbor, or perhaps just those dendrites expressing these channels, even when the somatic action potential was evoked by EPSPs generated in one or a few dendrites. Both of these factors can have dramatic effects on synaptic integration, and it will thus be of considerable interest to determine whether thalamic neurons also have these channels along their dendrites.

More recently discovered conductances now recognized as playing a major role in controlling the firing properties of relay cells and thus modifying the relay of information through the thalamus are described next. Most of these conductances operate through voltage dependent ion channels in the membrane of the soma and/or dendrites, although processes other than membrane potential control some of them. Some of these, such as the high threshold Ca^{2+} conductance, described below, can be initiated by the large depolarization of the action potential itself. Because most of the other conductances are voltage dependent, much like the Na^+ and K^+ conductances of the classical action potential, they are affected by postsynaptic potentials. That is, postsynaptic potentials often turn other membrane conductances on or off, resulting in additional membrane currents that ultimately affect the membrane potential at the axon hillock. This, in turn, means that these other conductances can have a quite dramatic effect on the pattern of action potentials fired by the postsynaptic cell. It is important to keep in mind that of all of the channels, only the voltage dependent Na^+ and K^+ ion channels underlying the action potential are always located along the axon, although other voltage dependent channels not considered further here are found in some axons. The only way that a thalamic cell can send a message to cortex is thus by the action potential, but the determinants of whether and how the cell fires depend heavily on the conductances that are considered next.

4.B.2.b. Low Threshold Ca^{2+} Conductance

Apart from the conductances underlying action potentials, the low threshold Ca^{2+} conductance is the most important voltage dependent conductance for thalamic relay cells. It occurs in relay cells in all dorsal thalamic nuclei of all mammals studied to date (Deschênes et al., 1984; Jahnsen & Llinás, 1984a, 1984b; Hernández-Cruz & Pape, 1989; McCormick & Feeser, 1990; Scharfman et al., 1990; Bal et al., 1995), so it is clearly a key to understanding the function of the thalamic relay. This conductance controls which of two distinct response modes, *tonic* or *burst*,[3] is operative when a thalamic relay cell responds to afferent input. The tonic mode of firing occurs when the low threshold Ca^{2+} and certain other associated conductances are inactivated. The relay cell then responds approximately in the same manner as the linear neuronal integrator described by cable modeling: its response to input is characterized by a steady stream of action potentials of a frequency and duration that correspond fairly linearly to input strength and duration. Other contributors to this linear relationship are discussed below. During the burst mode, which occurs when the low threshold Ca^{2+} conductance is de-inactivated and thus able to be activated, the neuronal response to a depolarizing input consists of brief bursts of action potentials separated by silent periods. As we shall see, there is a less linear relationship during burst firing between the amplitude or temporal properties of the input and the action potential response relayed to cortex. It is worth emphasizing that this response during burst mode bears no resemblance to the known firing patterns of afferent inputs, since, for instance, retinogeniculate axons show no evidence of burst firing. The further significance of these firing modes for understanding the way in which messages are relayed to cortex is the subject of chapter 6. Here we confine the discussion to the underlying membrane properties related to the production of tonic and burst firing.

As noted, the inactivation state of the low threshold Ca^{2+} conductance is responsible for whether the cell responds in tonic or burst mode, since the relay cell responds in tonic mode when this conductance is inactive and burst mode when it is first de-inactivated and then activated. The inactivation state itself is dependent on membrane voltage, much like the Na^+ conductance of the conventional action potential. However, the threshold for activating this conductance is at a lower, that is, more hyperpolarized, level than that for the action potential. When activated, it produces a spikelike, triangular depolarization of roughly 20–30 mV and lasting for roughly 50 msec: this is the *low threshold spike*.[4]

---

3. "Tonic" used in this sense refers to a response mode of a thalamic relay cell, and here it is paired with "burst." X and Y cells, two relay cell types found in the A-laminae of the cat's lateral geniculate nucleus (see chapters 2 and 3), display both response modes. This use of "tonic" should not be confused with another use of "tonic" when paired with "phasic" to refer to a cell type: "tonic" for X and "phasic" for Y. Throughout this account, we use "tonic" to refer only to response mode and not to cell type.

4. To avoid confusion between "spike" and "action potential," we refer to the voltage spike caused by activation of the voltage-sensitive Na^+ and K^+ channels as the "action potential" and that caused by activation of the T channels as the "low threshold spike."

Figure 4.5 illustrates the voltage dependency of this spike. The channel involved is known as the T (for transient) channel, and its voltage dependency is qualitatively precisely the same as that of the Na^+ channel involved in the action potential, although there are important quantitative differences. Thus the channel has the same two voltage activated gates. The starting point involves deactivation and de-inactivation of the channel (figure 4.5A). A suprathreshold depolarization then activates the channel (figure 4.5B), leading to an inward Ca^{2+} current called the T current (I_T). Like activation of I_{Na}, this leads to an all-or-none spike, which in this case is a Ca^{2+} spike. The resultant depolarization eventually causes inactivation of the T channel (figure 4.5C). This plus activation of various K^+ channels causes repolarization (figure 4.5D), and this repolarization eventually leads to de-inactivation of the T channel (back to figure 4.5A).

As noted, there are several important differences between the T channel and aforementioned Na^+ channel.

• The T channel is slower by roughly an order of magnitude so that, while activation is very fast, it takes roughly 100 msec to switch between inactivation states. Thus, if the T channel is de-inactivated, as in figure 4.5A, a sustained depolarization is required for inactivation. This means that a fast EPSP of 10 msec or so or even an action potential is insufficient for this purpose. Likewise, if the channel is inactivated, as in figure 4.5C, a sustained hyperpolarization is required to remove the inactivation, and thus a fast IPSP is insufficient. These issues of timing are considered again in the next chapter. However, as for the Na^+ channel, because the operation of the T channel is a complex function of voltage and time (Jahnsen & Llinás, 1984a; Smith et al., 2000), a larger shift in voltage results in a faster switch between inactivation states.

• The T channel operates in a slightly more hyperpolarized regime than does the Na^+ channel, so that the thresholds for the various activation and inactivation states are roughly 10 mV lower. Because I_T can thus be activated at a lower threshold than the action potential, the resultant Ca^{2+} spike is called the *low threshold spike*. Thus the low threshold spike and I_T refer to closely related phenomena.

• T channels are found in the soma and dendrites, but not to any appreciable degree in the axon. Thus the low threshold spike propagates through the dendritic arbor but not up the axon to cortex. T channel activity can certainly affect action potential firing in a thalamic relay cell, but action potentials represent the only message to reach cortex from thalamus.

The Low Threshold Ca²⁺ Spike

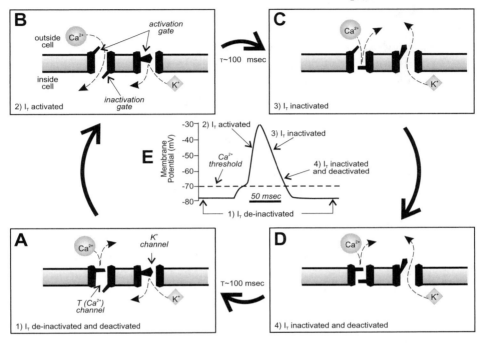

Figure 4.5

Schematic representation of actions of voltage dependent T (Ca²⁺) and K⁺ conductances underlying low threshold Ca²⁺ spike; conventions as in figure 4.4. Note the strong qualitative similarity between the behavior of the T channel here and the Na⁺ channel shown in figure 4.4, including the presence of both activation and inactivation gates with similar voltage dependency. The sequence of events is shown clockwise in *A–D*, with the membrane voltage changes shown in *E. A.* At a relatively hyperpolarized resting membrane potential (roughly −70 mV), the activation gate of the T channel is closed, but the inactivation gate is open, and so the T channel is deactivated and de-inactivated. The K⁺ channel is also deactivated. *B.* With sufficient depolarization to reach its threshold, the activation gate of the T channel opens, allowing Ca²⁺ to flow into the cell. This depolarizes the cell, providing the upswing of the low threshold spike. *C.* The inactivation gate of the T channel closes after roughly 100 msec (roughly, because as for the Na⁺ channel in figure 4.4, closing of the channel is a complex function of time and voltage), inactivating the T channels, and the K⁺ channel also opens. These combined actions repolarize the cell. *D.* Even though the initial resting potential is reached, the T channel remains inactivated, because it takes roughly 100 msec of hyperpolarization to de-inactivate it; it also takes a bit of time for the various K⁺ channels to close. *E.* Membrane voltage changes showing low threshold spike.

• Finally, because both channels can inactivate, in a depolarized state they play no role in the cell's activity. In principle, for the Na^+ channel, this means that continuous sufficient depolarization would render the cell silent, but healthy neurons are thought never to be so continuously depolarized. However, the amount of depolarization needed to inactivate the T channel—to about $-60\,mV$—is well within a cell's physiological range. Thus, sustained inactivation of the T channels is common for thalamic neurons, whereas sustained inactivation of the Na^+ channels is not.

Figure 4.6 shows results obtained from in vitro intracellular recordings from a geniculate cell in a cat, and this demonstrates how T channel behavior can affect action potential generation and thus the signal relayed to cortex. A depolarization of only about $5\,mV$ from rest for more than $100\,msec$ (figure 4.6A) is sufficient to inactivate the T channels, which then play no role in the cell's firing. Here the cell fires in tonic mode: the response to a sustained, suprathreshold depolarizing current injection is a stream of unitary action potentials that lasts as long as the suprathreshold stimulus. If, however, the cell has been hyperpolarized by about the same amount for more than $100\,msec$ (figure 4.6B), the T channels de-inactivate and are primed for action. The same depolarizing current injection that promoted tonic firing in figure 4.6A now activates the all-or-none low threshold Ca^{2+} spike, which is sufficiently large to evoke a high-frequency cluster of action potentials that rides its crest; this is burst firing. In this way, I_T and the resultant low threshold spike provide an amplification that permits a hyperpolarized cell to generate action potentials (typically two to ten; the reason for this variable number is explained below) in response to a moderate excitatory synaptic input.

It should be noted from figure 4.6A and B that precisely the same activating input results in a very different signal relayed to cortex, depending on the recent voltage history of the cell. Similarly, the same EPSP from a retinal afferent can lead to a very different signal relayed to cortex, depending on the cell's firing mode, tonic or burst. (Chapter 6 explores these differences more thoroughly.) Note also that only a few millivolts of depolarization or hyperpolarization sustained for a fraction of a second is sufficient to switch firing modes. Such changes are well within the physiological range of thalamic neurons, and thus it is common for each neuron to express both firing modes at different times and to switch freely between them. The next chapter describes how thalamic circuitry controls the firing mode of these cells.

Figure 4.7 represents a more complete and quantitative description of the voltage dependency of I_T measured from six different relay cells in the ventral posterior lateral nucleus of the rat, each indicated by a different set of symbols (Huguenard & McCormick, 1992). Similar data have also been found for relay cells in other nuclei and in other species (Deschênes et al., 1984; Jahnsen & Llinás, 1984a, 1984b; Hernández-Cruz & Pape, 1989; McCormick & Feeser, 1990; Scharfman et al., 1990; Bal et al., 1995), including the ventral anterior nucleus, medial geniculate nucleus, lateral geniculate nucleus, pulvinar, and other unspecified thalamic regions from ferrets, guinea pigs, hamsters, or cats. These data are based on measuring the actual I_T during voltage clamp recording.[5]

---

5. Voltage clamp is a useful technique, but there are problems associated with it that should be kept in mind. The main one is that it is difficult to maintain equipotential conditions throughout the cell at all times. Even when the electronics are sufficiently fast to keep pace with fast transient conductance changes, there remains the problem that neurons with extensive dendritic arbors act as cables do. Thus, if current is injected into the cell at the soma, say, to depolarize and clamp it to a specific membrane potential, some of this current will leak across the membrane as it travels out through the dendritic arbor. There is then less current available to depolarize the membrane as one proceeds further out along the arbor, and the result is a gradient in clamped membrane voltage rather than true isopotentiality throughout the neuron. The same problem exists with attempts to hyperpolarize the cell. If T type Ca^{2+} channels exist throughout the soma and dendrites, as seems to be the case (Destexhe et al., 1996; Destexhe et al., 1998a), then they will experience different membrane voltages at different locations. This in turn means that they will contribute differently at different locations during voltage clamp, because the differing voltages produce different levels of inactivation. There are several ways to deal with this problem. The most common is to record from acutely dissociated thalamic relay cells, because the dissociation removes most or all of the dendrites. Maintaining isopotential recording in such cells during voltage clamp is much more likely without the extensive dendritic arbor, but the problem here is the assumption that a cell with its dendrites ripped away will reveal normal physiological properties. Another implicit assumption is that the behavior of channels in the soma, which in theory can be studied more rigorously in dissociated cells, is identical to that of channels in the missing dendrites. This assumption seems reasonable, but it would still be necessary to know the distribution of channels in the dendrites to reconstruct completely how the cell would behave with respect to the channels under investigation (see Destexhe et al., 1996, and Destexhe et al., 1998a, for examples of how this may be done). It is thus important to understand the limitations of the voltage clamp method, although it is frequently used because it is still judged to be the best technique available to address these issues. The data in figure 4.7 are in fact taken from acutely dissociated cells.

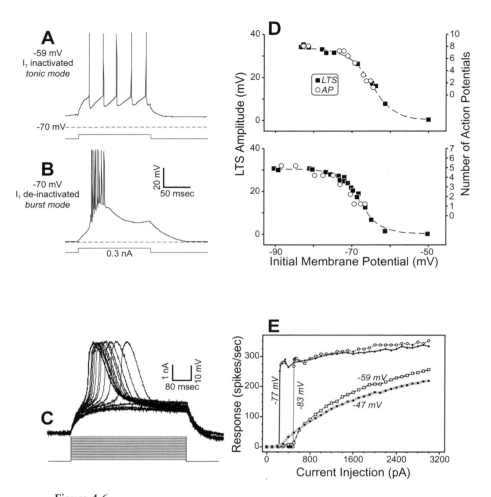

Figure 4.6

Properties of I_T and the low threshold spike (redrawn from Sherman, 2001). All examples are from relay cells of the cat's lateral geniculate nucleus recorded intracellularly in an in vitro slice preparation. *A* and *B*. Voltage dependency of the low threshold spike. Responses are shown to the same depolarizing current pulse delivered intracellularly but from two different initial holding potentials. When the cell is relatively depolarized (*A*), I_T is inactivated, and the cell responds with a stream of unitary action potentials as long as the stimulus is suprathreshold for firing. This is the *tonic mode* of firing. When the cell is relatively hyperpolarized (*B*), I_T is de-inactivated, and the current pulse activates a low threshold spike with eight action potentials riding its crest. This is the *burst mode* of firing. *C*. All-or-none nature of low threshold spikes measured in the presence of tetrodotoxin in another geniculate cell (from Zhan et al., 1999). The cell is initially hyperpolarized, and current pulses were injected starting at 200 pA and incremented in 10-pA steps. Smaller (subthreshold) pulses led to pure resistive-capacitative responses, but all larger (suprathreshold) pulses led to a low threshold spike. Much like conventional action potentials, the low threshold spikes are all the same amplitude regardless of how far the depolarizing pulse exceeded activation threshold, although there is latency variability for smaller suprathreshold pulses. *D*. Voltage dependency of amplitude of low threshold spike and burst response (from Zhan et al., 2000). Examples for two cells are shown; the upper is the same as shown in C. The more hyperpolarized the cell before being activated (Initial Membrane Potential), the larger the low threshold spike (filled squares and curve) and the more action potentials (AP) in the burst (open circles). The number of action potentials was measured first, and then tetrodotoxin was applied to isolate the low threshold spike for measurement. *E*. Input/output relationship for another cell. The input variable is the amplitude of the depolarizing current pulse, and the output is the firing frequency of the cell. To compare burst and tonic firing, the firing frequency was determined by the first six action potentials of the response, since this cell usually exhibited six action potentials per burst in this experiment. The initial holding potentials are shown, and $-47\,mV$ and $-59\,mV$ reflect tonic mode, whereas $-77\,mV$ and $-83\,mV$ reflect burst mode.

This technique pumps just the right amount of current into or out of the cell during recording to balance any activated currents (like I_T), thereby keeping the membrane voltage constant, or "clamped," at a predetermined voltage. The amount of current pumped in or out provides a measure of the actual membrane current activated by I_T, and this value can be converted to a measure of the related membrane conductance, which is actually plotted.[6] In figure 4.7, I_T is activated in two analogous experiments, one to measure the "inactivation" of I_T, and the other to measure the "activation" of I_T.

The insets in figure 4.7 illustrate the voltage regimens used to determine the points for the activation and inactivation curves. To obtain each inactivation curve (shown by the dashed lines), the cell is first clamped at different levels aimed to partly inactivate I_T, which is then assessed by measuring the membrane current evoked by a sudden clamping of the cell to a new depolarized level ($-42\,mV$) sufficient to activate any de-inactivated I_T. To measure activation (shown by the solid lines), the cell is first clamped at a very hyperpolarized level ($-110\,mV$) to completely de-inactivate I_T, and the current evoked by suddenly clamping the cell to various depolarized levels is determined. These curves of relative

---

6. Some authors simply plot I_T directly for these curves. However, the actual I_T flowing into the cell via Ca^{2+} is a function of both the number of open T channels and the driving force, which is the difference between the reversal potential for Ca^{2+} (roughly $+150\,mV$) and the membrane potential at which I_T is evoked. Thus the more positive the potential at which I_T is evoked, the lower the driving force. Some authors thus convert the current recorded during current clamp to an estimate of membrane conductance, which is not influenced by the driving force and does reflect the number of channels opened.

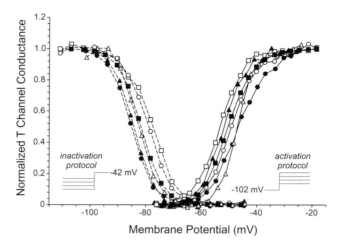

Figure 4.7
Voltage dependency of activation and inactivation of I_T for six cells of the ventral posterior nucleus in rats. The cells were recorded in vitro and in isolation after acute dissociation, which usually leaves the soma and stumps of primary dendrites. Recordings were made in voltage clamp mode to measure I_T, and from these measurements, the underlying conductance could be computed. The ordinate shows the conductance measures after each curve was normalized with respect to the largest conductance evoked. On the left are shown the *inactivation* curves (dashed lines). The points for these curves were obtained by first holding the membrane at various hyperpolarized levels (which are plotted on the abscissa) for 1 sec and then stepping up to −42 mV. The voltage protocol for this is shown at lower left. Note that the more hyperpolarized the initial holding potential, the more I_T is evoked, because more hyperpolarization produces more de-inactivation of I_T. On the right are shown the *activation* curves (solid lines). Here the points were obtained by initially holding at −102 mV, which would completely de-inactivate I_T, and then stepping up to the various membrane voltages plotted on the abscissa. The voltage protocol for this is shown at lower right. Note that larger depolarizing steps activate more I_T. (Data kindly supplied by J. R. Huguenard for replotting from Huguenard & McCormick, 1992.)

conductance lie between 0 and 1. The intermediate levels reflect partial activation or inactivation of I_T, and this reflects the probabilistic percentage of T channels being in a given state during these experiments. During the inactivation experiments, the more hyperpolarized the initial holding potential, the more T channels switch from the inactive state to become de-inactivated. Likewise, during the activation experiments, the larger the depolarizing pulse, the more T channels become activated and opened.

There are two points to note about these curves. First, there is very little overlap between activation and inactivation curves. An overlap is a sort of voltage "window," or a membrane voltage range in which I_T is constantly present, because it is both partially de-inactivated and partially activated, but this actually seems not to occur to any significant extent in these relay cells of the ventral posterior lateral nucleus in the rat. However, the extent to which this is also true for other relay cells in other species or thalamic nuclei is an open question. This question is an important one to address, because the presence and extent of such a window are important for understanding how a relay cell fires (Tóth et al., 1998; Hughes et al., 1999). That is, if a window exists and if the membrane voltage lies within it, the relay cell may begin to discharge spontaneously and rhythmically; furthermore, if a more depolarized relay cell is hyperpolarized (e.g., via an inhibitory synaptic input) into the voltage window, it may begin to burst rhythmically, which might seem to be a counterintuitive response to a hyperpolarizing input. However, for this to happen, relay cells must have an abnormally high input resistance brought on by blocking much of the K^+ "leak" conductance (Tóth et al., 1998; Hughes et al., 1999), so that relay cells in a more physiological state would not show bursting or other responsiveness upon entering the voltage window (Gutierrez et al., 2001). Second, while the activation curve appears to be fairly steep, there is nonetheless an *apparent* dynamic voltage range of about 20 mV in which partial depolarizing steps will evoke a partial I_T. This, however, is largely due to the conditions of voltage clamp recording. Thalamic relay neurons in the working brain are not voltage clamped. In such a cell, an EPSP might activate only a partial I_T, but without the voltage clamped, this partial I_T would further depolarize the cell, activating more I_T, and so on in the form of a positive feedback process (Zhan et al., 1999).

The result is a much narrower dynamic range than might be deduced from the activation curve of figure 4.7. By dynamic range we mean the range of depolarizations over which a graded low threshold spike can be evoked. The dynamic range is effectively zero or, more accurately, so narrow that it usually cannot be measured in practice, because the positive feedback means that most depolarizations either are too small to activate any low threshold spike (i.e., they are below threshold) or are so large that they evoke the maximum low threshold spike (i.e., they are above threshold). This is effectively an "all-or-none" response, like that of the action potential, and it is illustrated in figure 4.6C–E, which shows data from relay cells in the cat's lateral geniculate nucleus recorded in the "current clamp" mode without any attempt to clamp the voltage.

Figure 4.6C shows the result of injecting small, incremental steps of current into the cell from an initial membrane potential sufficiently hyperpolarized to de-inactivate a significant number of the T channels. For this experiment, tetrodotoxin has been added to block the Na$^+$ channels underlying conventional action potentials, allowing better visualization of the low-threshold Ca^{2+} spike (Zhan et al., 1999). Small current injections produce a simple resistive-capacitative response, but as the threshold voltage for the Ca^{2+} spike is reached, the first suprathreshold current injection activates a Ca^{2+} spike. Large suprathreshold injections activate Ca^{2+} spikes that are not significantly larger, although they do occur with shorter latency. Thus, in terms of amplitude, the Ca^{2+} spike behaves like an "all-or-none" spike with a voltage threshold, again much like the action potential.

While the low threshold spike is activated in an all-or-none manner, its size can vary depending on the initial membrane potential. This is because the more hyperpolarized the cell is before activation of I_T, the more T channels are de-inactivated and thus available to contribute to the low threshold spike. This is shown in figure 4.6D for two cells, the upper being the same cell as in figure 4.6C (Zhan et al., 2000). In these experiments, the amplitude of the low threshold spike is measured in the presence of tetrodotoxin as a function of the initial membrane potential. From any of these initial potentials, the low threshold spike is evoked in an all-or-none manner, as in figure 4.6C, but it is larger for more hyperpolarized starting points. Also shown in figure 4.6D are data using the same protocol in each cell but before tetrodotoxin is applied, so that the measure is the number of action potentials riding the crest of each low threshold spike. Note the close correlation between the number of action potentials and amplitude of the low threshold spike. This means that the size of the signal in number of action potentials relayed to cortex in burst mode can vary depending on the extent of hyperpolarization prior to arrival of the activating input. It is important to understand that, although these experiments were carried out with current injections to depolarize the cell enough to evoke low threshold spikes, this would also happen with any synaptic input (e.g., from retina) that produced sufficiently large postsynaptic responses.

Since the action potentials represent the only signal sent to cortex by thalamic relay cells, they are thus the only output of the relay cell seen by cortex. We can begin to ask how burst and tonic firing affect the input/output relationships of the relay cells. One important difference is illustrated in figure 4.6E for another cell. During burst firing, after activation from initial membrane potentials of −77 or −83 mV that are levels of significant de-inactivation of the T channels, a sudden jump in firing frequency is seen that corresponds to the threshold activation of Ca^{2+} spiking (Zhan et al., 1999). Thereafter, larger current injections have only a modest effect on the initial firing frequency. This can be contrasted to tonic firing after activation from initial membrane potentials of −47 or −59 mV, which are levels that inactivate most of the T channels. Now the relationship between input (i.e., the current steps) and output (i.e., the firing frequency) is much more linear, without a sudden jump or discontinuity as seen with burst firing.

Another linearity difference in firing modes is shown in figure 4.6. During tonic firing (figure 4.6A), the response lasts as long as the injected current, but during burst firing (figure 4.6B), the response does not faithfully represent the duration of the injected current. Fourier analysis of results of injecting sinusoidal currents into geniculate relay cells of the cat confirm that burst firing provides a significantly more nonlinear input/output relationship than does tonic firing (Smith et al., 2000).

Since the de-inactivation of I_T is relatively slow, its full inactivation takes on the order of 100 msec or longer. In principle, this is qualitatively like the refractory period for action potentials, except it lasts much longer. Thus the low threshold Ca^{2+} spike is followed by a refractory period that limits the rate of such Ca^{2+} spiking to 10 Hz or less. Also, since low threshold Ca^{2+} spikes are evoked from relatively hyperpolarized levels, since the depolarization caused by the low threshold spike is itself sufficient to inactivate much of I_T, and since the depolarization and/or Ca^{2+} entry into the cell associated with I_T leads to voltage- and/or Ca^{2+}-dependent K^+ conductances that act to hyperpolarize the cell, the cell rapidly returns to its hyperpolarized state following each low threshold spike. This prohibits tonic responses, and, given the relative refractory period of I_T, the result is relative silence between low threshold spikes. This silent period between low threshold Ca^{2+} spikes enhances the burstiness of the response.

Finally, while I_T activates very quickly, recent evidence in cats indicates that activation requires a moderate rate of depolarization

(Gutierrez et al., 2001). If the rate of depolarization is too slow, a tha-lamic relay cell can be taken from a hyperpolarized state in which I_T is fully de-inactivated to a depolarized state in which I_T is fully inactivated and tonic firing ensues without ever firing a low threshold Ca^{2+} spike. The rate of rise of most postsynaptic responses (e.g., from retina) is fast enough to activate I_T, but some postsynaptic responses via metabotropic receptors (described in chapter 6) may be slow enough to convert the firing mode of the relay cell from burst to tonic without evoking a burst.

4.B.2.c. Conductances Associated with I_T

As just noted, activation of the low-threshold Ca^{2+} spike itself leads to voltage- and/or Ca^{2+}-dependent K^+ conductances, which repolarize the cell to its former hyperpolarized level, thereby initiating the process of I_T de-inactivation. Another conductance often associated with the low threshold Ca^{2+} conductance is activated by membrane hyperpolarization and deactivated by depolarization. This *hyperpolarization-activated cation conductance* leads, via influx of cations, to a depolarizing current, which is called I_h (McCormick & Pape, 1990a, 1990b). It is sometimes called the sag current because it is activated by hyperpolarization and causes the membrane potential to drift back, or sag, toward the initially more depolarized level. Activation of I_h is slow, with a time constant of >200 msec. The combination of I_T, the above-mentioned K^+ conduc-tances, and I_h can lead to rhythmic bursting, which is often seen in recordings from in vitro slice preparations of thalamus (McCormick & Pape, 1990a, 1990b; Huguenard & McCormick, 1992; McCormick & Huguenard, 1992).

Figure 4.8 illustrates the series of conductances leading to trans-membrane currents associated with I_T (McCormick & Pape, 1990a, 1990b; Huguenard & McCormick, 1992; McCormick & Huguenard, 1992). This is almost certainly an oversimplification of the actual con-ductances involved. The sequence in this schematic diagram starts with a hyperpolarization sufficient in amplitude and duration to de-inactivate I_T (1). (The actual starting point in the cycle is arbitrary.) This will later activate I_h (2), providing a depolarization that activates I_T (3) and the associated burst of conventional action potentials (4). The low thresh-old Ca^{2+} spike and action potentials initiate the above-mentioned K^+ con-ductances that hyperpolarize the cell (5). However, until the cell has been hyperpolarized for some time (~100 msec for I_T and ~200 msec for I_h), I_T is inactivated and I_h is deactivated (6, 7). The prolonged hyperpolariza-tion will eventually activate I_h, but this activation is so slow that, before

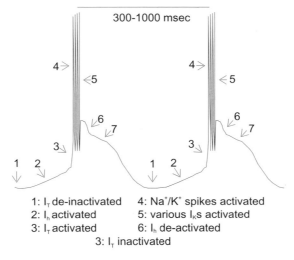

Figure 4.8
Schematic illustration of various voltage dependent conductances thought to contribute to cyclic burst firing of thalamic relay cells. Starting at a hyperpolarized membrane potential, I_T is de-inactivated (1), then I_h becomes activated (2), depolarizing the cell to activate I_T (3), which in turn activates action potentials (4). Several voltage dependent K^+ conductances then become activated (5), and after a variable period of time, I_T becomes inactivated (6) and I_h deactivates (7). Passive repolarization enhanced by the active K^+ conductances repolarize the cell, which starts a new cycle.

it begins, I_T becomes fully de-inactivated (1), and the process is repeated. This leads to prolonged rhythmic activation of low threshold Ca^{2+} spikes and bursts of action potentials. The Ca^{2+} spiking can occur at a variety of frequencies, typically at 1–3 Hz, the actual value depending on other parameters, including the presence of local feedback inhibitory circuits that may become involved during rhythmic bursting. This bursting can be interrupted only by a sufficiently strong and prolonged depolarization to inactivate I_T and prevent I_h from becoming activated. Appropriate membrane voltage shifts can thus effectively switch the cell between rhythmic bursting and tonic firing. Such rhythmic bursting may be seen during in vitro recording or during sleep and may require local circuitry, especially connections between thalamic reticular cells and relay cells, in addition to the conductances shown in figure 4.8. The rhythmic bursting seen during sleep is largely synchronized among relay neurons, a process that requires local circuitry, particularly the involvement of the thalamic reticular nucleus (Steriade et al., 1985; Steriade et al., 1993b), but the processes suggested by figure 4.8 do not imply any such synchrony among cells.

These associated conductances have been most thoroughly studied in vitro, and the following relationships have been proposed on the basis of these studies (Huguenard & McCormick, 1992). When the cell starts off relatively depolarized, it fires in tonic mode, because I_T is inactivated. When initially hyperpolarized, either by increased activity in inhibitory inputs, decreased activity in EPSPs, or both, the cell fires in burst mode or not at all, because any sufficiently strong activating (i.e., depolarizing) input will activate I_T. This burst firing would always be *rhythmic*. According to this proposal, random or arrhythmic bursting does not occur. Switching between these two modes is effected by changing membrane potential: depolarized cells will respond in tonic mode with a stream of unitary action potentials, and hyperpolarized cells will respond in burst mode with rhythmic clusters of two to ten action potentials. This proposal has also been extended to the more physiological in vivo condition, implying that, depending on membrane potential, relay cells will respond either tonically or with rhythmic bursting, the former being the condition during awake, alert behavior and the latter occurring during various phases of sleep or drowsiness. The idea here is that the sequence of conductances activated during burst firing (see figure 4.8) are much more powerful than those produced by synaptic activation via the driving inputs. In this sense, tonic firing would be the *only* relay mode for a thalamic nucleus, and burst firing would represent a functional disconnection of the relay cell from its driving inputs. As we show in chapter 5, this is not strictly correct, because arrhythmic bursting appears to be a prominent response mode of relay cells during waking behavior and can be a genuine relay mode. We shall be discussing three forms of bursting: (1) arrhythmic; (2) rhythmic and synchronized, meaning that large populations of thalamic cells fire with the same rhythm and in synchrony, which occurs during slow-wave sleep and certain forms of epilepsy; and (3) rhythmic and nonsynchronous. Obviously, to distinguish between the last two requires recording activity in populations of thalamic cells.

One final and particularly interesting feature of I_h is that it can be modulated by serotonin, noradrenalin, and histamine (McCormick & Pape, 1990a, 1990b; McCormick & Williamson, 1991). Application of any of these neuromodulators increases the amplitude of the evoked I_h, and it does so by altering the voltage dependency of the underlying ion channels. The detailed mechanisms of this effect have not yet been elucidated.

4.B.2.d. I_A

I_A is generated by a voltage dependent K^+ conductance (or several related K^+ conductances) found in most cells throughout the central nervous system (Adams, 1982; Rogawski, 1985; Storm, 1990; McCormick, 1991b). It is different from the K^+ conductances described above in terms of kinetics, and it also has a much lower activation threshold. One of the problems in dealing with intrinsic membrane properties is that there are often several different conductances using different ion channels that can involve the same ion. As we shall see, K^+ is not the only example of this.

There are certain similarities between I_A and I_T. For instance, I_A has the same three states, activated, inactivated, and de-inactivated. In thalamic relay cells, the voltage dependence of I_A is rather similar in shape to that of I_T but shifted in the depolarized direction (figure 4.9A; Pape et al., 1994). Thus, the I_A is inactivated at depolarized membrane potentials and activated by a depolarization from a hyperpolarized membrane potential. As for I_T, the activation of I_A occurs with a much faster time course than does the inactivation or de-inactivation. There is an important distinction between I_T and I_A: the I_T is carried by Ca^{2+}, which flows *into* the cell and *depolarizes* it, while the I_A is carried by K^+, which flows *out of* the cell and thereby *hyperpolarizes* it. When I_T is activated by a small depolarization, it produces a large depolarizing Ca^{2+} spike, which, as noted earlier, can be viewed as a nonlinear amplification of the activating depolarization. When the I_A is activated, it hyperpolarizes the cell, which tends to offset the original, activating depolarization. The result is a slowing down and reduction of the initial depolarization. If the cell responds in tonic mode, I_A will delay and reduce the frequency of action potentials. However, the effects of I_A during burst mode are more complex and less well understood. If I_T is activated by a strong depolarization, it will activate very quickly and from a more hyperpolarized level than needed to activate I_A; it thus appears that a low threshold Ca^{2+} spike will be fully activated before I_A has much chance to affect it. However, as noted earlier (see figure 4.6C), I_T activated by just suprathreshold stimuli has a longer latency, slower component before the all-or-none, autocatalytic, low threshold Ca^{2+} spike fires. We would expect I_A to be activated during this longer latency, which would further delay and perhaps reduce the size of the low threshold Ca^{2+} spike. Although this has to be experimentally verified, it remains the case that I_A can affect burst firing only for a narrow range of activating stimuli for I_T that are barely suprathreshold.

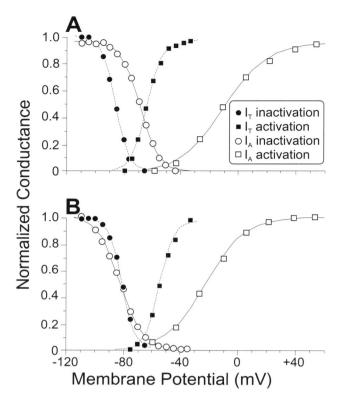

Figure 4.9
Activation and inactivation curves for both I_T and I_A in cells of the rat's lateral geniculate nucleus, generated in the same fashion as described in figure 4.7, with voltage clamp recording after acute dissociation. *A.* Curves for a relay cell. Note that the curves for I_T are shifted in a hyperpolarized direction with respect to those for I_A. *B.* Curves for an interneuron. Note that the inactivation curves for I_T and I_A are largely overlapped. See text for significance of these differences between relay cells and interneurons.

The similarity in the voltage dependencies of I_T and I_A suggests that these currents may frequently interact. Because I_T depolarizes the cell and I_A hyperpolarizes it, they would tend to offset one another if both were activated. Whether a postsynaptic potential activates one or both depends critically on the initial membrane voltage and temporal properties of voltage changes. If the membrane starts off sufficiently hyperpolarized to completely de-inactivate both conductances, then a depolarization would activate I_T before activating I_A, and the result would be a low threshold spike with a burst of action potentials riding its crest, and this pattern would be only subtly affected by the later activation of I_A. Notice also from figure 4.9A that there is a limited membrane potential near $-70\,mV$ for which I_T is thoroughly inactivated but I_A is still slightly de-inactivated. An excitatory synaptic input (or other depolarizing event) elicited within this range of membrane potentials will activate a small I_A without any I_T, so only tonic firing is possible. However, as noted above, the I_A will serve to slow down the build-up of the EPSP, which will delay and reduce the level of tonic firing. Finally, because the de-inactivation kinetics are much faster for I_A than for I_T, brief hyperpolarizations followed by depolarizations will selectively activate I_A and not I_T.

It is not clear what function I_A serves. One suggestion is that it extends the dynamic range of input/output relationships for neurons by reducing its slope (Connor & Stevens, 1971). That is, I_A, when activated by an EPSP, would sum with that EPSP to reduce the overall level of depolarization, and this enhances the range of EPSPs that evoke firing before saturation, or the maximal firing frequency, is reached. By opposing the build-up of an EPSP, activation of I_A would ensure that low to moderate stimuli would not maximally depolarize a cell, thereby preventing such stimuli from driving the cell to response saturation. The cell is thus able to signal the presence of stronger stimuli, and its dynamic range is enhanced. For relay cells, such a proposed function only makes sense for tonic mode, because the response of low threshold spikes in burst mode already has a limited dynamic range, and the low threshold spike will be evoked before I_A can influence it much.

4.B.2.e. High Threshold Ca²⁺ Conductances

In addition to the Ca^{2+} conductance underlying I_T are two or more much higher threshold Ca^{2+} conductances that are located in the dendrites and synaptic terminals (Llinás, 1988; Johnston et al., 1996; Zhou et al., 1997). One involves L type Ca^{2+} channels ("L" for "long lasting," because it slowly inactivates) and the other, N type channels ("N," wryly, for "neither," being neither T nor L type; it inactivates more rapidly than the L type channel). Other types of high-threshold Ca^{2+} channels also exist (Wu et al., 1998). The higher threshold than for T channels means that a much larger depolarization (to about $-20\,mV$) is needed to activate these Ca^{2+} conductances, and they are the reason that Ca^{2+} enters the cell as a result of an action potential. In synaptic terminals, these conductances represent a key link between the action potential and transmitter release, since the action potential will activate these channels, and the resultant Ca^{2+} entry is needed for transmitter release. Less is known about these Ca^{2+} conductances in dendrites, but by providing a regenerative spike that can travel between the site of an activating EPSP and the soma, they may help ensure that distal dendritic inputs that are strong enough to activate this conductance will significantly influence the soma and axon hillock. These channels might also play a role in the backpropagation of action potentials that depend on Na^+ channels through the dendritic arbor.

4.B.2.f. Ca^{2+} Dependent K^+ Conductances

Several K^+ conductances can be activated by increased Ca^{2+} concentrations. These commonly occur as the result of activation of low threshold spikes or action potentials, or both, which activates the high-threshold Ca^{2+} channels described in the preceding paragraph, and the increased Ca^{2+} concentration that results can activate Ca^{2+} dependent K^+ conductances, which will produce a hyperpolarization. Some of these conductances are fast to activate and will help to repolarize the cell. Others that are slower to activate will build up with more and more action potentials, leading to spike frequency adaptation (Adams et al., 1982; Powers et al., 1999). This phenomenon results in the slow reduction of the firing frequency of a neuron to a constant stimulus, and the higher the frequency of initial firing, the more adaptation that occurs. Spike frequency adaptation has been demonstrated for thalamic cells (Smith et al., 2001).

4.B.2.g. Persistent Na^+ Conductance

Finally, a persistent and noninactivating Na^+ conductance that is activated by a strong depolarization exists in thalamic relay cells, creating a plateau depolarization (Jahnsen & Llinás, 1984a, 1984b). When activated, it promotes sustained, tonic firing. This plateau potential involves different ion channels from those subserving the conventional action potential, because those related to action potentials are blocked by tetrodotoxin, while those related to the plateau potential are not.

4.B.3. Interneurons

Interneurons, possibly because of their relatively small size, are much more difficult to record than are relay cells. Until recently, functional criteria to distinguish interneurons from relay cells during recording were lacking. Several such criteria now exist (see Cox et al., 2003), especially for the in vitro preparation. However, except for these very recent experiments, few physiological data have been published regarding interneurons, and much less is known about their membrane properties.

4.B.3.a. Action Potentials

The important issue as to whether all thalamic interneurons exhibit action potentials was discussed in chapter 2. As we noted earlier, it is possible that axonless interneurons exist and that these do not fire action potentials, but clearly some (if not all) possess axonal outputs and fire action potentials. In any case, recent evidence indicates that the output from presynaptic dendritic terminals can be activated without an action potential (Cox et al., 1998; Cox & Sherman, 2000).

4.B.3.b. I_T and I_A

It had been thought that, unlike relay cells, most interneurons do not possess any measurable I_T, although evidence for some I_T was found in a few interneurons (McCormick & Pape, 1988). A subsequent analysis (Pape et al., 1994) suggested that interneurons do indeed actually exhibit I_T and can discharge low threshold Ca^{2+} spikes, but that the interaction of I_T and I_A in interneurons frequently obscures the former. The reason this happens in interneurons but not in relay cells probably relates to subtle differences between cell types in the voltage dependencies and peak amplitudes of these conductances. The relevant voltage dependencies are summarized in figure 4.9B. For relay cells, inactivation and activation of I_T is shifted to more hyperpolarized membrane potentials relative to I_A, and this is also true for activation of these currents in interneurons; however, inactivation of both conductances largely overlap in interneurons. Nonetheless, this implies that in both cell types, I_T will be activated before I_A by a depolarizing input. However, in relative amplitude terms, the I_A to I_T ratio is much larger in interneurons than in relay cells (not shown), so I_A can swamp I_T in interneurons, preventing a low threshold Ca^{2+} spike, if the activating depolarizing input is large enough. This might explain why I_T is generally more difficult to observe in interneurons than in relay cells. However, other evidence suggests that bursting may be as common in interneurons as in relay cells (Zhu et al., 1999), so the issue of how readily interneurons may express burst mode firing in behaving animals remains unresolved.

4.B.4. Cells of the Thalamic Reticular Nucleus

Reticular cells, in addition to conventional action potentials, also display a collection of conductances related to a low threshold Ca^{2+} conductance (Huguenard & Prince, 1992). The low threshold Ca^{2+} conductance is qualitatively similar to that seen in relay cells with a similar voltage dependency, and thus reticular cells also display burst and tonic response modes. However, there are some interesting quantitative differences between relay and reticular cells regarding this firing property.

4.B.4.a. I_T
One difference is in the temporal domain (Huguenard & Prince, 1992). Reticular cells show much slower activation and inactivation kinetics than do relay cells.[7] Furthermore, the inactivation of I_T in reticular cells is voltage independent, so that it remains slow to inactivate even during the low threshold spike. This contrasts with relay cells, which inactivate more quickly as the low threshold spike develops. The result of the slow kinetics and voltage independent inactivation is much more prolonged low threshold spikes in the reticular cells, giving rise to many more action potentials.

This pattern of burst firing of reticular cells has a dramatic effect on their target relay cells. Reticular cells are GABAergic and thus inhibit relay cells, and the slow kinetics of I_T in reticular cells means that de-inactivation and thus the refractory period following a low threshold Ca^{2+} spike is prolonged. It follows that the long bursts in reticular cells will produce powerful and prolonged inhibition of relay cells, and this in turn serves well to de-inactivate I_T in relay cells. After the burst of the reticular cell, the inhibition in the relay cell ceases because of the silence of the reticular cell, so passive repolarization of the relay cell will ensue, and this is further promoted by activation of I_h (see above). This relative depolarization can trigger I_T in the relay cells. In chapter 7 we come back to this property of how bursting in reticular cells can affect relay cells.

---

7. This current for reticular cells is sometimes designated I_{Ts}, where the subscripted "s" stands for "slow."

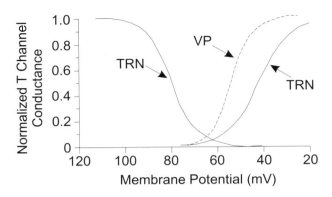

Figure 4.10
Activation and inactivation curves for a typical thalamic reticular cell (solid curves) of the rat. For comparison, an activation curve for a typical relay cell from the ventral posterior nucleus of the rat is shown (dashed curve). (Redrawn from Huguenard & McCormick, 1992.)

Another feature distinguishing I_T in reticular cells is the depolarization needed for activation. Figure 4.10 compares I_T activation curves for relay and reticular cells (Coulter et al., 1989; Huguenard & McCormick, 1992; Huguenard & Prince, 1992). These examples are from the rat; the relay cells are from ventral lateral posterior nucleus, and the reticular cells are from the adjacent, connected sector of the thalamic reticular nucleus. Note that not only is the activation curve for the reticular cells shifted toward more depolarized values than that for the relay cells, it is also shallower. This mean that larger depolarizing potentials are needed to activate I_T in reticular cells than in relay cells. There may be many reasons for this difference, but one suggested by modeling relates to the finding that many of the actual T type Ca^{2+} channels are located on peripheral dendrites of both cell types (Destexhe et al., 1996; Destexhe et al., 1998b). The larger electrotonic structure of reticular cells in the rat (noted above) compared to relay cells suggests that attempts to activate I_T from current injected in the soma, as in voltage clamp experiments such as shown in figure 4.10, would require more current and more depolarization for reticular cells if the channels to be activated are electrotonically more distant. This may thus be an artifact of the voltage clamp method, since the more physiological way of activating dendritically located T channels may involve EPSPs generated from synapses on the dendrites close to the channels.

There is another implication of having the T type Ca^{2+} channels located peripherally in reticular cells. This could permit peripheral synaptic inputs to control I$_T$ locally, perhaps to amplify an EPSP from a specific synapse by generating a low threshold Ca^{2+} spike there, and this synapse could then have a more powerful effect at the axon hillock. This would also allow synaptic inputs to control I$_T$ locally in different parts of the dendritic arbor. Thereby, a complex pattern of activated, inactivated, and de-inactivated patches of I$_T$ could result.

There is one important proviso to this discussion of I$_T$ and burst firing in reticular cells: the activity of these cells has rarely been recorded in awake animals. Although we know from such studies of relay cells that burst firing is seen during the waking state (see above and chapter 5), it is not yet completely certain whether reticular cells exhibit both response modes during normal, alert behavior. However, a recent study in unanesthetized but "lightly narcotized" rats described both tonic and burst firing in response to whisker deflections in the rat (Hartings et al., 2003). Whether the lightly narcotized state is truly representative of the normal waking state needs to be resolved.

4.B.4.b. Other Conductances

Above we described how, for relay cells, the combination of I$_T$, I$_h$, and probably one or more K$^+$ conductances combine to create rhythmic bursting in relay cells. There are at least two analogous but different conductances in reticular cells that combine with I$_T$ to produce rhythmic bursting (Bal & McCormick, 1993). Interestingly, these are triggered not by altered membrane voltage but by increased intracellular Ca^{2+} caused by the activation of I$_T$. One is a Ca^{2+} dependent K$^+$ conductance that produces a current known as I$_{K[Ca]}$. By opening K$^+$ channels, I$_{K[Ca]}$ allows K$^+$ to exit and thereby hyperpolarize the cell. The kinetics of I$_{K[Ca]}$ are quite slow, but it is sufficiently powerful to produce a marked afterhyperpolarization in the reticular cell following each low threshold spike. This hyperpolarization de-inactivates I$_T$, and the slow inactivation of I$_{K[Ca]}$ allows the cell to repolarize, triggering another low threshold spike, and so on. In many reticular cells, only a few burst cycles are seen, as the cell slowly depolarizes to inactivate I$_T$ and produce tonic firing. This is because the low threshold spikes produce another Ca^{2+} dependent conductance, called I$_{CAN}$, that seems to be nonspecific for cations. These cations enter the reticular cell, thereby depolarizing it. I$_{CAN}$ has much slower kinetics than does I$_{K[Ca]}$, so several burst cycles are expressed before I$_{CAN}$ slowly depolarizes the cell sufficiently to switch firing mode from burst to tonic.

There have been few published studies attempting to define voltage- or ion-sensitive membrane conductances for reticular cells other than that cited above regarding conductances underlying the low threshold spike, so it remains unclear how many others may exist. For instance, I_A seems to be a ubiquitous property of neurons throughout the brain, but there are no published reports, positive or negative, regarding the presence of I_A in reticular cells. Obviously the firing patterns of reticular cells are important to thalamic relays, since these cells provide powerful inhibition to relay cells, so understanding their intrinsic properties is an important goal. We need more study of this problem.

4.C. Summary and Conclusions

If we want to understand how nerve cells communicate with each other, then an essential question that needs to be addressed is how a neuron's cellular properties—or, more specifically, the passive and active properties of its dendritic (and somatic) membranes—affect its responses to synaptic input. This obviously applies for thalamic neurons. Indeed, the interplay between a relay cell's cellular properties and the nature of its synaptic inputs (described in chapter 5) is at the heart of understanding the functioning of thalamic relays.

Computed cable properties of relay cells, as suggested by consideration of their dendritic arbors, indicate relatively little electrotonic attenuation along the dendrites, meaning that synaptic inputs even on the most distal dendritic locations will have significant impact at the soma and axon hillock. However, it must be remembered that attenuation along a cable is frequency dependent, meaning that faster events, or faster postsynaptic potentials, will attenuate more during conduction to the soma than will slower ones. The cable properties of interneurons, in contrast, may be quite different. These cells have two outputs: a conventional one via the axon and another via terminals from peripheral dendrites. Cable modeling suggests that the latter are electrotonically isolated from the soma and axon, suggesting that interneurons might "multiplex," having two routes for input/output computations. Reticular cells seem to be electrotonically extensive, and they, like interneurons, may have dendritic as well as axonal outputs.

All of these thalamic neurons have numerous voltage dependent conductances in their dendritic membranes, and such active conductances can override issues related to cable properties. For instance, if interneurons have enough voltage dependent Na^+ channels in their dendrites, they can allow peripherally located synapses to have strong effects at the soma. The voltage dependent channels of relay cells have been studied in most detail. These include channels that underlie a variety of membrane currents, including I_T, I_A, and I_h, among others, and interneurons and reticular cells seem to have a similar complement of such channels. The state of these channels, especially their inactivation or activation, can strongly affect how the relay cell responds to driver input and thus how it relays information to cortex. Understanding how these voltage dependent channels are controlled by various synaptic inputs and how they might interact with one another is an ongoing challenge for students of the thalamus.

4.D. Unresolved Questions

1. To what extent do the properties described in this chapter apply to thalamic cells in general? Are there important differences between thalamic nuclei, species, or relay cell types?

2. How do voltage dependent conductances interact with one another and with the cell's cable properties to affect how the cell responds to various inputs?

3. What is the complete pattern in dendrites of thalamic relay cells, interneurons, or reticular cells regarding Na^+, Ca^{2+}, and K^+ channels? What effect do these channels have on synaptic integration. Does back-propagation of action potentials occur, and if so, what is the significance of this for synaptic integration?

4. How functionally isolated are dendritic F2 outputs of interneurons from each other and from the soma? Are there any interneurons that lack action potentials? Do the action potentials of interneurons invade the dendrites, affecting the F2 terminals? If they do, what is the functional effect?

5. Given the apparent importance of voltage dependent conductances seen with in vitro methods, what is the range of membrane potentials typically seen in thalamic cells of awake, behaving animals?

6. How general are presynaptic dendrites in reticular neurons? Do they function like those of interneurons, or differently? For any one species, do they exist, what is their distribution, and how does their distribution relate to the definable cable properties of these cells in different species?

5 Synaptic Properties

5.A. Properties Common to Synapses Throughout the Brain

In chapter 3, we described the main synaptic inputs to thalamic cells. The axon terminals of these inputs release transmitters that bind to postsynaptic receptors and thereby affect their postsynaptic thalamic targets. Exactly how these synaptic inputs affect the postsynaptic cell is crucial to understanding the functional circuitry of the thalamus. Not long ago, this seemed a relatively simple task: an action potential in an afferent axon leads to release of transmitter from its synaptic terminals; this affects the postsynaptic cell by producing a stereotypical, fast EPSP or IPSP (excitatory and inhibitory postsynaptic potential, respectively), the sign of the postsynaptic potential depending on the transmitter delivered; and the postsynaptic cell then linearly sums all of these postsynaptic potentials, much as a passive cable would, and the resulting membrane potential determines the postsynaptic firing frequency.

We now appreciate that the functioning of synapses is much more complicated. For one thing, a transmitter can have very different postsynaptic effects on any one cell, depending on the specific postsynaptic receptors activated. For another, as described in chapter 4, the postsynaptic cell does not act in the same fashion as a linear cable but instead exhibits a variety of voltage dependent, transmembrane ionic conductances. Thus, in addition to or even instead of seeing synaptic inputs as having a fairly simple and direct effect on the postsynaptic cell's firing rate, we must think in terms of the effects such inputs have on this cell's voltage dependent conductances, among which the Na^+ and K^+ conductances underlying the action potential are special cases. The most important of the other conductances for thalamic relay cells, emphasized in chapter 4, is the voltage dependent Ca^{2+} conductance underlying I_T, since this conductance determines whether the cell fires in burst or tonic mode, and the final response state plays a crucial role in the nature of the thalamic relay. Other complicating but important variables include presynaptic regulation of transmitter release involving activation of receptors on presynaptic terminals and active involvement of glia in synaptic functioning. In this chapter we summarize many of the key functional features of the several different types of afferent in the thalamus, with a focus on how synaptic activation affects both the firing rate and the response mode of relay cells.

5.A.1. *Ionotropic and Metabotropic Receptors*

One property common to many pathways in the brain and to most of the major inputs to the thalamus, regardless of the transmitter they use, is that they can activate two very different kinds of postsynaptic receptor. These are *ionotropic* and *metabotropic* receptors, and both are found on relay cells, interneurons, and reticular cells. These receptor types, when activated, produce profoundly different actions on the postsynaptic cell.

5.A.1.a. Different Types of Metabotropic and Ionotropic Receptors

Among the major transmitters released by afferents to the thalamus are glutamate, GABA, and acetylcholine. Each of these transmitters can bind to ionotropic and metabotropic receptors. Other transmitters involved in thalamic circuitry include noradrenaline, serotonin, and histamine. The nature of the receptor types activated in the thalamus by these other transmitters is not yet completely known, but preliminary evidence indicates that they activate mostly and in some cases only metabotropic receptors. Figure 5.1 schematically shows the main differences between an ionotropic and a metabotropic receptor (Nicoll et al., 1990; Mott & Lewis, 1994; Pin & Bockaert, 1995; Pin & Duvoisin, 1995; Recasens & Vignes, 1995; Brown et al., 1997; Conn & Pin, 1997; Molnar & Isaac, 2002; Conn, 2003; Huettner, 2003; Jingami et al., 2003), and the examples illustrated include the major ones in the thalamus involving receptors for glutamate, GABA, and acetylcholine.

It should be noted that most transmitters can activate several functionally distinct types of receptor within each of the ionotropic or metabotropic categories. These different actions are often first appreciated on the basis of differential sensitivity to specific agonists or antagonists, and once the different receptor types are recognized, further study usually reveals subtle differences in other properties. Receptors sensitive

Ionotropic Receptor (AMPA, GABA_A, Nicotinic)

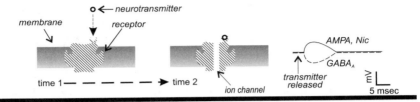

Metabotropic Receptor (mGluR, GABA_B, muscarinic)

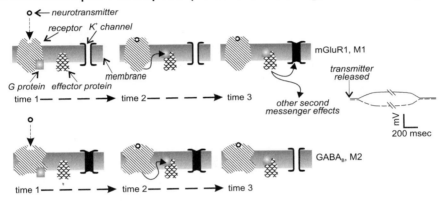

Figure 5.1

Schematic depiction of an ionotropic and a metabotropic receptor, each shown repeatedly at different times (time 1 and time 2 for the ionotropic receptor, and time 1, time 2, and time 3 for the metabotropic receptor). The actual receptor protein complexes are shown with hatching. For the ionotropic example, time 1 represents the period before binding to the transmitter, and time 2 is the period after binding. The binding causes a conformational change that opens the ion channel, which forms the central core of the receptor complex. For the metabotropic receptor, time 1 is the period before transmitter binding, and just after binding (time 2) a G protein is released, which reacts with an effector protein to produce a cascade of biochemical reactions, eventually resulting in opening or closing of an ion channel (time 3). Not shown is the possibility that for some receptors the G protein can directly affect the ion channel. See text for details.

to glutamate serve as an example of this heterogeneity. Three major ionotropic glutamate receptor types are recognizable on the basis of their sensitivity to different agonists: AMPA,[1] kainate, and NMDA[1] (Mayer & Westbrook, 1987; Nakanishi et al., 1998; Ozawa et al., 1998; Kidd & Isaac, 2001; Molnar & Isaac, 2002; Qian & Johnson, 2002; Binns et al., 2003; Huettner, 2003). Likewise, a variety exists for the metabotropic glutamate receptors. In addition to differing with regard to agonist and/or antagonist sensitivity, some of these metabotropic receptors are associated with different second messenger pathways. To date, eight different types classified in three groups have been described in brain tissue (Pin & Bockaert, 1995; Pin & Duvoisin, 1995; Recasens & Vignes, 1995; Conn & Pin, 1997; Molnar & Isaac, 2002; Conn, 2003; Huettner, 2003; Jingami et al., 2003). However, in the thalamus, there appear to be only two main groups of receptors: Group I, which includes types 1 and 5, and Group II, which includes types 2 and 3 (Godwin et al., 1996a) (these receptors are considered further in section 5.B.1). The above examples can, in general, be extended to receptors activated by other transmitters used by afferents to thalamus, including GABA, acetylcholine, noradrenaline, serotonin, and histamine.

5.A.2. Functional Differences Between Ionotropic and Metabotropic Receptors

As shown in figure 5.1, when the transmitter binds to an ionotropic receptor, it acts in a fairly direct fashion through a conformational change in the receptor to open a specific ion channel, which is actually embedded in and thus part of the receptor. Flow of ions into or out of the cell through these channels leads to the evoked postsynaptic potential. Because of the direct linkage between receptor activation and opening of the ion channel, the evoked potentials are fast: they have a short latency, a fast rise to peak, and generally last only 10 or so msec. The same is true for IPSPs evoked after activation of ionotropic (GABA$_A$) versus metabotropic (GABA$_B$) receptors: the former are considerably faster.

When the transmitter binds to a metabotropic receptor, a much more complicated series of events is triggered. The conformational change in the receptor ends in the activation of a G protein, which in turn leads to a cascade of biochemical reactions in the membrane and/or

---

1. AMPA is (RS)-α-amino-3-hydroxy-5-methyl-4-isoxazolepropionic acid, and NMDA is N-methyl-D-aspartate.

cytoplasm of the relay cell (see figure 5.1). This process is known as a second messenger pathway, because the postsynaptic effects of the transmitter are carried indirectly through second messengers by these processes. Several chains of reaction result, and one of these reactive chains eventually causes specific ion channels to open or close. In the thalamus, it appears that K^+ channels are affected in this way by activation of metabotropic receptors to glutamate, GABA, and acetylcholine. Note that either effect on ion channels, opening or closing, may occur, whereas ionotropic receptor activation usually produces only ion channel opening. Activation of the metabotropic glutamate receptor (mGluR1) or muscarinic receptor (M1) closes the K^+ channel, stopping a loss of positive charge and thus resulting in an EPSP; activation of the $GABA_B$ M2 type of muscarinic receptor opens the K^+ channel, increasing the loss of positive charge and thus resulting in an IPSP. Postsynaptic potentials produced in this way by metabotropic receptors are quite slow. They begin with a long and somewhat variable latency, usually much longer than 10 msec, take tens of milliseconds to reach their peak, and remain present for a long time, typically hundreds of milliseconds to several seconds or longer. Figure 5.2C shows an example of an EPSP generated in a thalamic relay cell from activation of a metabotropic glutamate receptor by stimulation of a cortical layer 6 input. Here, low frequency stimulation fails to activate an EPSP when ionotropic glutamate receptors are blocked (top trace), but higher frequency stimulation does evoke a prolonged EPSP (middle two traces). As noted below, it is a common feature of metabotropic receptors that they require relatively high levels of afferent activity for activation. This EPSP is not blocked by MPEP, a specific antagonist to the type 5 metabotropic glutamate receptor (third trace), but is blocked by LY367385, a specific antagonist to the type 1 metabotropic glutamate receptor (bottom trace).

Metabotropic receptor activation can lead to other, more subtle postsynaptic effects not simply linked to ion channel opening or closing. For instance, in chapter 4, section 4.B.2.c, we pointed out that serotonin, noradrenalin, and histamine can affect the amplitude of I_h in a relay cell, and that this effect involves activation of the appropriate metabotropic receptors. Also, metabotropic receptor activation in other parts of the brain can often produce effects through the second messenger systems that act on the cell nucleus to change gene expression. For instance, metabotropic receptors have been implicated in long-term plastic changes in neocortex and hippocampus that may underlie

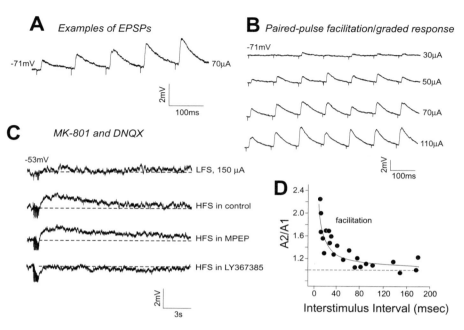

Figure 5.2
Corticothalamic EPSPs evoked from stimulation of layer 6 of barrel cortex of the mouse in a cell of the posterior medial nucleus of the thalamus. *A.* Example of evoked EPSPs. *B.* Paired-pulse facilitation and graded response of EPSPs. *C.* Evidence of an mGluR1 component. The EPSPs evoked by low frequency stimulation (LFS, 13 Hz for 600 msec; for all traces, stimulation intensity was 150 μA) are blocked with application of MK-801 and DNQX (top trace). With these antagonists present, high frequency stimulation (HFS, 125 Hz for 600 msec) evoked a sustained EPSP (second trace) that is not blocked by MPEP, an mGluR5 antagonist (30 μM, third trace), but is blocked by LY367385, an mGluR1 antagonist (50 μM, bottom trace). *D.* Time course of paired-pulse facilitation showing the ratio of amplitudes of the second EPSP divided by the first (A2/A1) as a function of interstimulus interval.

such phenomena as learning and memory and various developmental processes (Gereau & Conn, 1994; Reid et al., 1997; Huber et al., 1998; Thomas, 2002; Gomes et al., 2003; Otani et al., 2003; Riedel et al., 2003). However, while both immunocytochemical and pharmacological data indicate that metabotropic receptors are richly distributed in the thalamus, we have as yet little idea what effects, other than postsynaptic potentials or changes in I_h, result from their activation. This is clearly an issue that requires attention. In contrast, after ionotropic receptor activation, the postsynaptic potential is usually the only effect seen postsynaptically. However, in some cases an entering ion can trigger secondary effects. The NMDA receptor is a good example. Activation of this ionotropic glutamate receptor generates an EPSP that depends in part on Ca^+ entry into the cell, and this change in the internal Ca^+ concentration itself can often produce other long-term changes, such as long-term potentiation in neocortex and hippocampus (Collingridge & Bliss, 1987; Cotman et al., 1988). However, the NMDA receptor is ionotropic and produces a relatively rapid EPSP, in terms of duration and latency, that does not itself require a second messenger link. This EPSP, while longer in duration and latency than that associated with AMPA receptors, is still much faster than that produced by activation of metabotropic glutamate receptors. If it were proven that changes in internal Ca^{2+} concentration in thalamic relay cells can lead to long-term effects on their responsiveness, then it might become necessary to ask whether the burst firing considered in the previous chapter, which involves activation of I_T and a consequential Ca^{2+} entry, could also trigger second messenger pathways and produce long-term effects.

Finally, there is good evidence from other brain regions and limited evidence in the thalamus that the patterns of presynaptic stimulation needed to activate ionotropic versus metabotropic receptors are quite different (e.g., McCormick & Von Krosigk, 1992; Govindaiah & Cox, 2004). Single action potentials that invade the presynaptic terminal or a few closely spaced in time are generally able to activate ionotropic receptors. However, activation of metabotropic receptors typically requires bursts or trains of multiple action potentials (see figure 5.2C). One explanation for this is that metabotropic receptors tend to be further away from the synaptic junction than are ionotropic receptors, forming an annulus around the junction, as has been shown in the hippocampus (Lujan et al., 1996), and thus activation of metabotropic receptors requires more transmitter because of the extra diffusion (and dilution) involved. Whatever the explanation, this is particularly interesting for the pathways that can activate both types of receptor in the thalamus, and several examples are provided below. Such pathways can be expected to function in a way that depends critically on activity patterns of the inputs: low levels of brief activity may activate only ionotropic receptors, and as the activity levels increase in frequency or duration, metabotropic activation may be added. Unfortunately, this property has not yet been systematically studied in the thalamus.

5.A.3. Short-Term Synaptic Plasticity: Paired-Pulse Effects

Many synapses in the brain, including thalamic and cortical synapses, behave in a frequency dependent manner (Thomson & Deuchars, 1994, 1997; Lisman, 1997; Beierlein & Connors, 2002; Chung et al., 2002). This is because the presynaptic interspike interval can strongly influence the size of the evoked postsynaptic potential. This is often explored by comparing the sizes of postsynaptic potentials evoked by a first action potential to one evoked by the next action potential as a function of the intervening time interval. Different paired-pulse effects are shown in figures 5.2 and 5.3, where the former represents features found in a modulator input and the latter in a driver input. *Paired-pulse facilitation* (see figure 5.2A, B, and D) occurs when the second postsynaptic potential is larger than the first for interspike intervals smaller than a certain value. *Paired-pulse depression* (see figure 5.3B and E) is the opposite: the second evoked postsynaptic potential is smaller for a range of interspike intervals. The effective interspike intervals for both depression and facilitation are similar, with time constants of several tens of milliseconds that vary among synapses; with longer intervals, there is no facilitation or depression (figures 5.2D and 5.3E).

There may be many different cellular mechanisms for these phenomena, and there is still considerable debate about this. One idea is that the mechanisms are largely presynaptic and that they relate to the probability that a single action potential will cause transmitter release. The essential point here is that not every action potential causes transmitter release in any synapse; instead, there is a probability between 0 and 1 associated with this cause-and-effect relationship, and it is possible that the probability for any given synapse can change over time. Note that most axons contribute multiple synapses, sometimes hundreds, to one or more postsynaptic target cells, and that a probability less than 1 does not mean that an action potential often has no postsynaptic effect. That is, if the probability for release for each synapse, on average, is 0.5,

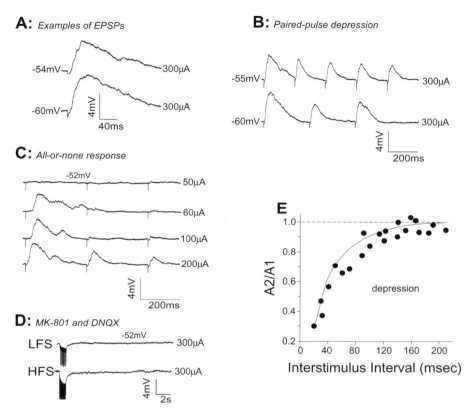

Figure 5.3
Corticothalamic EPSPs evoked from stimulation of layer 5 of barrel cortex in a cell of the posterior medial nucleus of a mouse. *A*. Example of evoked EPSPs. *B*. Paired-pulse depression. *C*. All-or-none response of EPSPs is apparent from responses to increasing stimulation intensities. *D*. Lack of mGluR component. After adding DNQX and MK-801, which block all AMPA and NMDA receptors, neither low-frequency stimulation (LFS, 50 Hz for 855 msec, top trace) nor high frequency stimulation (HFS, 125 Hz for 855 msec, bottom trace) evoked an mGluR response. *E*. Time course of paired-pulse depression, showing the ratio of amplitudes of the second EPSP divided by the first (A2/A1) as a function of interstimulus interval.

and an axon with several thousand terminals contacting many cells contacts a given cell with 50 synapses, then an action potential will cause 25 synapses on that target, on average, to release transmitter and produce a postsynaptic potential. The point is that for any one pair of synaptically linked cells, the larger the probability of release, the larger the resultant postsynaptic potential will be.

Depression is least likely to occur in a synapse if the preceding action potential fails to elicit transmitter release, since, as noted, this release is always a probabilistic occurrence. Such failure naturally will occur most commonly in synapses with low probability of release. This probability may be closely related to the Ca^{2+} concentration inside the synaptic terminal, since the probability of release is monotonically related to internal Ca^{2+} concentration (Dunlap et al., 1995; Matthews, 1996; Reuter, 1996). Synaptic terminals contain high threshold Ca^{2+} channels (described in chapter 4, section 4.B.2.e; see Dunlap et al., 1995; Matthews, 1996; Reuter, 1996) that differ from the T type channels involved in the low threshold Ca^{2+} spike. However, although these T channels, like those in terminals, are voltage dependent, they have a much higher (i.e., depolarized) threshold for activation. An invading action potential depolarizes the terminal sufficiently to activate these channels, leading to Ca^{2+} entry, and, as the internal Ca^{2+} concentration increases, so does the probability of transmitter release. However, when a single action potential and the subsequent Ca^{2+} influx fails to promote transmitter release, the Ca^{2+} concentration will remain elevated for several milliseconds. If a second action potential follows the first while the internal Ca^{2+} concentration remains elevated, it will cause a second wave of Ca^{2+} entry that will sum with what remains from the first, much like temporal summation in postsynaptic potentials. Since transmitter release increases with internal Ca^{2+} concentration nonlinearly as a power function with a power of 3–4 (Landò & Zucker, 1994), the result will be a higher probability of transmitter release for the second action potential. Since a typical axon innervates any target with many synaptic terminals, as long as the average probability of release for all these synapses is very low (in many connections within cortex this has been computed as <0.1), then most synapses will fail to release transmitter in response to the first action potential. However, the probability of release from each terminal may be significantly enhanced for the second action potential if it follows the first within tens of milliseconds or so.[2] This can result in

---

2. Just how low this probability must be for this to occur is a complex function of many factors. Consider an afferent axon with 20 synapses on one of

more transmitter release and thus a larger postsynaptic potential for the second action potential, thus producing paired-pulse facilitation.

Depression occurs, because once transmitter is released, it takes time (often hundreds of milliseconds) before the probability of release to another action potential returns to baseline levels. This may be partly due to depletion of transmitter stores or to other effects. The result is that for some time after transmitter release, the probability of release is reduced. This will result in paired-pulse depression in afferents having an average probability of release for their synapses high enough that many release transmitter to the first action potential.

It follows from the above that if an axon contacts a postsynaptic cell with synapses having a low probability of release (i.e., "low-p" synapses), these synapses are more likely to show paired-pulse facilitation. This is because most of the synapses will not release transmitter but will instead show an increased probability for some time because of an increased internal Ca^{2+} concentration. Conversely, if the contacts are made with synapses having a high probability of release (i.e., "high-p" synapses), they are more likely to show paired-pulse depression, because more synapses will release transmitter and show relative refractoriness until their transmitter pools are restored.

Note that this explanation for paired-pulse effects is based on the assumption that they are related to *presynaptic* factors involving the probability of release. However, it is possible that postsynaptic factors also play a role, perhaps even a dominant role. For example, if the probability of release were unchanged by paired-pulse effects, then one could simply consider the probability that an evoked EPSP sufficiently depolarized the postsynaptic cell to fire an action potential. Paired-pulse effects are then related to the nature of temporal summation of the EPSP and activation of NMDA receptors; often a single EPSP does not depo-

---

its target cells. If the average baseline probability of release is 0.1, only two synapses will release transmitter, creating a postsynaptic potential of proportional amplitude. The 18 synapses failing to release transmitter will have a greater probability of release to a second action potential if it arrives soon enough, and the two synapses that released transmitter will, in turn, have a much lower probability (near zero) of release. For the second action potential to create a larger EPSP than the first (i.e., to result in paired-pulse facilitation) would require that more than two synapses released transmitter, and this would happen if the average probability for the remaining 18 were $\geq 2/18$. Thus the phenomenon of paired-pulse facilitation depends on the initial probability of release, as well as on the increase seen in those terminals failing to release initially. The phenomenon of paired-pulse depression described later in the test has a similar dependence on these variables.

larize the postsynaptic cell sufficiently to overcome the Mg^{2+} block of the NMDA receptor, but two summed EPSPs could do so. Whatever the explanation for paired-pulse facilitation or depression, the fact that many synapses onto relay cells and thalamocortical synapses show one or the other behavior, as described more fully below, underscores the importance of these phenomena in thalamic functioning.

Perhaps the most important point about these paired-pulse effects is that they play a key role in the relationship between firing patterns of an afferent and the efficacy of synaptic transmission. For a synapse showing paired-pulse facilitation, low firing rates in the afferent would be relatively ineffective in influencing the postsynaptic cell, because such low rates would not lead to facilitation of the synapse. The result would be no or a very small postsynaptic potential evoked from most afferent action potentials. Such a synapse would be most effective when the afferent fired at rates high enough to elicit paired-pulse facilitation. For a synapse showing paired-pulse depression, a different pattern of firing evokes the greatest postsynaptic potential. That is, if the afferent fired at high rates, the synapse would be persistently depressed. The largest postsynaptic potential would result for an afferent action potential that followed a silent period long enough to ameliorate synaptic depression. Thus, for such a synapse, very low firing rates actually evoke the largest individual postsynaptic potentials. This point is reiterated below and in chapter 6.

5.B. Synaptic Inputs to Relay Cells

Figure 5.4 illustrates the transmitters and postsynaptic receptors for the best understood inputs to relay cells of the lateral geniculate and ventral posterior nuclei. This is further summarized in table 5.1 (the details of which can be found in Sherman & Guillery, 1996), which shows inputs that are common to many thalamic nuclei and thus exclude ones such as the inputs to the lateral geniculate nucleus from the pretectum and superior colliculus.

5.B.1. Driving Inputs to Relay Cells

5.B.1.a. Basic Features of Driving Synapses
As noted previously and considered in more detail later in chapter 7, by driving inputs we mean the inputs containing the main information to be relayed to cortex. For first order relays, this is carried, for example,

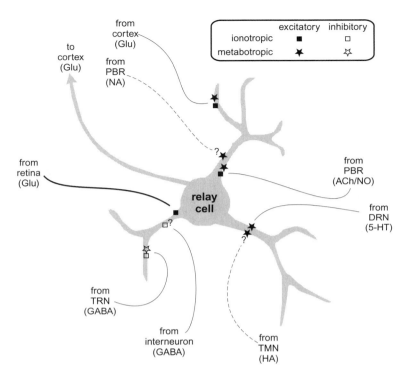

Figure 5.4
Inputs to thalamic relay cell showing transmitters (in parentheses) and ionotropic or metabotropic types of postsynaptic receptors. The question mark indicates uncertainty about the structural characteristics of the histaminergic input (see text for details). In the actual cell, any dendrite can receive any or all of the inputs. Abbreviations: 5-HT, serotonin; ACh, acetylcholine; DRN, dorsal raphé nucleus; GABA, γ-aminobutyric acid; Glu, glutamate; NA, noradrenaline; HA, histamine; NO, nitric oxide; PBR, parabrachial region; TMN, tuberomamillary nucleus; TRN, thalamic reticular nucleus.

by retinal axons to the lateral geniculate nucleus and by axons of the medial lemniscus to the ventral posterior nucleus; in higher order relays, this is carried by cortical layer 5 cell inputs to various thalamic nuclei, such as parts of the pulvinar.

Studies of transmitter actions of these driving inputs have largely been limited to certain rodents (rats, guinea pigs, hamsters) and to cats and ferrets, and mostly to subcortical inputs to the lateral geniculate and ventral posterior nuclei and layer 5 inputs to the posterior medial nucleus. The detailed summary below is based on

Table 5.1
Inputs to Replay Cells of Lateral Geniculate Nucleus and Ventral Posterior Nuclei, Including Transmitters and Receptor Types

Source	Transmitter	Receptor Type
Retina or medial lemniscus	Glutamate	Ionotropic
Cortex (layer 6)	Glutamate	Ionotropic and metabotropic
Parabrachial region	Acetylcholine	Ionotropic and metabotropic
Parabrachial region	Noradrenaline	Metabotropic
Dorsal raphé nucleus	Serotonin	Metabotropic
Tuberomamillary nucleus	Histamine	Metabotropic
Thalamic reticular nucleus	GABA	Ionotropic and metabotropic
Interneurons	GABA	Ionotropic and metabotropic

For details, see Sherman and Guillery (1996).

these observations. These driving inputs all use an excitatory amino acid (most probably glutamate) as a transmitter, and this activates ionotropic glutamate receptors. Evidence from the lateral geniculate nucleus in cats suggests that the receptors activated directly by retinal inputs are AMPA and NMDA receptors and that *every* retinal axon can activate both on relay cells (Scharfman et al., 1990); medial lemniscal inputs to the ventral posterior nucleus in rats also can activate both AMPA and NMDA receptors (Turner & Salt, 1998). As noted above, kainate receptors are the other ionotropic glutamate receptor (along with AMPA and NMDA receptors), but they do not seem to be involved in direct postsynaptic processing. A rather different role of kainate receptors in thalamic relays is considered below in section 5.B.5.a.

Whereas all modulatory inputs to the lateral geniculate nucleus that have been studied in cats and rats can activate metabotropic receptors, and most also activate ionotropic receptors (reviewed in Sherman & Guillery, 1996, 2001; Salt, 2002), the two driver afferents that have been studied from this point of view, the retinal afferents to the lateral geniculate nucleus and cortical layer 5 afferents to the posterior medial nucleus, activate only ionotropic, AMPA and NMDA, receptors (McCormick & Von Krosigk, 1992; Reichova & Sherman, 2004). Figures 5.2C and 5.3D illustrate this. It would be of great interest to know how general this property is for driver inputs in other thalamic nuclei, because the difference may be crucial to the distinction between drivers and modulators (see Sherman & Guillery, 1998, and chapter 7).

Activation of the AMPA receptors produces a prototypical, fast EPSP due to entry of Na^+ and perhaps other cations. The response associated with NMDA receptor activation is unusual, for three reasons. First, it has a voltage dependency, so that the more hyperpolarized the cell, the less that receptor activation produces an EPSP. This is because the ion channel portion of the NMDA receptor becomes clogged with Mg^{2+} ions, preventing influx of cations to depolarize the cell. The extent of this voltage dependent Mg^{2+} block varies among NMDA receptors (Kuner & Schoepfer, 1996), but this block has not been much investigated yet in thalamus. Nonetheless, prior depolarization of the cell prevents this Mg^{2+} block, and then activation of the NMDA receptor produces an EPSP. This EPSP is slower than that produced by activation of the AMPA receptor but much faster than metabotropic receptor action. Second, and as noted above, although NMDA receptors are ionotropic, their activation involves considerable influx of Ca^{2+}, and this in turn can activate certain second messenger pathways, providing other postsynaptic effects. Third, activation of NMDA receptors requires the presence of a cofactor in addition to glutamate (Kawajiri & Dingledine, 1993; Hashimoto & Oka, 1997; Banke & Traynelis, 2003; Gibb, 2004). That is, the receptor complex also contains a site activated by glycine, and both sites, that associated with glycine and that associated with glutamate, must be activated for the NMDA receptor to function. This is an unusual glycine site, because the more common glycinergic receptor associated with inhibition elsewhere in the brain is blocked by strychnine, but the NMDA glycine site is unaffected by strychnine. What is particularly odd about this glycine requirement for NMDA activation is that there is no known source of glycinergic input to thalamic relay cells. However, there is evidence that this glycine site is effectively activated by D-serine provided by glia (discussed in more detail in section 5.B.5.b).

Several other features characterize synaptic properties of driving inputs to relay cells, as demonstrated by studies of the driving afferents to the lateral geniculate, ventral posterior nucleus, and posterior medial nuclei in rodents and cats (Salt & Eaton, 1996; Turner & Salt, 1998; Castro-Alamancos, 2002; Chen & Regehr, 2003; Reichova & Sherman, 2004). These drivers respectively are the optic tract, the medial lemniscus, and the layer 5 pathway to the thalamus from the somatosensory cortex, and stimulation of any one of these showed the results illustrated in figure 5.3A–C. The synapses formed by drivers show fairly large EPSPs with paired-pulse depression. The EPSPs also can be evoked in an all-or-none manner, meaning that the EPSP evoked by electrical stimulation goes from nothing to maximum amplitude over a very narrow range of stimulation strength. This means that there is a very limited range of stimulation strength over which the evoked EPSP goes from zero to full strength, and this in turn suggests that very few—possibly one—axons provide the bulk of driver input to the cell in question.

5.B.1.b. Effect of Driving Afferents on the Response Mode of Relay Cells

We normally think of synaptic inputs as excitatory or inhibitory based on whether the evoked postsynaptic potential is more or less likely to activate action potentials or, more specifically, to activate the voltage dependent Na^+ and K^+ conductances that produce action potentials. However, we must also consider the effects of synaptic inputs on other conductances, particularly the low threshold Ca^{2+} conductance. Clearly, the response mode of relay cells, burst or tonic, strongly affects their responses to inputs and thus will affect their relay of driving inputs to cortex. The question here is: can the pattern of activity in driving inputs by themselves change the response mode of their postsynaptic relay cell targets? Unfortunately, we do not yet have a clear empirical answer to that question, but theory and indirect experimental evidence suggest that driving inputs do not play a major role in directly controlling the response mode.

The theoretical reason is that driving inputs to relay cells activate only ionotropic and not metabotropic glutamate receptors. These inputs clearly produce EPSPs, and thus the issue becomes whether this depolarization can convert a relay cell mode from burst to tonic, which would require the EPSP to inactivate I_T. The problem lies in the kinetics. EPSPs from ionotropic glutamate receptors are fast, typically decaying to low levels after 10–20 msec. As noted above, the activation of I_T is fast and requires the rate of depolarization (dV/dt) to be above a certain minimum, so such an EPSP could (and in fact does) readily activate I_T. However, inactivation is much slower, and the EPSP would be over and done before inactivation proceeded very far, and the cell would repolarize to its former value. The balance of T channels between inactivation and de-inactivation would thus be little affected, and the cell would again be primed to respond to inputs in burst mode. To switch to tonic firing by inactivating I_T would require a much longer depolarization than would be expected via a single EPSP from activation of ionotropic glutamate receptors. However, a sufficiently prolonged depolarization might be possible even with ionotropic glutamate receptor activation if a long, high frequency train of EPSPs were evoked, permitting temporal summation that would sustain the depolarization for roughly 100 msec or more.

One might then ask whether a train of EPSPs via ionotropic glutamate receptors[3] (e.g., via retinal synapses) could produce temporal summation that would sustain the depolarization sufficiently to inactivate I_T. If the retinogeniculate EPSP lasts for, say 25 msec, then summation will begin with firing rates exceeding 40 spikes/sec, certainly a reasonable rate for retinal afferents (Bullier & Norton, 1979). The potential problem here is that electrical activation of retinal afferents produces multisynaptic IPSPs that significantly shorten the monosynaptic EPSP to ≪10 msec (Suzuki & Kato, 1966). If this happens with natural visual stimulation, which seems plausible but has not yet been rigorously documented, then much higher rates of retinal firing (>100 spikes/sec) would be required to inactivate I_T. But even if such rates occurred, the resulting polysynaptic IPSPs might limit the sustained depolarization and thus limit the extent to which retinal input can inactivate I_T.

Another difficulty is that, for a cell starting off with I_T de-inactivated, any EPSP with a sufficiently fast rise time will activate I_T before inactivating it, so that a burst will be evoked; if the EPSP is relatively small in amplitude, only the burst will be evoked, but if it is sustained and strong enough, the burst may be followed, after a pause, by tonic firing. This is in fact seen when geniculate cells of the cat are activated either in vivo by visual stimuli (Lu et al., 1992) or in vitro with current injection (Smith et al., 2000). The point here is that EPSPs with a very fast rise time may, with temporal summation, inactivate I_T, but not before activating I_T and an associated burst of action potentials relayed to cortex. Thus with prolonged driver input one often sees a burst followed by tonic firing (Smith et al., 2000). Only a prolonged EPSP with a slow rise can inactivate I_T without activating a burst (see chapter 4, section 4.B.2.b). The obvious way to do this is by activating metabotropic receptors (see also below). Another might be to activate many EPSPs unsynchronized temporally from many convergent sources to produce a composite depolarization with a slow rise time. This could be possible through modulatory inputs, because there seems to be large convergence

3. For this consideration, we assume only AMPA receptors are involved. A consideration of any role of NMDA receptors in this process is complicated by the fact that they are voltage dependent and will not contribute to an EPSP unless the cell is already fairly depolarized. What role NMDA receptors might play in this process is not clear.

of these inputs to relay cells, but driving inputs from the retina to individual relay cells mostly derive from one or a very small number of axons with little convergence (Sherman & Guillery, 1998).

The preceding paragraphs suggest that driving inputs via ionotropic glutamate receptors cannot readily inactivate I_T. However, it is important to realize that only some thalamic relays (i.e., the lateral geniculate nucleus in guinea pigs, rats, and cats and the posterior medial nucleus of mice) has to date been tested for the type of receptor (ionotropic or metabotropic glutamate receptor) activated by the driving (retinal or cortical) input (McCormick & Von Krosigk, 1992; Godwin et al., 1996a; Turner & Salt, 1998; Li et al., 2003a; Reichova & Sherman, 2004). It is tempting to generalize this to other thalamic nuclei in other species, but more empirical evidence here is important.

Actual evidence regarding any role of driving inputs in the control of response mode of relay cells would be better than theoretical constructs. The evidence available to date is at best circumstantial, but it does suggest that activation of metabotropic receptors is a more efficient way to control response mode than is activation of ionotropic receptors (Godwin et al., 1996b). Two recent papers do show that visual stimulation of geniculate cells in an anesthetized in vivo preparation can affect firing mode (Alitto et al., 2005; Denning & Reinagel, 2005). Specifically, inhibitory stimuli, such as a dark region in the center of an on-center cell, can de-inactivate T channels and lead to bursting when that stimulus is replaced by an excitatory one, but this seems likely due to eventual effects of modulatory inputs from reticular cells or interneurons rather than any direct driver input. On teleological grounds, one might argue that it is better to control response mode through the modulatory inputs so that response mode is never confused with peripheral stimuli. Unfortunately, teleological grounds are often treacherous, and actual data are needed instead.

5.B.2. Inputs to Relay Cells from Interneurons and Cells of the Thalamic Reticular Nucleus

5.B.2.a. Basic Properties of Synapses from Interneurons and Reticular Cells

Both interneurons and reticular cells use GABA as a transmitter, and both of these "GABAergic" cells innervate relay cells (see figure 5.4). Based on the available evidence, GABA acts in the thalamus in an inhibitory manner. That is, relay cells exhibit IPSPs when inputs from either interneurons or reticular cells are activated. These potentials are generated through two different receptors—GABA$_A$, which are ionotropic, and GABA$_B$, which are metabotropic (see Table 5.1).[4]

Reticular cells, as a population, activate both receptors on relay cells (Sanchez-Vives & McCormick, 1997), although it is not clear if individual reticular axons or axon terminals activate both receptors or are more selective. The situation for interneurons is less clear. There is indirect evidence that at least some if not all of their dendritic terminals activate GABA$_A$ receptors on relay cells (Cox & Sherman, 2000; Govindaiah & Cox, 2004). However, there have as yet been no specific tests for GABA$_B$ responses for these synapses; nothing has been reported on the receptors activated by the axons of interneurons, and this is a particularly difficult problem to solve because there is no straightforward way to exclusively activate these axons.

Activation of the GABA$_A$ receptor opens Cl$^-$ channels (Nicoll, 1988; Nicoll et al., 1990). This inhibits the cell, but not very much by the amplitude of the IPSP, since the reversal potential and thus maximum hyperpolarization produced by an increased Cl$^-$ conductance are only to about -70 to -75 mV. Instead, GABA$_A$ activation creates such a large increase in the Cl$^-$ conductance that any tendency to depolarize the cell by opening other conductances, say, via an EPSP, would be offset by moving more Cl$^-$ into the cell. This effectively decreases neuronal input resistance and serves to shunt any EPSPs. In this way, activation of GABA$_A$ tends to clamp the cell near the Cl$^-$ reversal potential, around -70 to -75 mV, far from the activation threshold for action potentials, and thus the cell is effectively inhibited.

Activation of GABA$_B$ receptors is different (Nicoll et al., 1990; Nakayasu et al., 1995). It involves an increase in conductance to K$^+$,

---

4. Although it happens that GABA in thalamus of adult animals nearly always acts solely in a hyperpolarizing manner, there are exceptions to this action of GABA in other parts of the brain. In the suprachiasmatic nucleus, which is involved in diurnal rhythms, the effects of GABA are themselves diurnal, depolarizing by day and hyperpolarizing by night (Wagner et al., 1997). This neat trick is accomplished by diurnal changes in internal Cl$^-$ concentration of suprachiasmatic cells: this concentration is higher by day, high enough that activation of the GABA receptor causes Cl$^-$ to exit the cell, thereby depolarizing it. Also, GABA can act as a depolarizing transmitter in some developing neural systems and outside of the thalamus in adults. Transmitters should no longer be classified as excitatory or inhibitory, because their action depends not so much on the transmitter as on the specific postsynaptic receptor and ion channel combination with which it is related. Indeed, most transmitters in thalamus are both excitatory (i.e., depolarizing) and inhibitory (i.e., hyperpolarizing). Examples are given later in this chapter.

probably by increasing the K$^+$ "leak" conductance described in chapter 4. Increasing this conductance by GABA$_B$ activation causes K$^+$ to leave the cell, thereby hyperpolarizing it. Compared to activation of the GABA$_A$ receptor, this more strongly hyperpolarizes the cell toward the K$^+$ reversal potential of roughly $-100\,$mV but has much less effect on membrane conductance or neuronal input resistance. Thus GABA$_B$ inhibition acts not by shunting the membrane to a subthreshold level, as happens with GABA$_A$ activation, but by strongly hyperpolarizing the cell. Another way of looking at this difference in response is that GABA$_A$ activation actually reduces, or "divides," the EPSP, while GABA$_B$ activation has less effect on EPSP generation but provides a larger IPSP that is summed to any EPSP (Koch et al., 1982). In this sense, GABA$_A$ activation is multiplicative, whereas GABA$_B$ activation is additive. As noted above, activation of all other metabotropic receptors on relay cells, such as activation of GABA$_B$ receptors, also affects the K$^+$ "leak" conductance, some by increasing it and others by decreasing it.

Another difference between activation of the GABA$_A$ and GABA$_B$ receptors is the time course of the effect (Nicoll et al., 1990; Nakayasu et al., 1995). As noted above, the GABA$_A$ receptor is ionotropic, and so the IPSP associated with it is much faster in latency and duration than that associated with the metabotropic GABA$_B$ receptor. The GABA$_A$ IPSP is typically complete after a few milliseconds, while the GABA$_B$ IPSP typically lasts at least 10–100 times longer.

Finally, because GABA$_A$ is ionotropic, there is no reason to expect its activation to do anything more than transiently increase a Cl$^-$ conductance. Because the GABA$_B$ receptor is metabotropic, its activation turns on second messenger pathways. This, in addition to increasing a K$^+$ conductance, may also affect other cell properties that can have a prolonged effect on the postsynaptic relay cell. There is as yet no evidence in the thalamus for any such effects of GABA$_B$ activation beyond its IPSP, but this is clearly an important possibility that needs to be investigated specifically for the thalamus.

5.B.2.b. Effect of Interneuronal and Reticular Inputs on the Response Mode of Relay Cells

As above for driving inputs, we must consider the effects of these GABA-ergic inputs on the response mode, burst or tonic, of relay cells. It seems unlikely that brief, transient activation of the GABA$_A$ receptor will have much effect on response mode, although under special conditions considered below, GABA$_A$ activation can indeed promote burst firing in relay cells. Normally, GABA$_A$ activation drives the membrane toward about −70 to −75 mV. As shown in figure 4.6, this will at best partially de-inactivate I$_T$. Furthermore, de-inactivation of I$_T$ has a slow time course, and fairly complete de-inactivation requires hyperpolarization for at least 100 msec, whereas the GABA$_A$ response to a single input is largely over in 10–20 msec (see above). The brief hyperpolarization is also unlikely to activate I$_h$, so the return to the original resting potential following the GABA$_A$ IPSP is purely passive and not accelerated or amplified by I$_h$. Thus when the relay cell recovers from the brief GABA$_A$ IPSP and passively depolarizes to rest, that depolarization will not likely activate I$_T$. By this logic, activation of GABA$_A$ receptors alone by any one input under most normal conditions would seem an unlikely candidate to produce a low threshold spike. Of course, if multiple active GABAergic inputs converge onto a relay cell and produce extensive temporal summation of their GABA$_A$-activated IPSPs, this could well de-inactivate I$_T$.

Indeed, there is evidence that both GABA$_A$ and GABA$_B$ activation from reticular cells can produce low threshold spiking, i.e., burst firing in relay cells (Sanchez-Vives & McCormick, 1997). However, this result has been seen when large numbers of reticular cells burst synchronously, as happens during various sleep states, or during in vitro recording from thalamic slices, and thus it is not clear if it happens during the waking state. The prolonged bursts of action potentials produce a sufficiently prolonged and powerful IPSP to de-inactivate I$_T$ and activate I$_h$. This happens even when GABA$_B$ receptors are pharmacologically blocked, and thus it must partly represent activation of GABA$_A$ receptors (Sanchez-Vives & McCormick, 1997). Presumably, this example of GABA$_A$ inhibition producing burst firing is not likely to occur during periods of wakefulness, because it requires massive, prolonged activity of GABAergic afferents from the thalamic reticular nucleus, and such activity seems to occur only during sleep (Sanchez-Vives & McCormick, 1997).

Activation of GABA$_B$ receptors would seem better suited to produce burst firing in relay cells. This is because it produces a larger hyperpolarization, toward the K$^+$ reversal potential near −100 mV rather than the Cl$^-$ reversal potential. Also, because the response is metabotropic, it lasts much longer, typically for >100 msec. Thus the amplitude and duration of the GABA$_B$ IPSP are more likely to de-inactivate I$_T$ and activate I$_h$. Repolarization to rest after the IPSP decays, especially aided by I$_h$, should then activate I$_T$. For these reasons, GABA$_B$ inhibition should, in principle, play an important role in controlling the firing mode of relay cells. However, the precise roles of GABA$_A$ and

GABA$_B$ activation regarding response mode need to be more thoroughly investigated.

5.B.3. Inputs from Cortical Layer 6 Axons to Relay Cells

5.B.3.a. Basic Properties of Layer 6 Corticothalamic Synapses

In this section, by corticothalamic, we refer only to the layer 6 input. These corticothalamic axons, which provide an excitatory input to relay cells, use glutamate as a transmitter, and their synapses activate both ionotropic and metabotropic glutamate receptors on relay cells (see figure 5.4, page 191). Studies of this layer 6 corticothalamic input have been carried out in vitro in relay cells of the lateral geniculate, ventral posterior, and posterior medial nuclei in carnivores and rodents (McCormick & Von Krosigk, 1992; Godwin et al., 1996a; Turner & Salt, 1998; Castro-Alamancos & Oldford, 2002; Granseth et al., 2002; Li et al., 2003a; Reichova & Sherman, 2004), and the similarity of properties of these layer 6 inputs across species and nuclei is remarkable. The ionotropic receptors activated by corticothalamic axons are the same AMPA and NMDA types that are activated by driver inputs. However, because of the very different locations of their synaptic inputs upon the dendritic arbor—driver synapses are found proximally and corticothalamic, distally, with effectively no overlap (see figure 3.17)—driver and corticothalamic synapses are unlikely to activate the same individual receptors. It is particularly interesting that corticothalamic synapses also activate metabotropic glutamate receptors on relay cells, whereas driver synapses do not (see figures 5.2 through 5.4; see also McCormick & Von Krosigk, 1992; Godwin et al., 1996b; Turner & Salt, 1998; Reichova & Sherman, 2004). We do not yet know if every corticothalamic axon has access postsynaptically to both ionotropic and metabotropic receptors. That is, it is possible that some activate only ionotropic receptors, some only metabotropic, and some, perhaps, both types. The possibility that different corticothalamic axons can activate different mixes of receptor type means that different groups of these axons could produce quite different postsynaptic effects on the relay cell and thus subserve different functions. We saw in chapter 3 that there is evidence for heterogeneity of corticogeniculate axons from area 17, and, in addition, the pathway from cortex to the lateral geniculate nucleus involves several different cortical areas (Updyke, 1975), so different types of corticogeniculate axon might relate to differential postsynaptic activation of ionotropic and metabotropic receptors. Our lack of knowledge here is a severe limitation, because understanding corticogeniculate function requires such knowledge.

The available evidence suggests that corticothalamic synapses activate type 1 metabotropic glutamate receptors on relay cells (see figure 5.2C). The production of inositol phosphates resulting from this activation leads ultimately, through other biochemical pathways, to reduction of the K^+ "leak" conductance. This depolarizes the cell, creating an EPSP that is quite slow in onset ($\gg 10$ msec) and lasts for $\gg 100$s of milliseconds (McCormick & Von Krosigk, 1992; Li et al., 2003a; Reichova & Sherman, 2004). Also, corticothalamic activation of metabotropic glutamate receptors produces second messenger cascades and release of intracellular Ca^{2+} pools, which raises the possibility of long-term effects on relay cells. As noted earlier, this is an issue of fundamental importance that has yet to be investigated specifically for the thalamus.

Because of the slow and longlasting response to activation of type 1 metabotropic glutamate receptors (figure 5.2C), such a response is much better suited to maintain sustained changes in membrane voltage of relay cells than are those associated with ionotropic glutamate receptors. This in turn would control general cell excitability: the more depolarized the cell, the more excitable it would be. Also, because the EPSP resulting from activation of metabotropic glutamate receptors involves reduction of the K^+ "leak" conductance, this increases the neuronal input resistance, which in turn results in larger postsynaptic potentials, excitatory and inhibitory, via synaptic activation. Finally, such slow and prolonged membrane potential changes could be quite important in allowing cortex to exert control over voltage dependent conductances expressed by these relay cells (see below). The slow response, however, would act like a low-pass temporal filter in transferring information across the synapse so that specific firing patterns in the cortical afferents would not be imposed on the relay cells. In contrast, EPSPs evoked via ionotropic glutamate receptors, particularly AMPA ones, would be faster and perhaps permit better transfer of the firing patterns, but it would be less suitable for sustaining changes in membrane voltage.

Other properties of the corticothalamic synapse that contrast with those of driver inputs are that the electrically evoked EPSP tends to be small, shows paired-pulse depression, and is activated in a graded manner, meaning that the EPSP grows in amplitude with stimulation strength over a wide range of such strengths (Reichova & Sherman, 2004; see figure 5.2). This last feature suggests that numerous cortical axons converge onto each relay cell.

5.B.3.b. Effect of Corticothalamic Inputs on Response Mode of Relay Cells

On the basis of the evidence cited above, corticothalamic synapses in the lateral geniculate, ventral posterior, and posterior medial nuclei (and presumably elsewhere in the thalamus) can be seen to be particularly well suited to control the firing mode of the relay cells, because they can activate metabotropic glutamate receptors, and these provide a prolonged depolarization that would effectively inactivate I_T. Furthermore, as noted in chapter 4, to activate I_T requires that the depolarization exceed a minimal rate of rise, or *dV/dt*, and the rate of rise of the EPSP evoked via metabotropic glutamate receptors is too slow to activate I_T, but the ensuing depolarization is sufficiently prolonged to inactivate I_T (Gutierrez et al., 2001). Thus evoking a metabotropic EPSP can perform the neat trick of inactivating I_T without ever activating it. The result would be a strong bias toward tonic mode responses, and any bursting activity would be greatly reduced or eliminated. Evidence from in vitro studies of thalamus (both the lateral geniculate and ventral posterior nuclei) in guinea pigs and in vivo studies of the lateral geniculate nucleus in cats indicate that such a process does indeed occur (McCormick & Von Krosigk, 1992; Godwin et al., 1996b).

5.B.4. Brainstem Modulatory Inputs to Relay Cells

Brainstem modulatory inputs can vary quantitatively among thalamic nuclei (Fitzpatrick et al., 1989), and most of our detailed knowledge of these inputs stems from studies of the lateral geniculate nucleus. Thus the description in this section is limited to the lateral geniculate nucleus. Whether the same principles apply to other thalamic nuclei remains to be studied, as do many unanswered questions for the lateral geniculate nucleus.

5.B.4.a. Parabrachial Inputs

In the cat, most of the input to the lateral geniculate nucleus from the brainstem derives from cholinergic neurons in the midbrain and pontine tegmentum surrounding the brachium conjunctivum. We refer to this brainstem area as the parabrachial region (see footnote 3 in chapter 3). As is summarized by figure 5.4 (page 191), activation of this input usually produces an EPSP, due primarily to activation of two different receptors (McCormick, 1990, 1992). The first is an ionotropic nicotinic receptor that produces a fast EPSP by permitting influx of cations. The second is a metabotropic muscarinic receptor, known as an M1 type, that triggers a second messenger pathway, ultimately leading to a reduction in the K^+ "leak" conductance. This muscarinic response is a very slow, long lasting EPSP. In this regard, the effect of activating this muscarinic receptor is remarkably similar to the metabotropic glutamate response seen from activation of corticogeniculate input (see above). The possibility exists that both metabotropic receptors may be linked to the same second messenger pathways and K^+ channels, as appears to be the case for hippocampal neurons, although this has not yet been experimentally tested for thalamic neurons. As would be expected, activation of these parabrachial inputs by in vivo or in vitro application of acetylcholine effectively converts the firing mode of thalamic relay cells from burst to tonic mode (McCormick, 1991a; Lu et al., 1993).

In the above account, we stated that parabrachial input "usually" depolarizes relay cells. This seems true of all relay cells in first order relays, such as the lateral geniculate and ventral posterior nuclei. However, recent studies of the auditory thalamic relays suggest that, while this remains true for the first order relays, many or most relay cells in the higher order auditory relays are actually hyperpolarized by application of acetylcholine, presumably via activation of an M2 receptor (Mooney et al., 2004). Preliminary data suggest that this may be a general difference between first and higher order relays that includes the visual and somatosensory pathways (Varela & Sherman, 2004; see also chapter 8, section 8.C).

In addition to acetylcholine, these axons and their terminals in the lateral geniculate nucleus also release NO (figure 5.4; see also Bickford et al., 1993), a transmitter or neuromodulator with a widespread distribution in the brain (Boehning & Snyder, 2003). Relatively little is known concerning the action of NO in the lateral geniculate nucleus, and it is not yet clear what other thalamic nuclei, if any, also receive inputs that might release NO as a neuroactive substance. Two studies of the lateral geniculate nucleus suggest different but perhaps complementary roles for the release of NO from parabrachial terminals. In one in vitro study, application of NO donors depolarized relay cells and caused them to switch from burst to tonic firing (Pape & Mager, 1992), perhaps complementing the role of acetylcholine in this regard. In another in vivo study, similar application of NO donors promoted the activation of NMDA receptors via retinal afferents (Cudeiro et al., 1996; Rivadulla et al., 1996). This, too, could be related to depolarization of the relay cells, because such depolarization would relieve the NMDA receptor from the Mg^{2+} block. This study made no comment on the effect of NO on response mode, but we would expect that the depolarization that enables NMDA receptor activation would also promote tonic firing.

5.B.4.b. Other Inputs

Other sparse inputs to the relay cells of the lateral geniculate nucleus are shown in figure 5.4 and include noradrenergic axons from cells in the parabrachial region, serotonergic axons from cells in the dorsal raphé nucleus, and histaminergic axons from cells in the tuberomamillary nucleus of the hypothalamus (see chapter 3 for details). In most examples in the thalamus the dominant receptor type activated by these other inputs is metabotropic and the result is an effect on the K^+ "leak" conductance.

Noradrenaline has two very different effects on relay cells, and these effects result from activation of two different metabotropic receptors, known as α_1 and β adrenoreceptors (see Table 5.1). The first effect, via activation of the α_1 adrenoreceptors, increases excitability of relay cells in the lateral geniculate nucleus by reducing the K^+ "leak" conductance and thereby producing a long, slow EPSP. This has the additional result of promoting tonic firing (McCormick & Prince, 1988). This is much like the glutamate activation of metabotropic glutamate receptors or the cholinergic activation of muscarinic receptors just described. The other effect, which operates through the β adrenoreceptors, changes the voltage dependency of I_h in such a way as to increase this depolarizing, voltage dependent current, and this, too, has the effect of suppressing bursting (Pape & McCormick, 1989; McCormick & Pape, 1990b; Lee & McCormick, 1996). This latter effect was described in chapter 4.

Effects of serotonin are complex and somewhat controversial. In the in vivo preparation, application of serotonin or activation of the dorsal raphé nucleus, which contains the serotonergic cells that innervate the lateral geniculate nucleus, inhibits relay cells (Kayama et al., 1989). However, the picture from in vitro studies is very different. Here, application of serotonin has no conventional inhibitory or excitatory effect on relay cells (McCormick & Pape, 1990b). It seems plausible that the effects seen in vivo result from serotonergic excitation of interneurons or reticular cells, which would indirectly inhibit relay cells (Funke & Eysel, 1995). There is, nonetheless, an unconventional effect of serotonin on relay cells described from in vitro studies. By operating through an unknown but probably metabotropic receptor, serotonin has the same effect on I_h as described above for noradrenaline (McCormick & Pape, 1990b; see also chapter 4).

Finally, histamine clearly has effects on functioning of thalamic cells, but the anatomical substrate for this is not entirely clear (Manning et al., 1996). As noted in chapter 3, there is ample innervation of the thalamus by histaminergic axons from the tuberomamillary nucleus of the hypothalamus, but electron microscopic surveys of thalamus have revealed very few conventional synapses formed by these axons (Uhlrich et al., 1993). Perhaps this system works entirely without synapses by having the axon terminals release histamine into the extracellular space to diffuse to receptors on thalamic neurons. In any case, application to relay cells has nearly identical effects to noradrenergic application (McCormick & Williamson, 1991; Lee et al., 2004). One effect, operating through one metabotropic receptor (called H_1), reduces the K^+ "leak" conductance. This produces a long, slow EPSP that also promotes tonic firing. The other effect, which operates through a different metabotropic receptor (H_2), changes I_h in the same way that noradrenaline and serotonin do (see above and chapter 4).

5.B.5. *Other Synaptic Properties*

Among the major advances in recent years in the understanding of synaptic transmission are the elucidation of presynaptic modulation via activation of receptors on synaptic terminals and the dynamic role played by glia, namely astrocytes, in synaptic functioning. There is now evidence of both mechanisms in thalamic processing.

5.B.5.a. Presynaptic Receptors

It has long been appreciated that many presynaptic terminals throughout the central nervous system have receptors for various transmitters (Thompson et al., 1993; Wu & Saggau, 1997; Miller, 1998; MacDermott et al., 1999; Kullmann, 2001; Vitten & Isaacson, 2001). Recently, this observation has been extended to the retinogeniculate synapse in the mouse studied in vitro (Chen & Regehr, 2003). The presynaptic terminal contains receptors for both serotonin and GABA ($5HT_1$ and $GABA_B$, respectively), and both are metabotropic. Activation of either receptor acts to reduce transmitter release by reducing the presynaptic Ca^{2+} influx caused by the action potential invasion of the terminal. The result is that activation of either receptor will reduce the amplitude of the retinogeniculate EPSP. It remains to be determined both how common this is for other driver inputs and what other presynaptic receptors might be discovered.

Since there are no known synaptic inputs onto retinogeniculate terminals, these receptors must be normally activated by the presence of serotonin or GABA released by nearby terminals. As noted in chapter 3, many serotonergic terminals may not end in conventional synaptic contacts but rather discharge their transmitter load into the local extracellular spaces (de Lima & Singer, 1987a), and if the terminal is sufficiently near a retinal terminal, the result will be a reduction of the retinal EPSP. Terminals from interneurons, especially the dendritic terminals involved in triadic circuitry, are near retinal terminals, and even though they form conventional synapses, with sufficient transmitter release, they may well provide a source of presynaptic GABAergic modulation of the retinogeniculate terminals. Other GABAergic terminals, such as those from the axons of the reticular nucleus, relate to more distal relay cell dendrites (see figure 5.4), and so are less likely to act on the presynaptic receptors on the retinogeniculate terminals.

In a recent study, Binns et al. (2003) showed another role for modulation of presynaptic terminals, in this case, those of axons from the thalamic reticular nucleus contacting relay cells. Here, glutamate released from nearby terminals activates kainate receptors on these reticular terminals to reduce GABAergic release, providing disinhibition. Figure 5.4 shows that, of the two glutamatergic inputs to relay cells, driver and layer 6 cortical, only the latter are near enough to the peripherally located reticular terminals to play this role, and thus this seems another modulatory function carried out by corticothalamic inputs. However, this may be an oversimplified view, because single cells and their inputs lie amid many others in very complex arrangements, and so it is possible that a driver input to one cell actually lies close enough to reticular inputs onto a neighboring cell to have this effect.

5.B.5.b. Role of Glia

Glia can no longer be thought of as a sort of neuronal glue that serves a vaguely defined metabolic or supportive function for neurons. As indicated in chapter 3, it is now clear that glia, or more specifically astrocytes, which have processes that envelop many extraglomerular synapses, serve in the transport of K^+ ions, serve in the uptake of transmitters, have receptors to conventional transmitters, and can respond to these substances with changes, including increased internal Ca^{2+} levels, which in turn can cause these astrocytes to release transmitters[5] affecting

---

5. Now that we know that transmitters can affect glia and be released by them, the term "neurotransmitter" is not entirely correct. Perhaps the neuroactive substances affecting glia and released by them should be called something like "gliotransmitters." Despite this somewhat whimsical proviso, we have instead used the more general term of "transmitter" throughout.

local presynaptic terminals (reviewed in Haydon, 2001). Furthermore, astrocytes can communicate with one another via gap junctions, so this increase in internal Ca^{2+} can spread and affect more distant synapses (Haydon, 2001). These glial responses are relatively slow and sustained, lasting for several hundred milliseconds.

While there has been relatively little specific research devoted to glial activity in the thalamus, there are at least two recent observations relevant here. First is a study by Do et al. (2004), which provides evidence that glutamate released from nearby terminals activates astrocytes via a Group II or III metabotropic glutamate receptors, that this causes release of homocysteic acid from the astrocytes, and that this, in turn, presynaptically depresses terminals from the thalamic reticular nucleus. The end result is reduced inhibition, much like that involving kainate receptors on reticular terminals as noted earlier in section 5.B.5.a., and by the same logic, the source of glutamatergic input that starts this modulatory chain of events is likely to be corticothalamic.

The other observation that may have relevance for thalamic function involves the NMDA receptors. As noted earlier, this receptor has a glycine site, and for activation to occur, both this site and the glutamatergic site must be coactivated. The lack of a specific glycine input in the thalamus led to the suggestion that the glycine site, which is very sensitive and requires little glycine for coactivation, is constantly activated by metabolic levels present in the neuropil. While it may seem odd to have a receptor to an invariant substance, it may be that another function of glia is to locally adjust this glycine level and thus modulate the NMDA receptor, although there is no evidence for this function. An alternative view has been offered (reviewed in Hashimoto & Oka, 1997). Astrocytes adjacent to a glutamatergic synapse involving NMDA receptors themselves contain AMPA receptors that are activated by glutamate release, and this in turn leads to release of D-serine from the astrocytes, providing the necessary cofactor to activate the NMDA receptor. It is interesting that D-serine levels in the brain covary with NMDA receptors and are highest in the forebrain, including the thalamus (Hashimoto & Oka, 1997).

This new concept of glial function has implications for the glomerulus described in chapter 3. We showed in chapter 3 that an unusual feature of the glomerulus is that a cluster of complex synaptic connections, though surrounded by astrocytic processes, lacks astrocytic processes adjacent to the synapses. This configuration suggests that astrocytes are less able to influence synaptic processing within the glomerulus. This raises a further issue for those relay cells—mostly X—with glomerular inputs. As just noted, one possible function for astrocytes is to provide D-serine, a cofactor for the NMDA site, but this function does not seem plausible for the NMDA receptor postsynaptic to the retinogeniculate synapse in a glomerulus.

5.C. Inputs to Interneurons and Reticular Cells

Relatively few recordings have been made from interneurons and reticular cells. As noted above, interneurons have two distinct and functionally independent innervation zones that may be electrotonically isolated from each other: one is the soma and proximal dendrites, where firing of the axon and its F1 terminals is controlled, and the other is the region of (distal) dendritic F2 terminals. Thus in recordings from the soma of an interneuron, presumably only the former, soma-dendritic inputs are revealed. Although there is evidence for limited dendritic terminal output for reticular cells in some species (see chapter 2), for the most part these cells are organized in a conventional fashion, integrating synaptic inputs to produce an axonal output. Figure 5.5 summarizes the synaptic inputs to these cells and shows the types of postsynaptic receptors activated. The many question marks in figure 5.5 reflect the many gaps in our knowledge, even for such well-studied examples as the lateral geniculate and ventral posterior nuclei.

5.C.1. Glutamatergic Inputs

5.C.1.a. Driver Afferents
In chapter 2 we summarized evidence that interneurons receive synaptic inputs to both dendritic F2 terminals (controlling their local output) and to proximal dendrites and soma (controlling the axonal output). The inputs to F2 terminals control the output of these terminals and the inputs to proximal dendrites plus soma control the axonal output (Sherman, 2004). Recordings from cell bodies of interneurons reveal only the latter function. Such recordings indicate that retinal inputs produce EPSPs based on ionotropic glutamate receptors (Pape & McCormick, 1995; Cox et al., 1998). Indirect evidence, including immunocytochemistry and pharmacological studies of effects on relay cells attributed to interneuronal activation, indicate that retinal input to the dendritic F2 terminals activates metabotropic as well as ionotropic glutamate receptors (Godwin et al., 1996a; Cox et al., 1998; Cox & Sherman, 2000).

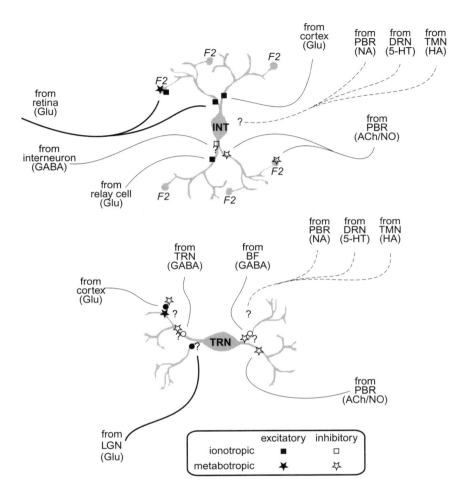

Figure 5.5
Inputs to interneuron (INT, upper) and cell of the thalamic reticular nucleus (tha-lamic reticular nucleus, lower), shown with the same conventions and abbre-viations as in figure 5.4. The question marks indicate uncertainty about the postsynaptic receptors involved due to lack of information; in some cases we know so little that no synaptic site is drawn, and in others, we have limited information about these sites and associated receptors. Note that the F2 termi-nals of the interneuron receive synaptic inputs.

The metabotropic glutamate receptors on these F2 terminals are type 5, which are subtly different from the type 1 metabotropic glutamate receptors activated by cortical axons on relay cells, but like them, their activation depolarizes the postsynaptic target by decreasing the K^+ "leak" conductance. Exactly how activation of these glutamate receptors controls the F2 terminals is not known, but it seems plausible that this acts by depolarizing these terminals. This, in turn, would lead to an influx of Ca^{2+} into the F2 terminal via a voltage dependent, high threshold Ca^{2+} conductance similar to that described in chapter 4 but perhaps employing different channel types. The resulting Ca^{2+} entry leads to transmitter release, GABA in this case. However, the small size of F2 terminals is a serious obstacle to obtaining direct recordings from them, and thus there is no direct evidence for voltage changes in the F2 terminal, and one can imagine other scenarios. For instance, activation of the metabotropic receptor on the F2 terminal can affect internal Ca^{2+} via second messenger pathways without having any effect of K^+ channels (and thus the membrane voltage), and a change in internal Ca^{2+} could influence transmitter release. Thus the details of precisely how metabotropic activation in the F2 terminal affects transmitter release are unresolved.

The result is that retinal input to the F2 terminal, as part of the triadic synaptic arrangement described in chapter 2, leads to feedforward inhibition of the relay cell through the F2 terminals. This is schematically shown in figure 5.6. Thus retinal inputs will evoke a monosynaptic EPSP and often a disynaptic IPSP in the relay cells that receive such triadic inputs and will evoke just a monosynaptic EPSP in those that do not.

However, since the retinal innervation of the F2 terminal involves a metabotropic receptor, but innervation of the relay cell does not, the operation of this circuit is likely to depend on activity patterns in the retinal afferent, since ionotropic and metabotropic receptors operate differently depending on these patterns (see above). That is, as noted earlier, metabotropic glutamate receptors respond relatively poorly to low rates of afferent input. Low rates or brief periods of retinal firing will activate only ionotropic receptors, leading to brief monosynaptic EPSPs (and brief disynaptic IPSPs in the relay cell due to the ionotropic glutamate receptors present on the F2 terminal); only with increasing rates or duration of firing will the metabotropic receptors on the F2 terminal become active, thereby producing a prolonged IPSP in the relay cell. Thus the inhibition relative to the excitation through the triadic circuit actually

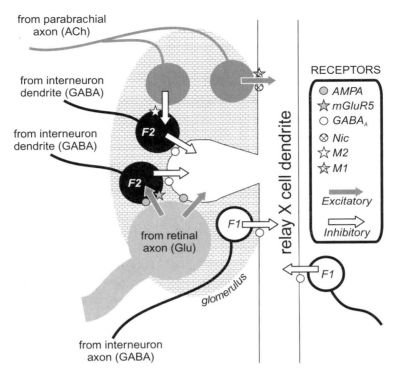

Figure 5.6
Schematic view of triadic circuitry showing transmitters and postsynaptic receptors. The triadic circuitry is in a glomerulus that also contains an appendage
from a relay cell. The arrows indicate the direction of each synapse from presynaptic to postsynaptic. Note that a single retinal terminal forms a triad with an
F2 terminal and the appendage of the relay cell dendrite, while two terminals
from the same parabrachial axon are involved in forming the same functional
sort of triad.

grows with increasing input strength. This may be important for
preventing response saturation in the relay cell for very strong inputs.
For retinogeniculate circuitry, this is a form of contrast gain control that
would enable the relay cell to continue to inform the cortex about
increasing stimulus strength or contrast over a wider dynamic range of
contrasts in the visual scene. Presumably, relay cells without triadic circuitry are less able to accomplish this.

Perhaps a similar function for the triad exists in other relays. For
example, in the medial geniculate or ventral posterior nuclei, this could

prevent response saturation as the sound or touch increased in amplitude. However, relevant data to address the general function of the triad in thalamus is lacking.

5.C.1.b. Cortical Layer 6 Afferents

Cortical axons from layer 6 innervate both interneurons and reticular cells. Their innervation of interneurons does not involve F2 terminals. Instead, cortical terminals innervate dendritic shafts of interneurons where they activate only ionotropic receptors that presumably produce only fast EPSPs (Pape & McCormick, 1995). It would thus appear that their main effect is to control axonal outputs of these cells, but there remains the untested possibility that action potentials from the soma can invade peripheral dendrites to influence F2 terminals.

There is ample evidence that, in general, activation of cortical or relay cell inputs excites reticular cells (but see below). However, the pattern of postsynaptic receptors associated with cortical or relay cell inputs to reticular cells is far from clear, partly due to lack of data and partly due to complexities unique to the reticular cells. One complexity is that these cells receive glutamatergic inputs from these two sources, and it is not yet known which glutamate receptors are associated with which glutamatergic inputs. Nor do we have clear evidence about exactly which types of glutamatergic receptors are found on reticular cells. There is immunocytochemical evidence (Godwin et al., 1996a) that these cells contain two types of metabotropic glutamate receptor: type 1 and type 2/3 (types 2 and 3 have currently not been distinguished from each other for the thalamus). This leads to another complication. Activation of the metabotropic type 1 receptor reduces the K^+ "leak" conductance, producing an EPSP, but activation of the metabotropic type 2/3 receptors increases the K^+ "leak" conductance, producing an IPSP (Cox & Sherman, 1999). The former response usually dominates, and the glutamatergic IPSP can be seen only when the excitatory responses are blocked or minimized. This may reflect the relative numbers of the receptor types, with type 1 outnumbering type 2/3, but no data are available at present. Thus, global activation of cortical or relay cell inputs or global application of agonists produces only the EPSP, swamping the IPSP. The distinct pos-sibility remains that, under some conditions, activation of perhaps some cortical or relay cell axons can actually inhibit reticular cells: perhaps only a small subset of these axons have terminals associated with type 2/3 receptors or perhaps only certain firing patterns activates these receptors. This clearly needs much more study.

5.C.2. Cholinergic Inputs

Based on recordings from cell bodies of interneurons and reticular cells, activation of the cholinergic inputs from the parabrachial region generally inhibits both cell types (McCormick & Prince, 1986; McCormick & Pape, 1988). This is interesting, because individual parabrachial axons branch to innervate both of these cell types as well as relay cells, and, as noted above, their action on relay cells is typically excitatory. This neat trick—a single axon exciting some targets (relay cells) and inhibiting others (interneurons and reticular cells)—is possible because different muscarinic receptors are activated on these different targets. This is illustrated schematically in figure 5.7. We have seen above that relay cells have nicotinic and M1 type muscarinic receptors, but another type of muscarinic receptor, a type 2, dominates on interneurons and reticular cells.

Activation of this M2 type of muscarinic receptor increases the K^+ "leak" conductance, leading to hyperpolarization of interneurons and reticular cells. However, cells of the thalamic reticular nucleus also respond to this cholinergic input via another, nicotinic receptor that leads to fast depolarization. Nonetheless, the main effect of cholinergic stimulation of these cells as seen at their cell bodies seems dominated by the muscarinic, inhibitory response. Since axonal outputs from these interneurons and reticular cells inhibit relay cells, activation of this cholinergic pathway thus disinhibits relay cells (see inset to figure 5.7).

An interesting aspect of cholinergic effects on interneurons is that parabrachial terminals innervate many of the dendritic F2 terminals of the interneurons in addition to the contacts nearer to or on the cell body mentioned above (Erişir et al., 1997a), and the effects of cholinergic activation of these terminals are likely to be invisible to somatic recording of the interneuron, just as the retinal innervation of these terminals is invisible. Typically, a retinal terminal and parabrachial terminal do not innervate the same F2 terminal. Indirect evidence based on recording from the relay cells postsynaptic to F2 terminals is that cholinergic afferents inhibit the F2 terminals and thereby disinhibit the relay cells (Cox & Sherman, 2000). This is illustrated in figures 5.5 through 5.7. It appears that the cholinergic parabrachial terminals contacting the F2 terminals activate only M2 muscarinic receptors, and this presumably increases the K^+ "leak" conductance, thereby hyperpolarizing the F2 terminal and reducing GABA release, although, as noted earlier, there is no direct evidence regarding how activation of these muscarinic receptors

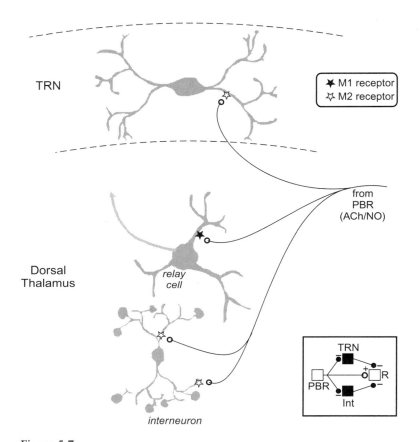

Figure 5.7
Pattern of innervation of thalamic cells by single parabrachial axon. All three
major cell types—relay cells, interneurons, and reticular cells—are innervated by
branches of the same parabrachial axon. However, the metabotropic (muscarinic)
receptors activated are not the same on these cells. For relay cells, an M1 type
of receptor is found, activation of which produces a slow EPSP. For interneurons
and reticular cells, an M2 type of receptor is found, activation of which
produces a slow IPSP. Not shown are nicotinic receptors, which appear to be
found on relay and reticular cells but not interneurons, and which produce fast
EPSPs. *Inset*: Schematic diagram of circuit properties. Inputs from parabrachial
region (PBR) inhibit (−) interneurons (Int) and cells of the thalamic reticular
nucleus (TRN), and these postsynaptic cells in turn inhibit relay cells (R). The
parabrachial axons excite (+) relay cells. Thus, the effect on relay cells of
increased activity in parabrachial afferents is direct excitation and indirect disinhibition, the latter via inhibiting inhibitory inputs to the relay cells.

reduces transmitter release in the F2 terminal. A sort of functional triad is formed by the parabrachial axons innervating relay cells and interneuronal F2 terminals, since the same axon contacts both, but usually with different presynaptic terminals (see figure 5.6). In this regard it differs from the triad formed from retinal terminals, where a single terminal contacts both an F2 terminal and an appendage of a relay cell dendrite (see figure 5.6), and it differs functionally, because the retinal input increases transmitter release from the F2 terminal, while the parabrachial input reduces this release. Thus the effect of firing in these cholinergic afferents from the parabrachial region is reduced inhibition in relay cells. This results because the cholinergic input affects the axonal F1 outputs by hyperpolarizing the cell body and/or it affects the dendritic F2 outputs, as described above.

5.C.3. GABAergic Inputs

The GABAergic pathway from the basal forebrain to the thalamic reticular nucleus (see chapter 2) likely inhibits the reticular cells, although there has been no published physiological or pharmacological study of this pathway. We noted in chapter 2 that this pathway does not directly innervate the lateral geniculate nucleus and thus does not innervate interneurons.

Reticular cells innervate each other by axon collaterals, and possibly in some cases by dendrodendritic synapses (Pinault et al., 1997; Jones, 2002a). Again, we can assume that these local interactions are inhibitory, but there is as yet no physiological confirmation of this assumption. It is thought that these local interconnections are important in synchronizing cells of the thalamic reticular nucleus, particularly during sleep, when they fire in rhythmic and synchronous bursts (see chapter 4; see also Steriade et al., 1993a, 1993b; Jones, 2002a).

Electron microscopic studies indicate that interneurons receive F1 terminals on their dendritic stems and branches and occasionally on their dendritic (F2) terminals (Guillery, 1969a, 1969b; Hamos et al., 1985; Erişir et al., 1998). These F1 terminals are GABAergic and are thought to be inhibitory, but to date we can account for the sources of only a few of these F1 inputs, and the physiology or pharmacology of these inputs has not been determined for any of them. In further electron microscopic studies of the axonal output of thalamic reticular cells to the lateral geniculate nucleus (Cucchiaro et al., 1991; Wang et al., 2001), these outputs were directed at relay cells, but a small minority innervated interneurons. There is also a GABAergic input from the pretectal region to the lateral geniculate nucleus that seems to target F2 terminals of interneurons (Cucchiaro et al., 1993). Presumably, this input inhibits F2 terminals, and rather indirect in vivo data are consistent with this possibility (Fischer et al., 1998). Such a pathway may be unique to the lateral geniculate nucleus. However, GABAergic inputs from areas other than the thalamic reticular nucleus have been described to other dorsal thalamic nuclei. In the ventral anterior nucleus of the monkey, a GABAergic projection from the globus pallidus and substantia nigra contacts both relay cells and interneurons (Ilinsky et al., 1997). In the rat's medial geniculate nucleus GABAergic inputs from the inferior colliculus contact relay neurons (Peruzzi et al., 1997), but since there are virtually no interneurons in the rat's medial geniculate nucleus (Arcelli et al., 1997), the possibility that interneurons in this nucleus might receive such input in other species remains open. Finally, the zona incerta projects a GABAergic input to various higher order thalamic relays (Barthó et al., 2002; but see Power & Mitrofanis, 2002; see also chapter 3), and this is again based on a study in rats with few interneurons in these nuclei, suggesting that most or all of such GABAergic inputs are onto relay cells.

5.C.4. Noradrenergic Inputs

Anatomical studies in the cat indicate that noradrenergic axons from the brainstem innervate the dorsal thalamus (see chapter 3), and here they may possibly innervate interneurons, although Pape & McCormick (1995) have shown that noradrenaline has no clear effect on interneurons. Some of these axons also innervate the thalamic reticular nucleus (Morrison & Foote, 1986; de Lima & Singer, 1987a; Fitzpatrick et al., 1989) where noradrenaline depolarizes reticular cells by reducing the K^+ "leak" conductance, presumably acting through a metabotropic receptor (McCormick & Wang, 1991).

5.C.5. Serotonergic Inputs

Anatomical data indicate that serotonergic axons from the dorsal raphé nucleus innervate the thalamic reticular nucleus and dorsal thalamus. However, the effects of serotonin are poorly understood. Serotonin depolarizes reticular cells by blocking the K^+ "leak" conductance, again presumably via metabotropic receptors (McCormick & Wang, 1991). The effects of serotonin on interneurons are confusing, since its application produces a slight depolarization of some interneurons while not clearly affecting others (Pape & McCormick, 1995).

5.C.6. *Histaminergic Inputs*

Very little published work is as yet available on the effects of histamine application to interneurons or reticular cells. Such application in vitro does depolarize interneurons, but the receptors involved are unknown. There is some evidence that this depolarization is an indirect result of activating excitatory inputs to interneurons and not a direct effect on interneurons (Pape & McCormick, 1995). Results from reticular cells indicate that histamine applied in vitro inhibits them by increasing a Cl⁻ conductance using an H_2 receptor (Lee et al., 2004).

5.D. Summary

In this chapter we have stressed the importance of the postsynaptic receptor in shaping the responses of neurons, and particularly of thalamic relay cells, to their afferent inputs. Two major classes of receptor are found on relay cells, ionotropic and metabotropic receptors. Activation of ionotropic receptors results in relatively fast postsynaptic potentials with a more rapid onset and briefer duration, while activation of metabotropic receptors produces postsynaptic potentials with a slower onset and longer duration. In addition, second messenger systems turned on when metabotropic receptors are activated could have other effects on relay cells beyond the creation of a postsynaptic potential, including such long-term effects as regulation of gene expression, but this possibility has not yet been studied for thalamic neurons.

The differential timing of activation of these receptor types has implications for the functioning of relay cells. Obviously, the sustained membrane potential changes associated with activation of metabotropic receptors will affect overall excitability of the cell. Furthermore, activation of these receptors seems particularly well suited to controlling the inactivation states of many of the voltage dependent conductances of relay cells, such as I_T, I_h, and I_A, because these have relatively long time constants for inactivation and de-inactivation. With I_T, for example, activation of excitatory metabotropic excitatory receptors (e.g., metabotropic glutamate, M1 muscarinic, and noradrenergic), will produce a long, slow EPSP ideally suited to inactivating I_T; and activation of metabotropic GABA$_B$ receptors will produce a long, slow IPSP that will effectively de-inactivate I$_T$. On the other hand, EPSPs and IPSPs activated via ionotropic receptors are too transient, without extensive temporal summation, to have much effect on the inactivation state of I$_T$. Thus activation of metabotropic but not of ionotropic receptors seems particularly appropriate for controlling I$_T$ and thus the response mode, burst or tonic, of relay cells. The importance of this response is emphasized in chapter 6.

In this context it is especially interesting that, for the lateral geniculate nucleus of the cat, the driver (retinal) input to relay cells activates only ionotropic glutamate receptors, while all other (modulator) inputs activate metabotropic receptors, although many also activate ionotropic receptors. Also, the layer 6 (modulatory) input to the ventral posterior and posterior medial nuclei in the mouse activates metabotropic glutamate receptors, while the layer 5 (driver) input to the posterior medial nucleus activates only ionotropic glutamate receptors (Li et al., 2003a; Reichova & Sherman, 2004). (It is of critical importance to determine if this distinction for driver and modulator inputs holds for the rest of thalamus.) This observation suggests that one of the important roles for modulatory inputs is to control the response mode of relay cells, and evidence for this role exists in studies related to corticogeniculate and cholinergic parabrachial inputs. This also suggests that retinal input is less effective in directly controlling response mode. By activating only ionotropic glutamate receptors, retinal axons would produce faster EPSPs, which avoids loss of high frequency visual information that would be com-promised by slower EPSPs via metabotropic receptors.

5.E. Unresolved Questions

1. Does the distinction between driver and modulator inputs with regard to the type of receptor activated, ionotropic or metabotropic, that is seen in some thalamic relays, namely the lateral geniculate, ventral posterior, and the posterior medial nuclei, apply to the rest of thalamus? That is, is it generally true that driver inputs activate only ionotropic (glutamate) receptors, while all modulatory inputs activate metabotropic receptors (and often ionotropic receptors as well)?

2. Do the metabotropic receptors in the thalamus have any long-term actions comparable to those seen in hippocampus or neocortex?

3. Do low threshold spikes from activation of I_T produce enough Ca^{2+} entry to generate similar second messenger cascades and perhaps other long-term effects?

4. What is the functional significance of the mix of receptor types, especially ionotropic and metabotropic, related to most afferent pathways to the thalamus? Do certain patterns of activity activate different receptors relatively selectively? Do individual axons in these pathways activate different combinations of receptors associated with the entire pathway? For instance, do all corticogeniculate axons from layer 6 activate metabotropic and ionotropic receptors, or do some activate just one or the other?

5. Do interneurons have two functionally independent synaptic input zones: one controlling F2 terminals and the other, the axon?

6. Can back propagation of the action potential invade dendrites of thalamic neurons to affect synaptic integration there? Can this occur in interneurons as a means of affecting the F2 terminals? Does normal synaptic activation of dendrites of thalamic cells produce action potential initiation in dendritic locations or only in the soma or axon hillock?

7. What is the function of the triad? Is it, as suggested in this chapter, a form of gain control for particular driver inputs?

8. How does the glomerulus affect synaptic function, particularly given new evidence for the role of glia in synaptic transmission and for the presence of presynaptic receptors, especially on retinal terminals?

9. What is the functional significance for information flow of the observation that driver inputs to thalamic relay cells show paired-pulse depression?

6 Function of Burst and Tonic Response Modes in the Thalamocortical Relay

As noted in chapter 4, thalamic relay cells display a variety of voltage dependent membrane properties. The best understood and undoubtedly the most important are those underlying conventional action potentials, because these represent the only way for thalamic relay cells to transmit information to cortex. Perhaps next in importance are those underlying the low-threshold Ca^{2+} spike, because the activation state of the conductance underlying this spike determines which of two response modes, burst or tonic, the relay cell will display. Since in each of these response modes the thalamic cells send a different pattern of action potentials to cortex, several obvious questions arise. What is the significance of the distinct burst and tonic response modes for thalamic relay functioning? How does local thalamic circuitry control firing mode? What is the behavioral significance of the different firing modes? There have been several different, although not mutually exclusive, answers proposed to these questions, and they are considered in this chapter.

6.A. Rhythmic Bursting

Initial studies from both in vitro slice and in vivo preparations have emphasized two features often associated with the burst response mode: (1) when relay cells exhibit burst firing, they frequently (but, as we shall see, not always) show rhythmic bursting, and (2) relay cells through large regions of thalamus become synchronized in their rhythmic bursting (Steriade & Deschênes, 1984; Steriade & Llinás, 1988; Steriade et al., 1993b; McCormick & Bal, 1997). Interactions between relay cells and cells of the thalamic reticular nucleus are critical for synchronizing such rhythmic bursting (Steriade et al., 1985). It is worth noting that detection of synchrony usually requires simultaneous recording from two or more cells, a technically difficult feat not often accomplished, so that most studies of rhythmic bursting have not directly assessed any synchrony among cells. The frequency of this rhythm (i.e., the inverse of the fairly constant time interval between bursts) can vary, depending on a variety of other factors, but typically is in the range of 0.3–10 Hz. While circuitry plays a role in rhythmic bursting, isolated relay cells also have some capacity to burst rhythmically. As noted in chapter 4, the combination of various membrane currents, including I_T, I_h, and various K$^+$ currents, can lead to rhythmic bursting in an isolated cell, which has been suggested as a mechanism for this property in some studies (McCormick & Huguenard, 1992).

The first in vivo studies of the response modes in cats demonstrated that, when an animal entered slow wave sleep,[1] individual thalamic relay cells began to burst rhythmically, and that such rhythmic bursting was not seen during awake, alert states (Livingstone & Hubel, 1981; Steriade & McCarley, 1990; Steriade et al., 1993b). The details of what underlies the pattern of synchronized, rhythmic bursting are not entirely known, but it seems to involve circuit features, with the thalamic reticular nucleus playing a key role (Steriade et al., 1985). This occurs as follows. After the burst in reticular cells, various K$^+$ conductances come into play (see chapter 4, section 4.C.1.b), and this, added to the strong IPSP activated in each cell from reticular interconnections, de-inactivates I_T in these cells. The subsequent passive repolarization after the IPSP decays plus active excitatory inputs from bursting relay cells activate low threshold spikes, and the cycle repeats. As long as the bursts of the relay cells are out of phase with those of the reticular cells, synchronous, rhythmic bursting will continue in both populations. Thus rhythmic bursting ensues and remains synchronized.

This led to the hypothesis that awake animals have depolarized thalamocortical cells that operate strictly in tonic mode and thus reliably relay information to cortex; during slow-wave sleep, the cells become

---

1. This is also called "synchronized" sleep and is characterized by rhythmic, low frequency, high voltage waveforms in the EEG. The other main stage of sleep is called "desynchronized" and is characterized by high frequency but low voltage waveforms in the EEG without much rhythmicity. Rapid eye movements also occur during this latter sleep phase, so it is also known as "REM" sleep. Relatively little is known specifically about thalamic relay properties during these sleep phases, although transmission through the thalamus seems somewhat depressed during synchronized sleep but not during desynchronized sleep. For further details about these sleep states and thalamic functioning, the reader is referred elsewhere (e.g., Favale et al., 1964; Dagnino et al., 1965, 1966, 1971; Ghelarducci et al., 1970; Marks et al., 1981; Llinás & Pare, 1991).

hyperpolarized and thus often burst rhythmically, which reduces relay of information to cortex. In this regard, rhythmic bursting is thought to represent a state during which normal driving inputs (e.g., retinal or auditory inputs for geniculate relay cells) have less impact on the firing patterns of their postsynaptic relay cells, and the relay of information to cortex is reduced or interrupted. (The reasons for this diminution are discussed more fully in chapter 7.) According to this view, information would be effectively relayed to cortex only during tonic firing. During rhythmic bursting, the firing pattern of the relay cells would be largely controlled by their intrinsic membrane properties plus the activity of reticular cells. However, it is important to note that tonic firing remains the dominant mode for relay cells, even during slow-wave sleep (McCarley et al., 1983; Ramcharan et al., 2000; Swadlow & Gusev, 2001; Massaux & Edeline, 2003). We still have much to learn about thalamic relay properties during sleep.

More important, we have much to learn about relay properties and the role bursting may play during the vigilant, wakeful state. Studies of sensory response properties of relay cells in the lateral geniculate, medial geniculate, and the ventral posterior nuclei of lightly anesthetized or awake, behaving animals suggest that bursting is not limited to sleep. Burst firing becomes relatively more common as the animal moves from alert wakefulness through drowsiness to sleep (McCarley et al., 1983; Ramcharan et al., 2000; Swadlow & Gusev, 2001; Massaux & Edeline, 2003). The data reviewed in the following paragraphs indicate that both tonic and burst response modes are normally used by thalamic relay cells to transmit sensory information to cortex.

6.B. Effect of Response Mode on Thalamocortical Transmission

6.B.1. *Visual Responses of Geniculate Relay Cells*

If the burst mode indeed represented a complete failure of relay through the thalamus, as suggested by earlier studies, it would follow that, in vivo, a geniculate relay cell sufficiently hyperpolarized to de-inactivate the Ca^{2+} conductance underlying its low threshold spike should either remain silent or begin bursting rhythmically, regardless of which visual stimuli, if any, are presented. Recording from lightly anesthetized cats in vivo shows that cells in burst mode in the absence of any visual inputs commonly fire arrhythmically, with randomly occurring bursts (Guido et al., 1992; Lu et al., 1992; Sherman, 1996). This general lack of rhythmicity seen in the awake state may explain why bursting was missed in earlier descriptions of thalamic cell responses during wakefulness. That is, the rhythmicity seen during sleep is nearly impossible to miss, since any regularities in responsiveness are relatively easy to detect, but the occasional appearance of bursts at unpredicted intervals might well be missed unless one were looking for them.

Not only is arrhythmic bursting seen during spontaneous activity (i.e., the cell firing when the visual stimulus is absent) in geniculate relay cells in vivo, but these cells, while still in the burst mode, also respond quite reliably to visual stimuli (Sherman, 1996). The bursts then follow the temporal properties of the visual stimulation rather than any intrinsic pacemaker frequency (figures 6.1 and 6.2). During burst firing, the response is in the form of bursts riding the crests of low threshold spikes rather than the streams of unitary action potentials that occur when the same cell responds in tonic mode (Guido et al., 1992; Mukherjee & Kaplan, 1995). The same response properties can be seen in the lateral geniculate nuclei of awake, behaving cats (Guido & Weyand, 1995) and monkeys (Ramcharan et al., 2000).

Thus, geniculate cells clearly respond to visual stimuli quite vigorously in either tonic or burst mode, the pattern of the response depending on the activation state of the underlying low threshold Ca^{2+}

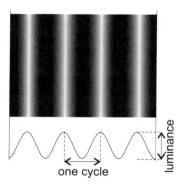

Figure 6.1
Sine wave grating used as a visual stimulus. The grating is shown at top and is vertically oriented in this example. Below it is its sinusoidal luminance profile. The grating may repeat over many cycles. Typically, such a visual stimulus would be temporally modulated in various ways, most simply by drifting the grating in a direction orthogonal to its orientation (horizontally in this example). When such a grating drifts, each point along its path is stimulated by light that sinusoidally varies in intensity.

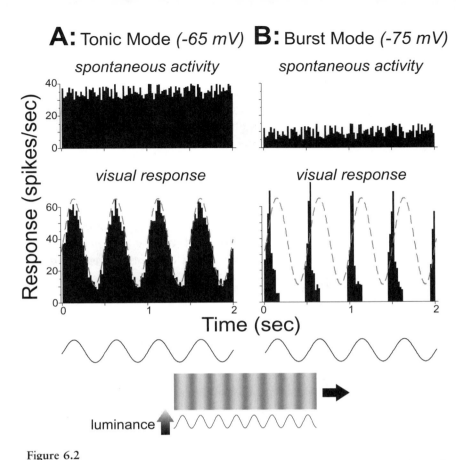

Figure 6.2
Responses of a single representative relay cell in the lateral geniculate nucleus of
a cat to a drifting sinusoidal grating like that shown in figure 6.1. The cell was
recorded intracellularly in a lightly anesthetized cat while the grating was drifted
across the cell's receptive field. Current was injected into the cell through the
recording electrode to alter the membrane potential. Thus, in A the current injection was adjusted so that the membrane potential without visual stimulation
averaged −65 mV. This represents tonic firing, because I_T is mostly inactivated at
this membrane potential. Shown are average response histograms, with the mean
firing rate plotted as a function of time averaged over many epochs of that time.
Also shown are the sinusoidal changes in contrast as the grating moves across
the receptive field; these are shown twice, once below the histograms and again
as a dashed gray curve superimposed over the lower histograms. In B the current
injection was adjusted to a more hyperpolarized level, permitting burst firing.
The bottom histograms in A and B reflect firing in response to four cycles of the
drifting grating; the bottom histograms in A and B reflect spontaneous activity
when the gratings have been removed. Note that the response profile during
the visual response in tonic mode (A, bottom) looks like a sine wave, but the
companion response during burst mode (B, bottom) does not. Note also that the
spontaneous activity is higher during tonic than during burst firing (A and B,
top).

conductance at the time the visual stimulus is presented. This state, in turn, depends on the recent status of the membrane potential (see chapter 4). Recent analysis of the pattern of burst and tonic firing in response to various visual stimuli indicates that both firing modes can convey roughly equal amounts of information (Reinagel et al., 1999). Burst firing conveys information more efficiently (with less noise), but other experiments show that tonic firing conveys information more linearly (Guido et al., 1992). That is, while the total amount of information relayed is roughly similar during both response modes, it should be clear from chapter 4 (figure 4.6) and figure 6.2 that burst and tonic response modes represent different types of stimulus/response transformation, and that these response modes almost certainly represent different forms of relay of information to cortex.

6.B.1.a. Functional Significance

The obvious question then is, What is the functional significance of the two modes for transmission of retinal information by geniculate relay cells? This key question can be broken down into two different but ultimately related questions. The first, considered in this section, asks, What is the possible significance of burst versus tonic firing in terms of the type of information each mode relays to cortex? The second, considered next in section 6.C, asks, What is the possible significance of the two firing modes in terms of the transmission of this information from thalamocortical axons to cortical cells?

One of the differences between burst and tonic firing involves linear summation of visual stimuli. Strictly speaking, linearity in the context of visual receptive field properties means that the response to two or more individual stimuli can be summed linearly, and the result is the same response that would be evoked in response to the combination of the two or more stimuli presented simultaneously; any departure from this indicates lack of linear summation, or nonlinearity, in the response.[2] Such linearity is frequently tested with a sinusoidal stimulus, such as a sinusoidal grating as illustrated in figure 6.1. This stimulus could be presented in several ways, but a common way discussed below is to drift it through the receptive field of the cell at a constant velocity in a direction orthogonal to the orientation of the grating. Such a sinusoidal stimulus makes it easier to apply Fourier techniques to the study of responses,

---

2. This definition of linearity can be extended to any neuron as follows: the response to a complex combination of inputs equals the sum of responses of the neuron to each component stimulus.

and this in turn offers a fairly straightforward way to assess the linearity of these responses.[3] Another advantage is that this is a stimulus that generally serves to activate geniculate cells.

Figure 6.2 shows examples of burst and tonic responses in the same cell to a drifting grating like that shown in figure 6.1, and this illustration suggests two prominent differences between tonic and burst mode. One is that the tonic mode displays much greater linear summation than does the burst mode. In this example, since the visual stimulus changes contrast in time with a sinusoidal wave form, a cell that responds linearly should show a response profile that is correspondingly sinusoidal. Thus the sinusoidal response profile during tonic mode firing (figure 6.2A, bottom) reflects a linear transformation between the visual stimulus and the response. In contrast, the response profile during burst mode firing (figure 6.2B, bottom) reflects a nonlinear distortion, since the response here is nonsinusoidal to the sinusoidal stimulus. This very likely results from the nonlinear amplification of the low threshold spike described in chapter 4 (see figure 4.6E, page 160), which provides a similar response regardless of the amplitude or duration of any suprathreshold stimulus. This would have the effect of creating a response to a sinusoidal stimulus that was dominated by an initial burst near the beginning of each cycle, and thus instead of the response during burst firing being graded in a sinusoidal fashion (as during tonic firing), it has a pronounced peak near the beginning of each cycle. These impressions of more linear summation for tonic than burst firing have been confirmed by Fourier analysis of the responses of the cells during the two response modes, as summarized in figure 6.3A (Guido et al., 1992, 1995) and also by analysis of responses to flashing spots (Mukherjee & Kaplan,

---

3. Fourier techniques refer to the analytical methods developed by the French mathematician, J. Fourier (1768–1830). He showed that any complex waveform could be synthesized or analyzed by the linear addition of pure sine waves appropriately chosen for amplitude, frequency, and phase. Determining the component sine waves of a complex waveform is called Fourier analysis, and creating a complex waveform from sine waves is called Fourier synthesis. A neuron can be tested for linearity by stimulating it with a sine wave input (e.g., a sinusoidally varying visual stimulus, such as shown in figure 6.1) and Fourier analyzing the response profile. The Fourier sine wave component that matches the input sine wave in frequency is the linear response component, and all other sine wave components of the response comprise nonlinear response components. Note that a linear response must have both the frequency and sinusoidal shape of a sine wave input: a departure from the sinusoidal shape indicates nonlinear distortion components of the response. For further details on this subject, see Shapley and Lennie (1985).

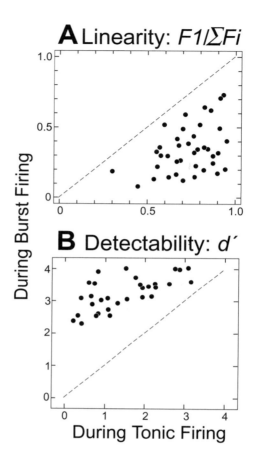

Figure 6.3
Measurements of linearity and detectability for population of relay cells recorded from the lateral geniculate nucleus of lightly anesthetized cats during both tonic and burst firing modes. A. Linearity. This was assessed by Fourier analyzing the response of each cell to a drifting grating and dividing the fundamental (F1) component, which is linear, by the sum of the first 10 nonlinear components. The denominator thus gives an estimate of the extent of nonlinearity in the response, and the larger this fraction, the more linear the response. Each point represents a single cell, and the abscissa reflects linearity during tonic firing, while the ordinate reflects linearity during burst firing. The line of slope 1 is also shown, and every cell falls below this line, indicating that tonic firing is always more linear. B. Detectability. This was assessed by ROC analysis (see text and figure 6.4 for details). As in A, each point represents a single cell, reflecting its ability to detect the same stimulus during tonic and burst firing. The line of slope 1 is also shown, and every cell falls above this line, indicating that burst firing is always better for stimulus detection.

1995). It should be noted that the difference in spontaneous activity contributes to the difference of the responses, because the higher level during tonic mode (figure 6.2*A* and *C*, top) helps to prevent nonlinearities due to half-wave rectification[4] in the response.

The other prominent difference between response modes illustrated by figure 6.2 is the difference between spontaneous and visually driven activity. That is, the lower spontaneous activity during burst mode coupled with vigorous visual responsiveness during either mode (Guido et al., 1995) suggests that the ratio between signal (visual response) and noise (spontaneous activity) is actually improved during burst mode. This, in turn, suggests that cells in burst mode might be more capable of detecting a stimulus than when in tonic mode. This possibility has been tested formally by using techniques of signal detection theory to create receiver operating characteristic curves for responses during tonic and burst mode; these curves test the ability of the cell to detect a visual stimulus against background noise (Green & Swets, 1966; Macmillan & Creelman, 1991). Figure 6.4 shows how this technique is used to assess stimulus detectability for burst and tonic firing. As shown in figure 6.3*B*, every geniculate cell so tested displays considerably better detection of the visual stimuli when in burst mode than when in tonic mode (Guido et al., 1995). Furthermore, the more difficult a stimulus is to detect (e.g., stimuli of lower contrast), the greater the detection advantage of the burst over the tonic mode. This is because a less salient stimulus would produce a smaller response during tonic mode, but such a stimulus, if detectable, would provide nearly the same response during burst mode as would a more salient stimulus.

---

4. A visual stimulus can be excitatory, inhibitory, or both. For instance, the sine wave grating in figure 6.1 would excite an on-center geniculate cell when the bright half of each cycle falls across the receptive field center, and it would inhibit the same cell when the dark half of each cycle falls across the receptive field center. Passage of a full cycle of the sine wave across the receptive field thus would produce an alternating increase and decrease in firing of the geniculate cell. To encode the full response to a complete cycle of the stimulus linearly would require that the spontaneous activity be high enough to permit a sculpting out of the inhibitory phase of the response. Put another way, negative firing rates (i.e., below zero) cannot be relayed to cortex, and if there is too little spontaneous activity, the inhibitory responses will be clipped and not relayed. In the extreme case of no spontaneous activity, only the responses to the excitatory half of the stimulus are relayed to cortex, and this is half-wave rectification, which is a significant nonlinearity.

*R*eceiver *O*perating *C*haracteristic Analysis

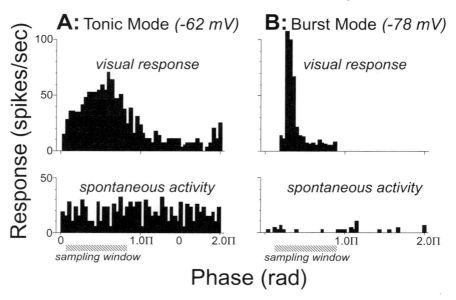

A: Tonic Mode *(-62 mV)*

B: Burst Mode *(-78 mV)*

visual response

visual response

spontaneous activity

spontaneous activity

sampling window

sampling window

Response (spikes/sec)

Phase (rad)

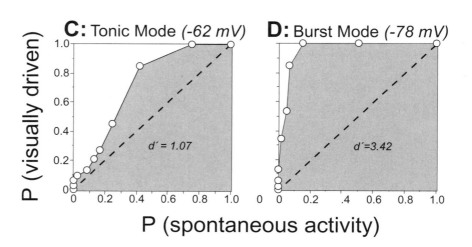

C: Tonic Mode *(-62 mV)*

D: Burst Mode *(-78 mV)*

$d' = 1.07$

$d' = 3.42$

P (visually driven)

P (spontaneous activity)

Figure 6.4

Example of signal detection estimate based on derivation of receiver operating characteristic (ROC) curves (Green & Swets, 1966; Macmillan & Creelman, 1991). This is another relay cell recorded intracellularly from the lateral geniculate nucleus of a lightly anesthetized cat. As in figure 6.2, current injection was applied to create either tonic firing (A, C) or burst firing (B, D). The histograms in A and B represent responses to a drifting grating and spontaneous activity based on averaging responses to many trials, as in figure 6.2. Under the histograms and roughly centered on the peak of the visual response are shown the sampling windows. These represent the time periods during each stimulus trial during which spikes are counted; an equivalent period is also used to count spikes during spontaneous activity. From these counts, the ROC curves in C and D are constructed. These curves represent the cumulative probabilities that at least a criterion number of spikes, from zero to the largest number found in any sampling window for any single trial, will be found in each window, and this is calculated for each of the criterion numbers of spikes. Thus, for a low criterion number of spikes (e.g., 0) the probabilities of finding at least that number are high (e.g., 1), and vice versa for a high criterion number. The probabilities seen during spontaneous activity are plotted against those seen during visual responses. The line of slope 1 is also shown in each ROC curve, and this represents the locus of probabilities for which the cell's responses to a visual stimulus are no better at signaling the presence of that stimulus than are the cell's responses during spontaneous activity, when no stimulus is present. The extent to which the curves lie above the line of slope 1 provides a reliable estimate of the ability of the cell to detect the specific visual stimulus used. From the area under the curve, a value (d') can be computed that reflects detectability (Green & Swets, 1966; Macmillan & Creelman, 1991).

Besides the differences in linear summation and signal detection, the response mode has an effect on temporal tuning. Geniculate neurons firing in tonic mode respond to a broader range of temporal frequencies than do the same cells firing in burst mode (Mukherjee & Kaplan, 1995). That is, in tonic mode, geniculate cells in the cat respond well to the lowest temporal frequencies of visual stimulation and continue to respond as temporal frequency increases until the resolution limit is approached; in burst mode, the cells respond poorly if at all to very low temporal frequencies (<1 Hz), respond best to middle frequencies (~4 Hz), and respond poorly if at all to higher frequencies (>10 Hz). This 10-Hz limit is determined by the time dependency of I_T de-inactivation, which is about 100 msec, thereby creating a 100-msec-long refractory period for the low threshold Ca^{2+} spike. In engineering terms, this means that cells in tonic mode behave as low-pass temporal filters, while those in burst mode act as band-pass filters. This difference suggests that, in burst mode, geniculate cells respond more selectively to sudden changes in the visual world and will not respond well to static images or gradual changes.

In any case, it is clear that both response modes efficiently relay visual information to cortex. Burst mode is better for initial detection of stimuli. This may be effective during visual search when the less accurate analysis permitted by the nonlinear responses is nonetheless sufficient for target acquisition. It may also be useful when attention is directed elsewhere (e.g., to another part of visual space or to another sensory modality or during drowsy periods of relative inattention) as a sort of "wake up" call for novel and potentially interesting or dangerous stimuli. This notion is in many ways similar to the "searchlight" hypothesis for burst firing first advanced by Crick (1984) in relation to the possible function of the thalamic reticular nucleus in attention.

The nonlinear distortion associated with burst mode suggests that, while the stimulus can be readily detected, it will not be as accurately analyzed while the relay is in this mode. Tonic mode, with its more linear relay of visual information, would permit more faithful signal analysis. The differences between these response modes in temporal tuning (Mukherjee & Kaplan, 1995) are also consistent with this hypothesis, because the low-pass tuning during tonic mode would effectively relay information contained in lower temporal frequencies that result from stimuli being fixated or tracked and thus imaged fairly stably on the retina, which would be expected for stimuli analyzed in detail. Sudden changes in the visual world (e.g., the appearance of a novel stimulus) or visual search would not have much representation of low temporal frequencies, so if cells in burst mode are concerned with such tasks, they need not be sensitive to these lower frequencies.

6.B.1.b. Extent of Bursting

As noted in the preceding discussion, bursting becomes relatively rare in thalamic relay cells during wakefulness, but there are two reasons why many estimates of burst levels may be low. First, data are often analyzed during periods when there is no visual stimulus for cells of the lateral geniculate nucleus (or equivalent stimulus for other relays), and so the only responses that permit identification of burst or tonic mode occur during what is known as spontaneous activity. However, the level of spontaneous activity is lower during burst mode (see figure 6.2 and Guido et al., 1995). This means that a cell in burst mode is generally silent during no visual (or other) stimulation, emitting rare bursts, and these periods of silence would not be counted as bursts. However, if the cell were presented with a visual stimulus during one of these silent periods, it would respond with a burst. Second, recent evidence indicates that natural scenes evoke considerably more bursting than do simple geometric visual stimuli or white noise (Lesica & Stanley, 2004). Therefore, in the more natural situation, when an animal is exploring visual space under more physiological conditions, bursting may be much more prevalent than current estimates suggest.

6.B.2. Responses of Relay Cells of Other Thalamic Nuclei

Such analyses of and speculations about firing modes for thalamic nuclei other than the lateral geniculate nucleus have not yet appeared in the literature. For other sensory relay nuclei, it is a fairly simple matter to extrapolate these ideas from vision to audition or somesthesis. For example, a change or sudden appearance in a somatosensory stimulus would be better detected during burst firing, but the detailed and accurate analysis of such a stimulus would be better accomplished when the relay cells fired in tonic mode.

Indeed, analysis of spontaneous activity in widespread areas of the thalamus, including somatosensory and motor relays, shows that arrhythmic bursting is present in ventral posterior cells of awake, behaving rats (Nicolelis et al., 1995; Fanselow et al., 2001; Nicolelis & Fanselow, 2002) and rabbits (Swadlow & Gusev, 2001; Swadlow et al., 2002), in medial geniculate cells of guinea pigs (Massaux & Edeline, 2003; Massaux et al., 2004), and in various thalamic relays in humans (Lenz et al., 1998; Radhakrishnan et al., 1999).

Furthermore, in addition to these analyses of spontaneous activity, there has been limited study of evoked responses in thalamic relays of behaving animals outside the lateral geniculate nucleus. For instance, auditory stimuli evoke bursts in the medial geniculate nucleus of behaving guinea pigs, and, as for lateral geniculate cells, these auditory neurons show more bursting as the animal's behavioral state moves from alert through drowsy to slow-wave sleep (Massaux & Edeline, 2003; Massaux et al., 2004). Also, these medial geniculate cells show tighter tuning for sound frequencies during burst firing than during tonic firing (Massaux et al., 2004), which is analogous to the above-mentioned difference for temporal tuning between firing modes for lateral geniculate cells (Mukherjee & Kaplan, 1995). Finally, bursts are associated with whisking in the ventral posterior medial nucleus of rats (Nicolelis et al., 1995; Fanselow & Nicolelis, 1999).

The above-mentioned hypothesis for lateral geniculate neurons, that burst firing is used as a "wake up call" to shift attention and that tonic firing is used for a more complete analysis of the visual scene, could even be extrapolated to thalamic relay nuclei in general. To the extent that all thalamic nuclei relay driving input to cortex, the hypothesis would suggest that any change in the pattern or sudden appearance of a novel or unexpected driving input would be detected better when the postsynaptic relay cells responded in burst mode, and that tonic firing provides more accurate representation of the driving patterns of input in information relayed to cortex. What is vitally needed is experimental testing of this idea to support or reject this notion of the possible role of response mode in relaying information to cortex. Indeed, experimental data on burst and tonic firing of thalamic relay cells during normal behavior are likely to prove crucial to our understanding of thalamic functions.

This idea can naturally be extended to higher order thalamic relays, which receive their driving afferents from layer 5 of cortex itself (see chapter 8 and figure 8.1 for further details). The higher order thalamic relays can be expected to use the burst and tonic modes in the same way as the first order relays, but now in the transfer of information passing from one cortical area to a second. A burst mode in a higher order relay might then represent a state that is ready for sudden shifts in the pattern of outputs coming from the relevant driver afferents that arise from layer 5 pyramidal cells in the first cortical area. These shifts would serve as a "wake up call" so that the second cortical area, the target cortex of the higher order thalamic relay, could then, via its layer 6 efferents, switch the mode of the relay to tonic firing so that a more faithful record of the message sent from the first cortical area via its layer 5 efferents could be transferred to the second cortical area. It is to be noted that this is a function that may be characteristic of the transthalamic corticocortical relay but not of the direct corticocortical relay. In this context, it is interesting that there seems to be more bursting in higher order than in first order relays (Ramcharan et al., 2005).

6.C. Effect of Response Mode on Transmission from Relay Cells to Cortical Cells

6.C.1. Paired-Pulse Effects in Thalamocortical Synapses

The previous section emphasized the possible effects of response mode on the different attributes of information that might be relayed to cortex:

better linearity during tonic firing and better signal detection during burst firing. An additional and potentially very important issue relates to the possible consequence of these two firing modes for transmission across thalamocortical synapses. This issue arises because interspike intervals differ in burst and tonic mode and, as described in chapter 5, there is evidence that many synapses in the brain, including thalamic and cortical synapses, behave in a frequency dependent manner (Thomson & Deuchars, 1994, 1997; Lisman, 1997; Thomson, 2000a, 2000b; Chung et al., 2002; Thomson & West, 2003; Reichova & Sherman, 2004). In particular, the geniculocortical synapses in layer 4 studied in vitro in the cat show paired-pulse depression (see chapter 5) (Stratford et al., 1996). Also, evidence exists for paired-pulse depression for the layer 4 thalamocortical synapses from in vivo studies of the pathway from the ventral posterior nucleus to somatosensory cortex in the rabbit (Swadlow & Gusev, 2001) and rat (Castro-Alamancos & Connors, 1996; Chung et al., 2002) and of the pathway from the ventral lateral nucleus to motor cortex in the rat (Castro-Alamancos & Connors, 1996). One in vitro study also described paired-pulse depression for layer 6 thalamocortical synapses in the rat somatosensory system (Beierlein & Connors, 2002).

Such paired-pulse depression for thalamocortical synapses becomes important in the context of response mode of thalamocortical cells. The issue is the size of the EPSP created by a thalamocortical synapse, and how this size might vary with the response mode of the thalamic cell. This has important implications, because the action that thalamic relay cells can have on their postsynaptic cortical cells will depend on the firing mode of thalamic relay cells.

6.C.2. Relationship of Response Mode to Paired-Pulse Effects

Of special interest here is the interaction of response mode, burst or tonic, and the paired-pulse depression seen at the thalamocortical synapse. To appreciate this, we must first consider the difference between response modes in the pattern of evoked action potentials. Figure 6.5 shows the difference in interspike interval patterns between firing modes. For burst firing, the first spike in a burst (lower right clusters in the histograms of figure 6.5, in gray shading) is characterized by a long silent interval preceding it and a short interval following it. The long silent preceding period occurs because the evoked burst results from a low threshold Ca^{2+} spike that requires activation of I_T; for this to happen, I_T must first be de-inactivated, which requires sustained hyperpolarization lasting for 100 msec or so; sustained hyperpolarization means no firing

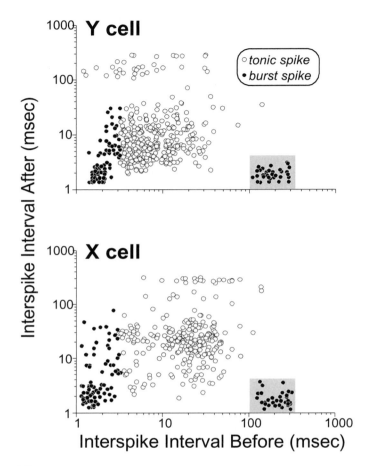

Figure 6.5
Examples of two-dimensional interspike interval plots for two representative cells, one X and one Y, of an anesthetized cat's lateral geniculate nucleus, based on extracellular recording. The abscissa plots the interval to the previous action potential, and the ordinate plots the interval to the next one, with each symbol representing an individual action potential. Action potentials during tonic and burst firing are shown separately. Note that there is distinct clustering in these patterns. See text for further details.

during that period, and thus the prior silent period can be explained. The short interval following is a reflection of the high firing rate of the burst. In any case, the important point here is that the long silent period before the burst ensures that any depression of the thalamocortical synapse will be relieved. That is, a glance at figure 5.3 (page 187) shows that depression in such synapses lasts for only about 100 msec or so. The end result is that a burst occurs only at times that the thalamocortical synapse shows no depression, and thus the EPSP evoked by the first spike in the burst will be of maximal amplitude. Following spikes in the burst will show depressed EPSPs, but they occur with such high frequency that temporal summation will occur, and the overall result is a very large composite EPSP resulting from a burst.

In contrast, the temporal properties of tonic firing (represented by open circles in the histograms) are such that they would result in depression of the synapse. Most of the interspike intervals during tonic firing are between 10 and 30 msec, and, as indicated by figure 5.3, these intervals would produce profound synaptic depression. Thus, while this analysis predicts that burst firing should produce a large EPSP in cortex, tonic firing would produce a relatively small one.

Evidence from the behaving rabbit shows this prediction to be valid for the input from the ventral posterior nucleus to somatosensory cortex. That is, during combined recording of a thalamic relay cell and its postsynaptic target in layer 4 of cortex, the probability that a presynaptic action potential elicits one in the postsynaptic cell is many times greater for the first action potential of a burst than for a tonic action potential, and when subsequent action potentials are factored in, the difference is even greater (Swadlow & Gusev, 2001). Furthermore, current source density analysis with the same behaving rabbit preparation indicates that a burst firing provides a much larger activation of cortex that extends further from layer 4 into other layers than does tonic firing (Swadlow et al., 2002). Thus, burst firing punches through to cortex more extensively than does tonic firing, and this is consistent with the above-mentioned hypothesis that burst firing serves as a sort of "wake up" call.

Note that this analysis and the experimental evidence relate to a thalamocortical synapse that shows paired-pulse depression. What if some of these synapses instead show paired-pulse facilitation? Although there is no evidence for this as yet, the point can be made that, even for such a synapse, burst firing is better. That is, the high frequency firing within a burst ensures that such a synapse will show maximum facilitation (see figure 5.2, page 184). Tonic firing, however, has interspike intervals (mostly 10–30 msec) that are mostly too long to provide much facilitation (see figure 5.3). The beauty of burst firing is that the silent period before the burst ensures that a synapse showing paired-pulse depression is not depressed, while the high frequency of the burst itself ensures that a facilitating synapse will be facilitated. For tonic firing, the interspike intervals are mostly too short to relieve depression and yet too long to provide much facilitation. By any measure, then, we predict that burst firing will provide a much stronger postsynaptic response in cortex than will tonic firing. This is considered further below in section 6.D.

The thalamocortical inputs to layer 6 cells are of particular interest, because layer 6 cells provide the feedback modulatory input from cortex to thalamus. It is not clear whether all thalamocortical axons contact layer 6 cells. Nor is it known whether the layer 6 cells that receive thalamic afferents are the ones that project to thalamus, since only some of the cells in layer 6 project to thalamus (see chapter 3). We also need to know how generally these synapses show paired-pulse depression (Beierlein & Connors, 2002) These are other issues that need experimental study. There has also been very little study of the synaptic properties of the thalamocortical input to layer 6, although one in vitro study in the mouse somatosensory system reported paired-pulse depression for these synapses (Beierlein & Connors, 2002), which is thus similar to the layer 4 thalamocortical input.

If any thalamocortical axons do innervate corticothalamic cells in layer 6, a particularly interesting possibility exists that is most simply described for geniculocortical interactions but would also work in a similar way for other thalamocortical systems. The topography of the corticothalamic projection, including reticular (or interneuron) involvement is critical here, and not completely understood. However, the study of Tsumoto et al. (1978) (see also chapter 3, page 127) offers an important clue here. They found that, when they recorded from a geniculate cell in a cat and activated layer 6 in visual cortex with glutamate delivered from a second recording pipette, the effect on the geniculate cell depended on the relative topographic arrangement of the cortical and thalamic sites. If the receptive fields at both sites overlapped, the effect of activating layer 6 on the geniculate cell was excitory; if the receptive fields were slightly offset, the effect was inhibitory; and if the receptive fields were entirely separate, there was no effect. This suggests a sort of arrangement of the corticothalamic input as described by figure 6.6C.

As noted in section 6.D.2 below, the layer 6 feedback from cortex is especially important in the control of response mode. Namely, the direct cortical input to relay cells looking at the same part of visual field activates metabotropic glutamate receptors, which would have the effect of inactivating the T channels and promoting tonic firing, and the indirect input via cells of the thalamic reticular nucleus could activate sufficiently strong inhibition in relay cells looking at the adjacent, surrounding part of visual field to remove inactivation of the T channels and promote burst firing (see section 6.D.2 and figure 6.7C).

If even part of the reciprocal connections between thalamus and layer 6 of cortex work this way, it suggests the following, albeit presently speculative, scenario (see figure 6.7). When a part of the visual field (region a in figure 6.7A) contains nothing novel or likely to activate receptive fields of geniculate cells looking there, but a neighboring region does (region b), the former evokes little activity in its associated cortical column (column a), while the neighboring region will promote strong firing in its cortical column (column b in figure 6.7A). Thus the layer 6 feedback pathway is relatively silent in column a but active in column b. There will also be some inhibition of cell a from column b through the TRN, and this will put cell a in burst mode. The result is that the geniculate relay cell innervating column a (cell a) is primed to fire in burst mode, while the nearby geniculate cell innervating column b (cell b) fires in tonic mode. This will have the effect that any significant excitatory stimulus suddenly appearing in the receptive field of cell a will evoke a low-threshold Ca^{2+} spike and a burst, which will readily be detected by column a. The burst strongly activates the layer 6 cell in column a, which in turn inactivates the T current in cell a, promoting tonic firing (figure 6.7B). This will also serve to hyperpolarize and promote burst firing in cell b as the activating stimulus for its receptive field diminishes. The result of this "wake up call" would be to switch the thalamocortical pattern to that illustrated in figure 6.7C.

6.D. Control of Response Mode

In the first section of this chapter we suggested that the different tonic or burst response modes provide different advantages in the relay of visual information through the lateral geniculate nucleus to cortex. Tonic firing enhances linearity in the relay and is thus better suited for signal analysis; burst firing enhances signal detection. We can thus suggest from

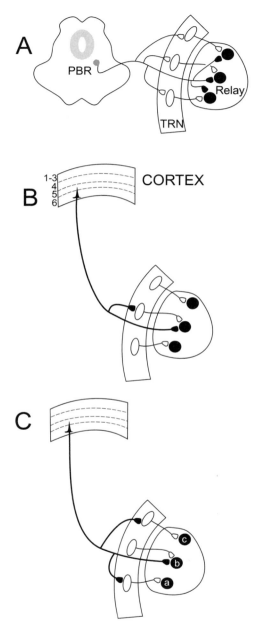

Figure 6.6
Functional circuitry of modulator inputs to thalamic relay cells (relay) from the parabrachial region (PBR) and cortex. These modulatory inputs also innervate the thalamic reticular nucleus (TRN). *A*. Parabrachial innervation. Because this

innervation has little topography for individual axons, and because the action of parabrachial input is to inhibit reticular cells and excite relay cells, the overall effect on relay cells is straightforward to predict. This is direct excitation and indirect disinhibition, leading overall to frank excitation. B. Feedforward inhibition from corticothalamic inputs. In this model, individual cortical axons excite a reticular cell and the postsynaptic relay cell target of that reticular cell. This leads to both direct excitation and indirect inhibition of the relay cell. While this might have little overall effect on membrane potential, the increased synaptic conductance will reduce the gain of the driver input (Chance et al., 2002). C. More complex corticothalamic circuitry. Here an individual corticothalamic axon innervates reticular cells and relay cells in a pattern where the latter is not targeted by the former. The result is direct excitation only for some relay cells and indirect inhibition only for others nearby. Evidence for this arrangement exists (Tsumoto et al., 1978). See text for details.

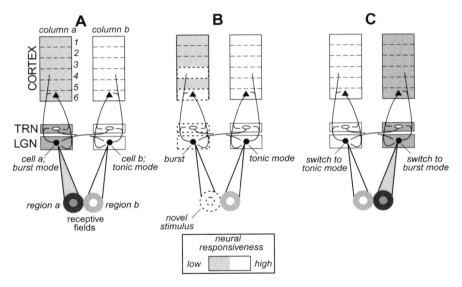

Figure 6.7
Speculative scenario for possible control of geniculate firing mode by visual cortex. Shown are two nearby columns (columns a and b) that are mapped to nearby regions (regions a and b) of the visual field. The geniculate relay cells innervating each column thus have receptive fields in the appropriate regions of the visual field. A. Cell b is in tonic mode and responding to ongoing visual stimulation, activating cortical column b, while nearby cell a is unstimulated and in burst mode, and thus cortical column a is relatively quiet. B. A novel stimulus to cell a elicits a burst, which then strongly drives cortical column a. C. The new activity in column a results in strong firing of the layer 6 corticogeniculate axons. This directly depolarizes cell a, causing it to switch to tonic mode, while it hyperpolarizes cell b through reticular circuitry, causing cell b to switch to burst mode. See text for further details.

the above that geniculate relay cells switch between tonic and burst firing modes depending on the state of the visual system or of the animal. That is, the response mode of the relevant geniculate relay cells would depend on whether that part of the animal's visual system is involved in signal analysis or detection, whether the animal is attending to other visual or other sensory stimuli, or whether the animal is more or less alert. This does not imply that detection of novel visual stimuli during burst mode is better but that burst mode helps overcome the reduced ability to detect such changes during inattention. When attention is focused on a target, detection is no longer a priority, and tonic mode dominates; this provides the advantages of a more linear, faithful thalamic relay. Tonic firing also reduces cortical activation compared to burst firing, on average, and this may be because a more linear signal varies between small and large to encompass a typical stimulus, while the nonlinear burst may always activate cortex maximally. This hypothesis about the functional significance of the burst and tonic modes can also be readily extended to other thalamic relays. For this to be plausible, there must be a ready means for modulatory inputs to control these response modes. This can be accomplished through effects on the membrane potential of relay cells, since the low-threshold Ca^{2+} conductance underlying the burst mode is voltage dependent. Both brainstem and cortical inputs can do this, although, as noted above, cortex does this with local sign, whereas brainstem acts more globally. Other factors, discussed below, could also contribute to control of the response mode, and these may also be influenced by brainstem or cortical inputs.

6.D.1. Brainstem Control

The largest brainstem input to the lateral geniculate nucleus derives from cholinergic cells in the parabrachial region, and this is the brainstem input that has been most studied. Electrical activation of the parabrachial region in vivo causes dramatic switching of geniculate relay cells from burst to tonic mode (Lu et al., 1993). Likewise, in vitro application of acetylcholine eliminates low threshold spiking, causing bursting cells to fire in tonic mode (McCormick, 1989, 1992). Since activation of parabrachial or cortical inputs switches firing mode from burst to tonic, it seems likely that inactivation of these pathways does the opposite, but this remains to be tested empirically.

As noted in chapter 5, parabrachial inputs to the lateral geniculate nucleus activate both ionotropic (nicotinic) and metabotropic (muscarinic) receptors on relay cells. Because membrane voltage changes must be maintained for ≥ 50–100 msec to produce a significant change in the inactivation state of the low-threshold Ca^{2+} conductance underlying burst firing, and because EPSPs produced by activation of the metabotropic receptors are sufficiently long to produce this inactivation state, but those activated via ionotropic receptors are not, it seems likely that it is activation of the metabotropic (muscarinic) receptors that is crucial to this control of response mode (see chapter 5).

Other brainstem inputs to thalamic relay cells that were noted in chapter 3 include noradrenergic axons from the parabrachial region, serotonergic axons from the dorsal raphé nucleus, and histaminergic axons from the tuberomamillary nucleus. These inputs appear to activate only metabotropic receptors on relay cells, so it seems likely that activation of these other inputs is also well suited to creating the lengthy changes in membrane potential needed to control response mode. As noted in chapter 5, activation of noradrenergic or histaminergic inputs evokes long, slow EPSPs in relay cells, and this promotes tonic firing. Also, in vivo activation of the tuberomamillary nucleus, the source of the histaminergic inputs, increases visual responsiveness of lateral geniculate cells in the cat and causes them to fire more in tonic mode (Uhlrich et al., 2002). Activation of serotonergic inputs may have the opposite effect by directly exciting interneurons and/or reticular cells, thereby producing IPSPs in relay cells that could promote burst firing. However, while it seems likely that these inputs can control response mode, there is as yet no direct experimental evidence that they actually do so.

Precisely how these inputs may act to control response mode is to an important extent related to their innervation patterns. That is, brainstem axons that diffusely innervate the entire thalamus will likely have global effects, with little ability to differentially control specific thalamic regions. Unfortunately, the relevant available evidence for the brainstem inputs, which must be at the single-axon level, is scarce. For instance, if many axons are labeled in a pathway from brainstem to thalamus, connections of individual axons cannot be resolved. The overall global pattern may appear to be diffuse and innervate the entire thalamus. However, it would still be possible that single axons have quite discrete and specific projection patterns, and it is this single-axon pattern that would determine whether or not the pathway can act with local sign (see chapter 3). However, there are some hints in the literature.

Evidence for parabrachial axons indicates that they have much less local sign than do corticogeniculate axons (described below), but they are more specific in innervation patterns than are axons from the dorsal raphé nucleus. In a study of parabrachial axons innervating the lateral geniculate nucleus in cats, Uhlrich et al. (1988) found that most of these axons branch to also innervate other visual thalamic structures (i.e., parts of the pulvinar), but they never innervate nonvisual thalamic nuclei (e.g., the ventral lateral posterior or medial geniculate nuclei). Perhaps others innervate only auditory, somatosensory, or other related thalamic nuclei, but this has not been explicitly demonstrated. The implication is that most parabrachial axons are unimodal in operation, and this is precisely what may be needed to switch firing modes in related thalamic nuclei so that, for instance, relay cells of the lateral geniculate nucleus could be maintained largely in tonic mode, whereas those of the ventral lateral posterior or medial geniculate nuclei would fire mostly in burst mode.

Parabrachial axons innervating the lateral geniculate nucleus typically branch to innervate interneurons and the adjacent thalamic reticular nucleus as well (Cucchiaro et al., 1988; Uhlrich et al., 1988). Figure 6.6A, which omits interneurons for clarity, shows these patterns of connectivity. Although the precise role of the interneurons and the thalamic reticular nucleus in controlling the switch between tonic and burst modes remains to be defined in the alert animal, it should be clear from their connections that they are likely to be intimately involved in the switch, presumably via their activation of metabotropic $GABA_B$ receptors on relay cells. Figure 6.6A shows that activation of parabrachial inputs has an unequivocal effect of depolarizing relay cells, thus promoting tonic firing. This is because these inputs directly excite relay cells and disinhibit them by inhibiting TRN inputs to relay cells (see chapters 3 and 7); although not shown in figure 6.6A, further disinhibition occurs via the inhibition of interneurons by parabrachial inputs.

Individual serotonergic axons from the dorsal raphé nucleus seem to be genuinely diffuse in that each seems to innervate most thalamic nuclei, including large regions of the thalamic reticular nucleus, rather indiscriminately (unpublished observations by N. Tamamaki and S. M. Sherman based on labeling individual axons from the brainstem to their thalamic terminal arbors). Thus this pathway is likely to have global effects on response mode throughout much of thalamus. This may be related to global levels of arousal that would have relatively uniform effects on response mode of relay cells throughout thalamus.

6.D.2. Cortical Control

The role of corticogeniculate input in the control of the response mode has been more difficult to assess in vivo, because electrical activation of this pathway also usually activates geniculocortical axons antidromically, obscuring the interpretation of any orthodromic effects. However, because corticogeniculate inputs are the only ones that activate metabotropic glutamate receptors (i.e., retinogeniculate inputs, which are the only other known glutamatergic input to geniculate relay cells, activate only ionotropic glumatate receptors; see chapter 5), it is possible to mimic activation of the corticogeniculate input fairly specifically by applying agonists for this receptor while recording from the relay cells. When this is done either in vitro (McCormick & Von Krosigk, 1992) or in vivo (Godwin et al., 1996b), geniculate cells switch firing mode from burst to tonic. This presumably results from the prolonged depolarization associated with activation of the metabotropic glutamate receptor, a depolarization that inactivates I_T.

Like brainstem axons, those from cortex also branch to innervate geniculate cells as well as reticular cells and interneurons, so that understanding the role of the corticogeniculate input in the behaving animal must also take into account neural circuits involving these local GABAergic circuits. By definition, the input from visual cortex to the lateral geniculate nucleus is visual in nature, and as far as we can tell, the layer 6 connections to other thalamic nuclei also represent the same modality (i.e., visual, somatosensory, motor, etc.) that is relayed through thalamus. This is probably different from the nature of many of the brainstem inputs to thalamus described above, which are not known to reflect single sensory modalities and may often relate to several modalities or to no identifiable modality, although some may be unimodal (see Uhlrich et al., 1988).

The action of corticogeniculate inputs is more complex and less well understood than that of the parabrachial inputs, and there are two related differences to consider. First, as shown in figure 6.6B and C, no matter what the fine details of corticothalamic innervation are, a widespread increase in corticogeniculate activity will directly depolarize relay cells, but this will also depolarize reticular cells and interneurons, thereby indirectly hyperpolarizing relay cells (see also chapter 3). The end result on relay cells is hard to predict from this alone, although the expected increase in synaptic conductance would have the effect of reducing the relay cell's response to driver input, and thus this acts like a gain control mechanism (Chance et al., 2002). Second, unlike the parabrachial and dorsal raphé inputs, those from cortex show considerable local sign or topographic fidelity (e.g., retinotopic fidelity in the lateral geniculate nucleus). This makes the local details of the connections with relay cells, reticular cells, and interneurons critical, but at present we do not know these details, on which the actual effect on relay cells will depend. Shown in figure 6.6B and C (see also page 127) are two plausible circuits (among many possibilities) to illustrate this point and also to show that we do not know enough about the cortical inputs to understand how they are organized to control response mode. For simplicity, the circuits shown do not include interneurons, but one could easily imagine how important it is to know details of their local connectivity as well. With the circuit of figure 6.6B, activation of the corticogeniculate axon would both directly depolarize and indirectly hyperpolarize the relay cell, so the final effect on membrane potential would be hard to predict, but, as just noted, the increased synaptic conductance will affect gain of the relay.

As noted earlier, the data of Tsumoto et al. (1978) favor the pattern of figure 6.6C. Thus, in terms of controlling response mode, this suggests that activation of layer 6 will promote tonic firing in relay cells looking at the same part of visual field, while near neighbors of these geniculate cells, looking at adjacent parts of the visual field, will be driven to burst firing, and more distant geniculate cells will be unaffected. That is, with the circuit of figure 6.6C, activation of any one corticogeniculate axon would have quite distinct effects on neighboring relay cells: for instance, activation of the corticothalamic axon would indirectly hyperpolarize relay cells a and c, promoting burst firing, while it would simultaneously directly depolarize relay cell b, promoting tonic firing.

Whatever the details of innervation pattern, the high degree of local sign in the corticogeniculate pathway means that it has the potential to control response mode differently for relay cells looking at different parts of the visual field. The pathway may be even more specific in the sense that individual cortical afferents may relate to unique geniculate cell types, such as X versus Y or M versus P, since the evidence presented in chapter 3 suggests that different subpopulations of layer 6 cells project to distinct geniculate layers. What is also potentially interesting about the corticogeniculate control of response mode is that, unlike brainstem inputs, the cortical input represents a sort of feedback pathway, although we do not know the extent of true feedback on a cell-by-cell basis (see figure 6.7*B* and *C*). This means that cortex can, in principle, control the response mode of its own afferent supply. The feedback pathway emanates from cortical layer 6, and relay cell axons terminate mainly in cortical layer 4 but with a substantial input into layer 6 as well. Thus the layer 6 feedback appears to lie very close in a hierarchical sense to thalamic inputs, and if we could close this loop—that is, follow in detail the processing steps between thalamic input and the layer 6 cells that innervate thalamus—we would likely to be able to understand more fully how the cortex controls the firing mode of its thalamic inputs.

6.E. Summary

We can now speculate on the possible role of burst and tonic response modes for vision and by extension for other thalamic relays as well. When the animal is not attending to a particular visual stimulus, either because it is searching for a stimulus, attending visually to a different stimulus, attending with another sensory modality, or not attending at all but in a drowsy state, the geniculate relay cells for that particular stimulus will be in burst mode. This suggests that the direct cortical and parabrachial inputs to these geniculate cells are relatively quiet; it could also imply strong activity in cortical inputs to reticular cells innervating these geniculate cells, in the case of topographically organized burst and tonic zones, as suggested by figure 6.6. Note that figures 6.6C and 6.7 suggest that the maps between cortex and the thalamic reticular nucleus may be slightly out of register (see Tsumoto et al., 1978; Pinault & Deschênes, 1998b), but this is still orderly and requires systematic mapping in accord with the published observations of maps in the reticular nucleus (see chapter 9). When in burst mode, the geniculate cell responds to a novel stimulus, one that is potentially interesting or threatening, in a manner that enhances detectability and activation of cortex. The enhanced detection, however, is associated with nonlinear distortion of the relayed signal and is thus unsuitable for accurate stimulus processing. Once novel stimuli or major components of a visual scene activate a previously quiescent cortical column, the layer 6 corticogeniculate neurons also become active and effect a switch in firing from burst to tonic in their geniculate targets, which may also be their geniculate afferents. The tonic firing now enhances linear processing, permitting the visual system to analyze the scene more faithfully, but this is at the expense of stimulus detectability and ability to activate cortex. There are two important further points. First, the enhanced detectability does not imply that an animal is more likely to detect a novel stimulus when attention is reduced (i.e., when bursting is more likely), but rather that burst mode helps overcome the potentially dangerous tendency to miss novel objects when inattentive. Second, the lower cortical activation in tonic mode may simply reflect the fact that, once attended, an object does not need overpowering activation of cortex to be properly analyzed.

Increases in activation of the cholinergic afferents from the parabrachial region would produce comparable results, although the circuitry shown in figure 6.6A suggests that the more active the parabrachial inputs, the more prone the target relay cells would be to fire in tonic mode. We know less about the effects of other afferents, such as serotonergic, noradrenergic, and histaminergic afferents, on response mode, although there is evidence that activation of the noradrenergic, and histaminergic inputs promotes tonic firing, while activation of the serotonergic inputs promotes burst firing. There is also very little evidence yet to suggest what controls the activity of these afferents, although changes between drowsy and alert states are generally associated with changes in activity of brainstem afferents. Although the details are not defined, the actions of these other afferents may serve to allow affective states to influence perception.

At the cellular level, both cortical and brainstem inputs have similar effects, producing long, slow postsynaptic potentials in relay cells via metabotropic receptors. Nonetheless, their roles in controlling response mode are probably quite different, and the difference depends on the connectivity each pathway establishes with thalamic circuitry. We can briefly reiterate some of the conclusions stated earlier as follows. The brainstem inputs, which probably lack local sign, are likely to have global effects on response mode. These inputs are thought to be involved in arousal and in general levels of attention, and as the level of activity in these pathways diminishes, with a related faltering of attention, thalamic relay cells may tend to respond more in burst mode and thus be ready to provide a "wake up call" if something changes significantly in the environment requiring attention. Some of the brainstem inputs may also be related to a single sensory modality, although we are basically ignorant of the specific sorts of messages conveyed by these afferents and just how some particular patterns of sensory stimulation activate these brainstem centers, while others leave them unaffected. Whatever the mechanisms may prove to be, some brainstem afferents described earlier as having a distribution limited to one sensory modality (Uhlrich et al.,

1988) may provide a basis for switching attention between sensory modalities so that when we attend, say, to auditory signals, many relay cells in the medial geniculate nucleus are in tonic firing mode, while most in the visual or somatosensory relays are in burst mode, primed to submit a "wake up call" if their sensory domain changes abruptly.

The cortical input to the lateral geniculate nucleus conveys strictly visual information, and, as noted, it is mapped with great retinotopic precision. Thus its control of response mode would be limited to attentional needs within the visual domain. For instance, if the animal were paying attention to one stimulus (e.g., likely with the fovea or area centralis, but conceivably in peripheral retina), some geniculate cells mapped to nearby regions (and perhaps to much of the rest) of the visual field would be maintained in burst mode, primed to detect any new stimulus of potential interest or danger. Once a group of these thalamic inputs signals a change in the visual scene with bursts, local processing within cortex might lead to increased firing in the layer 6 feedback pathway, and this, in turn, could lead to a switch in firing from burst to tonic for the specific group of relay cells that had been responding in burst mode. This same increased firing of the layer 6 cells might cause very different changes in response mode in nearby geniculate cells, depending on the details of corticoreticular-thalamic circuitry, as depicted in figure 6.6B and C. Indeed, more complex corticothalamic circuitry, such as but not limited to that depicted in figure 6.6C, permits highly specific and local control of response mode by corticothalamic afferents, biasing some relay cells toward burst mode and others toward tonic mode. One can even imagine that a highly active focus of layer 6 output representing a small region of visual space would maintain tonic firing in the retinotopically aligned geniculate relay cells while simultaneously maintaining burst firing in relay cells with receptive field surrounding the target of interest. This could mean that, while tonic firing related to the region of immediate interest optimizes detailed analysis of targets within that area, surrounding areas would be more sensitive to any changes that might require a shift of attention.

Many thalamic relay cells burst rhythmically and in synchrony during certain phases of sleep (Steriade & Llinás, 1988; Steriade et al., 1990; Steriade et al., 1993b), although the extent to which those of the lateral geniculate nucleus do is a matter currently unresolved (McCarley et al., 1983; Ramcharan et al., 2000). Rhythmic, synchronized bursting seems to imply a functional disconnection of these cells from their main afferents, interrupting the thalamic relay. Our suggested role for the burst mode of firing is not incompatible with this other role. We are suggesting that, depending on the animal's behavioral state (e.g., alert or drowsy versus sleeping), burst firing can subserve at least two quite different roles, or perhaps two extremes of one role. It can either provide a relay mode in the awake animal for detecting significant changes in specific afferent activity, and following detection, changes in cortical or brainstem inputs can then be used to switch the relay to tonic mode for more accurate analysis. In the sleeping animal, the burst mode may involve more complete functional shutting off of cortical and parabrachial inputs, more analogous to the in vitro situation where these inputs are physically removed. Then the switch from burst to tonic mode may occur only in response to major stimuli that are threatening or significant for other reasons, such as an infant's cry for the mother. The low levels of activity present in the cortical and parabrachial pathways during the awake state may permit single low threshold spikes and an associated burst of action potentials but prevent rhythmic bursting. Bursting, when rhythmic and synchronized, may provide a positive signal to cortex that nothing is being relayed despite the possible presence of sensory stimuli, and this is less ambiguous than no activity, which could mean either no relay or no stimulus. When the bursting is arrhythmic, cortex can interpret this arrhythmicity as representing responses evoked by sensory stimuli.

6.F. Unresolved Questions

1. What is the differential role of tonic and burst firing for thalamic relays, and what is the significance of this for behavior?

2. Although burst and tonic behaviors have now been found in many thalamic relays, how general is this behavior for relay cells? That is, are these firing modes characteristic of all thalamic relay cells, including those in intralaminar and midline nuclei?

3. What is involved in "closing the loop" between thalamic afferents and layer 6 corticogeniculate cells in feedback control of thalamic response mode? How do the details of corticogeniculate circuitry involving the thalamic reticular nucleus contribute to control of the response mode?

4. Related to question 3, do thalamocortical axons that innervate cells in cortical layer 6 innervate the cells that project back to the thalamus, or only a different subpopulation?

5. Since burst firing is much more effective in driving cortical circuitry than tonic firing, does this imply that bursting more effectively activates the layer 5 outputs that serve as drivers for higher order thalamic relays? In other words, are bursts particularly effective in initiating corticocortical communication through higher order thalamic relays?

6. If bursts indeed serve as a sort of "wake up call," how often would one expect to see bursting in behaving animals, given that such a function may be fairly rarely required?

7 Drivers and Modulators

7.A. Drivers and Modulators in the Lateral Geniculate Nucleus

In earlier chapters we introduced the distinction between drivers and modulators; this concept has also been presented previously (Sherman & Guillery, 1998). Examples of the former are retinal inputs to the lateral geniculate nucleus and medial lemniscal inputs to the ventral posterior nucleus; examples of the latter are various brainstem inputs, the feedback pathway from cortical layer 6, and inputs from local, GABAergic reticular cells and interneurons. Perhaps the most important aspect of this distinction is the now well-documented (see chapter 5) but often overlooked point that the many synaptic inputs to a neuron have distinct postsynaptic actions and that one cannot hope to understand the functional organization of a circuit just by mapping all of the inputs and outputs of that circuit. The nature of synaptic inputs, and in particular whether they are drivers or modulators, or perhaps even either one or the other under differing conditions, is key to this understanding. For example, if we could not identify drivers versus modulators among inputs to relay cells of the lateral geniculate nucleus, we might easily be misled by consideration of the relative numerical strengths of inputs. Since, as we have shown in chapter 3, the brainstem afferents provide more synaptic contacts on relay cells than do the retinal afferents, it would be easy to conclude, in the absence of other information, that the lateral geniculate nucleus relays brainstem information to cortex and not retinal information. In this chapter we attempt to explain more formally what we mean by drivers and modulators and consider the extent to which this distinction applies throughout the thalamus and perhaps even to other parts of the brain. We start by looking specifically at relationships in the lateral geniculate nucleus, because drivers and modulators are most clearly understood there.

It may seem unnecessary to define the driver input for the lateral geniculate nucleus, since it seems obvious to accept retinal afferents for this role, but if we stop to consider why we so readily believe this for the lateral geniculate nucleus, it will be useful in thinking about driver inputs to other, less well-defined thalamic relays. There are two major reasons to be confident that retinal input is the driver for the lateral geniculate nucleus. Both reasons relate to the concept that the driving input conveys to the thalamic nucleus the main form of information to be relayed to cortex.

First, it is clear from clinical and experimental evidence that striate cortex is primarily or exclusively involved with vision, and that its main thalamic innervation arrives from the lateral geniculate nucleus. It is also clear that of the potential sources of subcortical afferent systems innervating all relay cells of the lateral geniculate nucleus (which includes various brainstem sources described in chapter 3), only the retinal afferents are frankly visual. The tectal inputs, which innervate some geniculate laminae, fail the next criterion for identifying a driver, which is based on receptive field properties, because the directionally selective receptive fields of tectal cells cannot readily account for the center/surround properties of the geniculate cells that they innervate. Second, one way to determine the nature of information processed by a sensory neuron is by studying its receptive field properties, and where the receptive field properties can be mostly accounted for by any subset of afferents, these afferents must be considered the drivers. For geniculate relay cells, retinal input is clearly the driver, because the retinal afferents pass their receptive field properties to geniculate relay cells with only minor changes (reviewed in Cleland et al., 1971; Sherman & Spear, 1982; Cleland & Lee, 1985; Shapley & Lennie, 1985; Sherman, 1985; Usrey et al., 1998). It should be noted here that it is not necessary that the postsynaptic cell have virtually the same receptive field properties as their driver inputs, only that the drivers can account for these properties. It happens that geniculate relay cells have virtually the same center/surround receptive fields as do their retinal afferents (see chapter 2, section 2.A.3). However, as we describe later in this chapter, cells in visual cortex have receptive fields that are quite different from their geniculate afferents, but these afferents can nonetheless account for the cortical receptive field properties in layer 4, which is one reason we argue that the geniculate afferents are the drivers for their postsynaptic target cells in cortex.

Although retinal inputs are the only plausible subcortical source of driver input to the lateral geniculate nucleus, a major input to this structure derives from the visual cortex itself. Could corticogeniculate axons provide significant driver input? The best evidence that they do not comes from studies of ablating or otherwise silencing the visual cortex and thus this input. Such studies, and there have been many, have found rather subtle effects of removing this pathway on receptive fields of geniculate neurons (Kalil & Chase, 1970; Richard et al., 1975; Baker & Malpeli, 1977; Schmielau & Singer, 1977; Geisert et al., 1981; McClurkin & Marrocco, 1984; McClurkin et al., 1994; Sillito & Jones, 2002). More recent studies have suggested that the pathway affects temporal properties of relay cell discharges (McClurkin et al., 1994; Godwin et al., 1996b) or establishes correlated firing among nearby relay cells with similar receptive field properties (Sillito et al., 1994). Additional evidence for this conclusion comes from receptive field analysis: the corticogeniculate afferents have elongated receptive fields, with orientation and often direction selectivity, that, like the tectal afferents described above, are unlikely contributors to the center/surround receptive fields of geniculate cells. Overall, the available evidence indicates that the corticogeniculate pathway is modulatory and not a driver input.

If we accept retinal afferents as the drivers, we can begin to explore what other features distinguish drivers from modulators. Table 7.1 summarizes some of the differences between retinal and nonretinal afferents for the lateral geniculate nucleus of the cat. (It also includes information about cortical layer 5 input to higher order relays, an issue that will be taken up later in this chapter.) We shall go on to suggest that these differences between retinal and nonretinal inputs help to distinguish drivers from modulators throughout thalamus. Because of their importance, it is worth considering in detail the 13 criteria listed in table 7.1 for identifying drivers and modulators in the innervation of lateral geniculate relay cells (it should be noted that the driver inputs are the retinal afferents, and the modulator inputs shown are the various nonretinal inputs as listed). Left out for simplicity from modulator inputs to the lateral geniculate nucleus are the less common and less well-characterized modulator inputs, that is, the noradrenergic axons from the parabrachial region, serotonergic axons from the dorsal raphé nucleus, histaminergic axons from the tuberomamillary nucleus, and GABAergic axons from the nucleus of the optic tract (see chapter 3 for details). It is plausible, and perhaps likely, that, as we learn more about these other modulator

Table 7.1
Criteria for Identifying Drivers and Modulators in Lateral Geniculate Nucleus, plus Layer 5 Drivers to Higher Order Relays

Criteria	Retinal (Driver)	Layer 5 to HO (Driver)	Modulator: Layer 6	Modulator: PBR	Modulator: TRN and Interneurons
Criterion 1	Determines relay cell receptive field	*Determines relay cell receptive field	Does not determine relay cell receptive field	Does not determine relay cell receptive field	Does not determine relay cell receptive field
Criterion 2	Activates only ionotropic receptors	Activates only ionotropic receptors	Activates metabotropic receptors	Activates matabotropic receptors	TRN: Activates metabotropic receptors; Int: †
Criterion 3	Large EPSPs	Large EPSPs	Small EPSPs	†	TRN: small IPSPs; Int: †
Criterion 4	Large terminals on proximal dendrites	Large terminals on proximal dendrites	Small terminals on distal dendrites	Small terminals on proximal dendrites	Small terminals, TRN: distal; Int: proximal
Criterion 5	Each terminal forms multiple contacts	Each terminal forms multiple contacts	Each terminal forms single contact	Each terminal forms single contact	Each terminal forms single contact
Criterion 6	Little convergence onto target	Little convergence onto target*	Much convergence onto target	†	†
Criterion 7	Often thick axons	Often thick axons	Thin axons	Thin axons	Thin axons
Criterion 8	Glutamatergic	Glutamatergic	Glutamatergic	Cholinergic	GABAergic
Criterion 9	Synapses show paired-pulse depression (high p)	Synapses show paired-pulse depression (low p)*	Synapses show paired-pulse facilitation	†	†

Criterion 10	Well-localized, dense terminal arbors	Well-localized, dense terminal arbors	Well-localized, dense terminal arbors	Sparse terminal arbors	Well-localized, dense terminal arbors
Criterion 11	Branches innervate subtelencephalic targets	Branches innervate subtelencephalic targets	Subcortically known to innervate thalamus only	†	Subcortically known to innervate thalamus only
Criterion 12	Innervates dorsal thalamus but not TRN	Innervates dorsal thalamus but not TRN	Innervates dorsal thalamus and TRN	Innervates dorsal thalamus and TRN	TRN: both; Int: dorsal thalamus only
Criterion 13	Creates narrow cross-correlogram	†	Creates broad cross-correlogram*	†	†

* Very limited data to date.
† No relevant data available.
Abbreviations: HO, higher order; PBR, parabrachial region; TRN, thalamic reticular nucleus; Int, interneuron; p, probability.

inputs, we will find they share properties with the modulators shown in table 7.1. The criteria are listed in the table in a rough order of perceived importance.

7.A.1. Influence on Receptive Field Properties (Criterion 1)

It is clear that the basic receptive field properties of lateral geniculate relay cells are based on inputs from one or a small number of retinal afferents, and there is indeed little difference in these receptive field properties between retinal axons and relay cells (Hubel & Wiesel, 1961; Cleland et al., 1971; Cleland & Lee, 1985; Mastronarde, 1987a; Usrey et al., 1999; reviewed in Sherman, 1985). That is, the center/surround receptive field of a geniculate relay cell is more like that of its retinal afferent(s) than of afferents from visual cortex or thalamic reticular nucleus. It is very likely quite different from that of any brainstem or hypothalamic afferent, all of which almost certainly lack classical visual center/surround receptive fields. Thus, in terms of receptive field properties, retinal afferents dominate the output of a geniculate relay cell when it is transmitting visual information.[1] In contrast, all the other afferents have relatively little obvious effect on basic, qualitative receptive field properties of the relay cell but instead modulate the input/output relationships to control quantitative features of the relay.

Thus, for relay cells of the lateral geniculate nucleus, we can define drivers as primary transmitters of receptive field properties and modulators as inputs that do not provide the basic receptive field properties to the relay cell. This distinction may also serve for some of the other first order sensory thalamic relays (see chapter 8), such as the ventral posterior nucleus and the medial geniculate nucleus, where receptive field properties of the relay cells are well understood. However, this criterion will not serve to distinguish drivers from modulators in other thalamic nuclei where receptive fields have not been defined. Examples include the medial dorsal nucleus, midline and intralaminar nuclei, much of the pulvinar, and other nuclei. We must consider other features that distinguish drivers from modulators to develop more general criteria, and can again start by considering the lateral geniculate nucleus and using table 7.1 as a starting point.

---

1. This refers to receptive fields seen in the lightly anesthetized or awake preparations, since geniculate relay cells respond quite differently during certain phases of sleep (see section 7.E of this chapter and also Ramcharan et al., 2000).

7.A.2. Postsynaptic Receptors (Criterion 2)

One clear distinction between retinal and nonretinal inputs is that the former activate only ionotropic receptors, whereas the latter activate metabotropic receptors, often in addition to ionotropic receptors (reviewed in Sherman & Guillery, 1998, 2004). Of particular importance here is the observation that, in general, activation of ionotropic receptors evokes a brief postsynaptic potential, while activation of metabotropic receptors evokes a prolonged postsynaptic potential (see chapter 5). The fast, brief EPSPs activated by drivers enables an individual action potential in the driver input to be encoded by one EPSP in the relay cell up to rates of presynaptic firing that begin to evoke temporal summation postsynaptically. Such temporal summation obliterates the one-to-one relationship between action potential and EPSP, but the presence of ionotropic receptors in the absence of metabotropic receptors allows for this to occur at much higher rates of presynaptic firing than would be the case with metabotropic receptors. Put another way, the sustained postsynaptic potentials seen with metabotropic receptors act as low-pass temporal filters that result in the loss of temporal information. Thus, information flow is maximized by having ionotropic receptors only.

The sustained postsynaptic potentials evoked by nonretinal inputs are consistent with their role as modulators. Such sustained postsynaptic potentials imply that the effect on the relay cell is a prolonged shift in responsiveness, a clear modulatory role. Furthermore, as noted in chapter 4, relay cells (like neurons generally) possess a number of voltage and time dependent conductances for which the membrane voltage must be altered for sustained periods (e.g., ~100 msec); examples are I_T, I_A, and I_h. The fast postsynaptic potentials associated with ionotropic receptors are ill-suited to control these conductances, while the sustained postsynaptic potentials associated with the modulators are ideal for this control. Further details about how these metabotropic responses help control I_T are provided in chapter 6, and this serves as an excellent example of the significance of postsynaptic receptors for modulatory functions.

What is not clear, then, is why many modulator inputs also activate ionotropic receptors, nor is it clear whether individual modulatory inputs activate both receptor types or just one. One plausible explanation for the ionotropic receptors here is related to criterion 6 in table 7.1 (see also below): if modulator inputs to a relay cell show considerable convergence, and as long as their firing is not synchronized, their summed postsynaptic potentials should produce sustained changes in membrane potential, which then serve to complement the activation of metabotropic receptors. The advantage of this scenario is that the latency is much shorter for ionotropic receptors (see chapter 5), so the modulation can start earlier, and then the metabotropic response can kick in to sustain the change.

7.A.3. Postsynaptic Potential Amplitude (Criteria 3–5)

As noted in chapter 5, retinogeniculate EPSPs are large and those from corticogeniculate axons are small. In this context, the IPSPs activated from reticular inputs also tend to be small. To date, there have been no reported studies of EPSPs activated from parabrachial or interneuronal sources, and this applies to other thalamic relays as well. The point is that, because driver input represents information to be relayed, it should have secure postsynaptic activation, whereas the subtler modulatory effects of modulation may benefit from smaller postsynaptic potentials that can be more finely graded. It may seem odd at first that retinal input is so dominant in driving the relay cell despite the fact that, as noted in chapter 3, it produces only about 5%–10% of the synapses on the relay cell.

There are at least three ready explanations for the functional dominance of retinal inputs. First, sizes of the retinal contact zones on relay cells tend to be much larger than those of other inputs, and each retinal terminal produces many such zones, whereas most modulator terminals tend to produce only one, and some, such as the histaminergic terminals, seem not to have specialized contact zones at all. Larger, more numerous contacts might lead to more transmitter release and larger EPSPs. Second, retinal terminals are proximally located, where they are more likely to influence the soma and axon hillock, whereas modulator inputs can be distal, although some are proximal. Third, as noted in chapter 5, synapses can vary greatly with respect to the probability that an action potential invading the presynaptic terminal leads to transmitter release (reviewed in Lisman, 1997). Also, the discussion in chapter 5, section 5.A.2, makes the point that paired-pulse depression and facilitation are associated with synapses showing high release probability (high p) and low release probability (low p), respectively. If retinal synapses, which show paired-pulse depression, have, on average, much higher p values than other synapses, then the effective EPSP in a relay cell from an action potential in a retinal axon would consequently be relatively larger than expected from a source providing only 5%–10% of the inputs to that relay cell. For example, if a retinal axon produced, say, 600 synapses on a relay cell, but each had a probability of release of 0.9, then an action potential along that axon would generate release from 540 synapses. If several cortical axons together produced 600 synapses onto the same cell and fired together, but the probability of release of their synapses was only 0.1 (and, as reviewed by Lisman [1997], release probabilities of 0.1 or lower are common in hippocampus and neocortex), then only 60 synapses would be activated. Thus, before we can begin to relate relative synaptic numbers to functional properties, we must know more about synaptic physiology of these inputs than we do at present.

7.A.4. Convergence onto Postsynaptic Target (Criterion 6)

Evidence for the lack of convergence among retinogeniculate afferents is given in chapters 3 and 5. This includes evidence from paired recordings of retinal axons and their geniculate cell targets (Cleland et al., 1971; Cleland & Lee, 1985; Mastronarde, 1987b; Usrey et al., 1999) and evidence that activation of EPSPs from optic tract stimulation is all-or-none (Reichova & Sherman, 2004). Evidence for convergence for cortico-geniculate inputs comes partly from the observation that stimulation of the pathway evokes EPSPs in a graded fashion (Reichova & Sherman, 2004). Also, the fact that there are 10–100 layer 6 axons for each relay cell suggests that there must be considerable convergence (Sherman & Koch, 1986). Again, comparable evidence for parabrachial or reticular cells or interneurons is lacking.

There is a logical explanation for the large number of modulators and the smaller number of driver afferents impinging on any one relay cell. Neuromodulation is likely to be produced by afferents that come from many different sources and that act together to produce a finely graded effect linked to many aspects of the behavioral state, such as alertness and attention; this implies a large number of inputs, each contributing a relatively small effect. Drivers, on the other hand, need a relatively small number of units to carry the basic message to the target level. This is analogous to the situation in many brain structures where the main output message of complex neural computations is carried by very few cells. For instance, in cortex, the number of cells reflecting the output of a column (e.g., the subset of layer 5 cells carrying the results of the columnar computation to subcortical targets) represents a minority of cells in the column.

7.A.5. Axon Diameter (Criterion 7)

For known inputs to geniculate relay cells, the X and Y axons are clearly thicker than any of the modulators, but the retinogeniculate W axons are thinner than the X or Y. Because these observations are mostly qualitative and made at the light microscopic level, it is not clear whether or not the W axons are nonetheless thicker than the various modulator axons. In any case, all of the known modulator axons are thin, and many and perhaps all of the retinogeniculate axons are thicker, some considerably so. Axon diameter is clearly related to conduction velocity, and it may be argued that transmitting signals faster is more important for drivers than for modulators. Axon diameter, however, may have other implications as well, such as the rate that metabolic agents can be transferred from the cell body to the axon terminals, or the number and size of the terminals sustained by the axon, and this could conceivably also impact driver/modulator function. As we noted, the criteria in table 7.1 are listed in order of perceived relevance to the driver/modulator distinction, and it may be that axon diameter is not an important parameter in this context. Of course, this proviso applies increasingly for the other criteria described below.

7.A.6. Transmitters (Criterion 8)

The neurotransmitters involved were described in chapter 5. We argue later in this chapter that IPSPs, and thus inputs using GABA, are poorly suited for driver inputs because they limit the rate of information transfer (Smith & Sherman, 2002). We would thus expect only excitatory neurotransmission to be used by driver inputs. The putative drivers so far suggested are all glutamatergic, although so are some modulators, such as the corticogeniculate input. Whether other transmitters, such as acetylcholine, can be associated with driver inputs remains to be determined.

7.A.7. Paired-Pulse Effects and the Probability of Transmitter Release (Criterion 9)

Again, chapter 5 described paired-pulse depression for retinal inputs and paired-pulse facilitation for cortical inputs. Because these are so closely tied to probability of release (p), it is assumed here that paired-pulse depression is associated with high p values and paired-pulse facilitation, with low p values, and thus p values are not further discussed in this context. There have been no reported studies of paired-pulse effects for the parabrachial or GABAergic inputs. The finding of paired-pulse depression in driver inputs is not easily explained. However, one recent suggestion is that paired-pulse depression plays an important role in information processing by helping the system to adapt to ongoing levels of activity (Chung et al., 2002), and if so, this would be a useful property of driver inputs. As for modulators, since paired-pulse effects have been described so far only for layer 6 inputs (Granseth et al., 2002; Reichova & Sherman, 2004), it is not clear the extent to which this typifies modulators more generally.

7.A.8. Terminal Arbor Morphology (Criterion 10)

As noted in chapter 3, retinogeniculate arbors are relatively compact and dense with terminal boutons. Some modulator inputs, such as those from the parabrachial region, are quite diffuse, bouton-sparse, and spread out, while others, such as corticogeniculate and reticular inputs, are relatively focused. Where detailed information is available, such as for retinogeniculate and corticogeniculate arbors, the former are more compact. The reason for compactness of driver inputs seems clear: these inputs involve detailed mapping of peripheral information from relatively few cells onto relatively few cells, which is in keeping with the arbor morphology. Modulators that have diffuse action, such as the parabrachial axons, are better subserved by diffuse arbors, but the point here is that some modulatory action can be very topographic and require a compact arbor, as is the case with reticular or corticogeniculate inputs. Thus, a driver input requires a well-localized, dense arbor, whereas modulator inputs can have either type of arbor, depending on whether or not the modulatory effects are topographic.

7.A.9. Innervation of the Thalamic Reticular Nucleus (Criterion 11)

The evidence for innervation of the thalamic reticular nucleus was given in chapter 3. Retinal inputs innervate the main layers of the lateral geniculate nucleus but do not innervate the thalamic reticular nucleus. Both layer 6 corticogeniculate and parabrachial axons branch to innervate the lateral geniculate nucleus and thalamic reticular nucleus. The last column requires some explanation: reticular cells can have axons that branch to innervate their neighbors as well as the main layers of the lateral geniculate nucleus, so they fit this "modulator pattern," but interneurons only innervate locally.

That retinal input activates principally only relay cells within thalamus and generally not modulator circuits, such as those involving the thalamic reticular nucleus, suggests that the information to be relayed to cortex by itself does not control the transmission (i.e., modulatory) properties of the relay. Then, modulation becomes initiated only by the appropriate sources initiated in cortex or brainstem and partly played through the local GABAergic circuits. One problem with this view is that driver inputs to thalamus activate interneurons as well as relay cells.

7.A.10. Extrathalamic Targets (Criterion 12)

The evidence for this was raised in chapter 3 and is discussed further in chapter 10. Most or all retinal axons that innervate the lateral geniculate nucleus branch to innervate the midbrain. To date, layer 6 corticogeniculate axons have been found to innervate only the thalamus subcortically, although they also provide local branches within cortex. Both reticular cells and interneurons innervate only thalamus. The situation with parabrachial axons is less clear. The few single axons traced from the parabrachial region innervated thalamus only (Uhlrich et al., 1988). However, because of the widespread innervation by parabrachial cholinergic axons throughout the forebrain, the possibility exists that many such axons branch to innervate thalamus as well as other targets.

The significance of driver inputs branching to also innervate extra-diencephalic targets identified mostly as "motor" has been discussed elsewhere (see chapter 10; see also Guillery & Sherman, 2002b; Guillery, 2003). This gets to the very nature of driver inputs to thalamic relays, the suggestion being that they convey a copy of motor instructions. Modulators, in contrast, may largely be concerned only with acting on thalamic relays.

7.A.11. Cross-Correlograms Resulting from Input (Criterion 13)

The functional linkage between retinal afferents and their target geniculate relay cells involves more than the structure of their receptive fields. During simultaneous recording of a geniculate relay cell and one of its retinal afferents, a close temporal correspondence is seen in the action potentials in these connected cells (Cleland et al., 1971; Cleland & Lee, 1985; Mastronarde, 1987b; Usrey et al., 1999): most retinal action potentials are followed with a fixed latency by one in the relay cell. This is graphically evident when a cross-correlogram is constructed showing the temporal relationship between the action potentials in the two cells.[2] Such a cross-correlogram has a relatively narrow peak, with a latency of several milliseconds and a relatively low, flat baseline (figure 7.1A and C).

There are several criteria that the EPSPs from an afferent must meet to produce a sharp, narrow peak in the cross-correlogram. One criterion is that there be relatively little latency variation in the EPSP, because this would tend to smear the peak. Another concerns the relationship between the EPSP duration and frequency. As long as the EPSP duration is briefer than the interspike interval of the afferent, there will be no temporal summation in the evoked response. With no temporal summation, the peak of the cross-correlogram will be closely related to the duration of individual EPSPs, but if temporal summation occurs, the peak will again be smeared. Therefore, the briefer EPSP related to activation of ionotropic receptors (see table 7.1 and chapter 5) allows the production of a narrow peak with moderate rates of afferent firing, whereas the longer EPSPs related to activation of metabotropic receptors would smear already lengthy EPSPs to produce an even broader peak.

From the point of view of signal transmission, there is an important distinction to be drawn between a narrow peak and less temporal summation and a broader peak with more temporal summation. With more temporal summation, individual input spikes are no longer clearly resolved in the transmitted signal, since summation creates a single, broader EPSP. In fact, only if individual action potentials in the retinal

---

2. Such a cross-correlogram is constructed by computing for each retinal action potential the probability that an action potential is seen in the relay cell as a function of time, typically looking for several hundred milliseconds before and after the retinal action potential, which is set at time zero. This is repeated for every retinal action potential, and an average histogram is then constructed. This histogram is the cross-correlogram. Consider what would be expected if most retinal spikes evoked one spike at a fairly constant latency in the postsynaptic relay cell, and very few other spikes were seen postsynaptically. This cross-correlogram would have a large peak at a time after zero that reflects transmission time of the retinal action potential from the recording site to the terminals in the lateral geniculate nucleus plus synaptic delay (e.g., several milliseconds, depending on the recording site), and the width of the peak would reflect synaptic "jitter." There would be very few events in the cross-correlogram outside of this peak. See Fetz et al. (1991) and Nelson et al. (1992) for a further discussion of cross-correlograms.

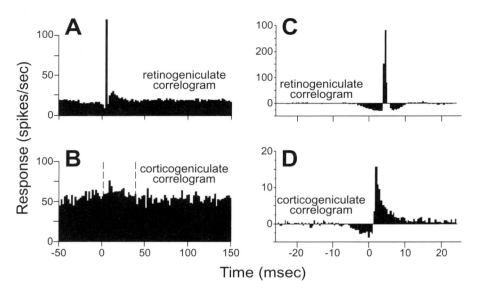

Figure 7.1

Cross-correlograms displaying the difference between drivers and modulators. Each is based on simultaneous recordings in cats from two neurons, one presynaptic to the other. The cross-correlograms represent the firing of the postsynaptic cells relative to a spike at time zero for the presynaptic cell. *A*. Retinogeniculate cross-correlogram based on spontaneous activity in both the retinal and geniculate neurons. Note the narrow peak rising out of a flat, low baseline that marks this as a driver connection. (Redrawn from figure 3*A* of Mastronarde, 1987a, by permission of the publisher.) *B*. Corticogeniculate cross-correlogram based on spontaneous activity in both a layer 6 cell in area 17 and geniculate neuron. Glutamate was applied to cortex to enhance the spontaneous firing of the afferent cell. Between the vertical dashed lines it is possible to discern a very gradual, prolonged, and small peak arising from a noisy, high baseline that marks this as a modulator connection. (Redrawn from figure 2*A* of Tsumoto et al., 1978, by permission of the publisher.) *C* and *D*. Cross-correlograms taken from the same laboratory using identical techniques for easier comparison. Both are based on visually driven activity and involve a "shuffle correction" (Perkel et al., 1967), and they are normalized against the firing level of the afferent, which is why some bins fall below zero. Both represent driver inputs and include another retinogeniculate pair (*C*) plus a geniculocortical pair (*D*). Note the difference in vertical scale, indicating that the retinal input accounts for more postsynaptic spikes in the geniculate cell (*C*) than does the geniculate input to the layer 4 cell of striate cortex (*D*). Note also that the time represented by these cross-correlograms is much briefer than that for *A* and *B*. Nonetheless, both cross-correlograms have narrow peaks rising from a flat, low baseline, marking them as driver inputs. Data were kindly provided by the authors for replotting. (*C* is redrawn from figure 2 of Usrey et al., 1998, and *D* is redrawn from figure 2 of Reid and Alonso, 1996).

afferent occur with long enough interspike intervals (i.e., during low-frequency firing) will each be correlated with a specific postsynaptic action potential and thus be individually recognized. What this all boils down to has already been mentioned in section 7.A.2: the longer the EPSP, as with metabotropic responses, the more high-frequency information is lost. Conversely, the fact that retinal input activates only ionotropic receptors preserves high-frequency information in the relay to cortex. This is akin to saying that the fast postsynaptic responses to the driver input that are produced by ionotropic receptors act as a broadband temporal filter passing a wide range of frequencies, whereas slower metabotropic responses act as a low-pass temporal filter that fails to pass higher frequencies.

This "driver" cross-correlogram with a narrow peak can be contrasted with the expected one between a relay cell and its modulator input. Unfortunately, examples from the literature of such cross-correlograms are exceedingly rare, and indeed only one is known to us. This is shown in figure 7.1B, and it is a cross-correlogram obtained from a concurrent recording of a layer 6 cortical cell and a target geniculate cell. This shows a small peak with a broad foundation on a high baseline. The difference between this and the retinogeniculate "driver" cross-correlogram of figure 7.1A and C is critical for the distinction between modulators and drivers. It may eventually be necessary to quantify the difference, but at present there is too little relevant evidence for this. We would also predict that other modulatory inputs to geniculate relay cells, such as from brainstem or local GABAergic cells, will exhibit cross-correlograms with relay cells that resemble that in figure 7.1B much more than those in figure 7.1A and C.

The difference between driver and modulator cross-correlograms shown in figure 7.1A–C probably relates to at least two factors. First, as noted earlier, the sharp peak of figure 7.1A and C depends in part on there being no (slow) metabotropic receptors, only ionotropic receptors, activated by retinal afferents on relay cells, whereas in figure 7.1B the corticogeniculate afferents from layer 6 activate metabotropic receptors as well as the ionotropic ones (see table 7.1 and chapter 5). This results in a prolonged EPSP with a long and relatively variable latency, and one would expect such an EPSP to promote prolonged firing of the relay cell, with individual action potentials in the postsynaptic cell not clearly related to specific action potentials in the cortical afferent. Second, there are likely to be many modulators but few drivers for any one relay cell. With little convergence of the driver retinogeniculate afferents, the postsynaptic responses of the relay cell to any one driver will be relatively strong and well synchronized to it. In contrast, the modulators, such as layer 6 corticogeniculate afferents, show significant convergence (see above), and the effect of any one modulator, possibly one of hundreds, may be minuscule. Furthermore, unless the modulator inputs from cortex fire in a highly synchronized manner, which seems unlikely in the normal, behaving animal, the postsynaptic action potentials will not be synchronized to those of any one corticogeniculate afferent. Either or both of these two factors can contribute to the differences seen between the driver cross-correlogram of figure 7.1A and C and the modulator example of figure 7.1B.

A driver, if it is to drive, must produce a distinct, measurable effect. The quantitative relationships of putative drivers to their postsynaptic neurons will almost certainly prove important, and the extent to which any one driver in any other thalamic relay can actually produce a cross-correlogram as sharp as that in figure 7.1A and C is untested and is likely to be a useful feature to explore. Since modulatory inputs far outnumber driver inputs in the thalamus, a numerically strong afferent pathway, which is sometimes (wrongly) interpreted as a pathway that must be important in information transfer, may instead often indicate modulatory influences. That is, one cannot simply assume a dominant (i.e., driver) input on the basis of large numbers, and understanding the functioning of thalamic circuits requires identifying drivers and modulators by criteria other than the numerical strength of the inputs.

In theory, this use of the cross-correlogram as a criterion for the driver/modulator distinction provides a relationship based on individual action potentials that can be applied to thalamic (and other) relays where receptive fields cannot be defined. Where, as in the transmission of many receptive fields, critical temporal relationships are a key function of the driver, any transmission not producing a sharp cross-correlogram (i.e., a narrow peak arising from a flat baseline) would lose all temporal information not contained in the lowest frequencies. This raises an important qualification for this criterion. Clearly, higher frequencies are important to vision, touch and kinesthesis, and hearing, so this criterion makes sense when applied to the thalamic relays for these sensory pathways. High frequencies may also be important for the transmission of most other types of information via thalamic relays, but this needs to be established. Smell, for instance, or taste are examples of sensory systems that may involve only slow processes and thus very low temporal frequencies, and perhaps the cross-correlogram reflecting the driver input relayed through the thalamic nuclei associated with smell or taste (i.e., respectively a part of the medial dorsal nucleus and a small-celled group related to the ventral posterior nucleus called VMb by Jones [1985]) may not resemble those of figure 7.1A and C. This is an issue that remains to be experimentally defined, and that may well differ for thalamic cells concerned with smell as compared to those that deal with taste. That is, the thalamic relay for taste is reasonably treated as a first order relay on the pathway to the cortical taste area (see Benjamin & Burton, 1968), where the ascending afferents must be the functional drivers. In contrast to this, the functional significance of the olfactory afferents to the medial dorsal nucleus is less clear, since these come from piriform cortex (Kuroda et al., 1992b), and we know of no morphological or functional evidence that would establish this pathway as a driver or a modulator of cells in the medial dorsal nucleus. Nor do we know that the messages coming from the piriform cortex are concerned with smell per se and not some other function related to smell.

The cross-correlogram seems like a very useful criterion to distinguish drivers from modulators, but there are serious qualifications to this conclusion that result in this being the last criterion listed in table 7.1. That is, while useful in theory, this criterion is difficult to test in practice. This is because the test requires recording simultaneously from a cell and one of its postsynaptic targets. Finding the second member of this pair is often like looking for a needle in a haystack. Only where there is very strict topography in connections and this topography is well documented is it practical to hunt for such pairs. This is practical for retinogeniculate, geniculocortical, and corticogeniculate pairs, as indicated in figure 7.1, but is generally not a practical endeavor for most pathways in the brain. Thus table 7.1 has many blank cells for this criterion. For this reason, we downgrade this criterion as a useful one to apply, but we describe it nonetheless because its theoretical applicability goes a long way toward defining a key functional difference between drivers and modulators.

7.B. Other Plausible Examples of Drivers Beyond First Order Thalamic Relay Cells

It is important to note that some other putative driver inputs to higher order thalamic relays and also to some relays outside thalamus are a small minority of the input as well. For instance, there is evidence that the large RL terminals that represent the driver inputs in the thalamus (see chapter 3) represent less than 4% of the synapses to their target relay cells in the pulvinar of the cat (Wang et al., 2002a). Also, only 5%–10% of the synapses to layer 4 cells in striate cortex come from the lateral geniculate nucleus, and the geniculate afferents can be regarded as the major (or only) source of driving afferents (Ahmed et al., 1994; Latawiec et al., 2000). The remarkable similarity in the relative synaptic numbers that retinogeniculate and geniculocortical drivers contribute to their postsynaptic cells may be a coincidence. Only a more widespread survey of the relative number of synapses that drivers form on their postsynaptic targets will address the generality of these numbers. It may well be relevant that morphological studies of spinal motoneurons suggest that Ia afferents, which constitute a major driver input, provide less than 5% of the synaptic terminals to these cells (reviewed on p. 462 of Henneman & Mendell, 1981). In considering other putative drivers, it is useful to refer to table 7.1, because with the exception of criteria 11 and 12, which are limited to thalamus, these criteria can be applied anywhere in the central nervous system.

7.B.1. Thalamic Reticular Cells

It is not clear whether, even if the driver/modulator distinction has general validity, all neurons necessarily have both input types. One can imagine that some cells, such as cells that serve as modulators, are themselves postsynaptic to modulators alone. Although this is certainly possible, the one example for which we have some evidence, namely the thalamic reticular cell, does seem to have both types of input. That is, there are at least three reasons to identify the relay cell input as the driver input to the reticular cell, with other inputs that dominate numerically, including layer 6 cortical and brainstem inputs, being the modulator inputs. First, the cells of the cat's perigeniculate nucleus, which we identified as part of the thalamic reticular nucleus in chapter 1, have receptive fields that can best be regarded as constructed from inputs from a few geniculate relay cells. That is, these receptive fields are restricted in size although larger than those of relay cells, and they respond to small flashing lights and to elongated targets such as gratings without evident orientation or direction selectivity. These properties are much more like those of relay cell receptive fields than cortical ones. Second, recent in vitro work on reticular cells of the rat somatosensory thalamus indicates that EPSPs from relay cells are larger and have a lower failure rate than those from cortex (Gentet & Ulrich, 2003, 2004). Third, there is evidence that terminals from relay cells are larger, rarer, and located more proximally on reticular cell dendrites than those from cortex (Ohara & Lieberman, 1981, 1985; Liu & Jones, 1999).

7.B.2. Layer 5 Input as a Driver to Higher Order Thalamic Relays

Evidence is presented in chapters 3 and 8 supporting the notion that cortical layer 5 afferents to higher order relays are drivers. This is well summarized by table 7.1, which shows that, for every one of the criteria listed except the last, for which no data are yet available, the layer 5 afferents resemble retinogeniculate input and not any modulator input. In particular, it is interesting to note the comparison between layer 5 and layer 6 inputs. By every criterion except the eighth and tenth, these two thalamocortical pathways differ. The morphological evidence for the driver nature of layer 5 inputs (i.e., criteria 4–7 and 10–12) is reviewed elsewhere (Guillery, 1995; Guillery & Sherman, 2002a; Sherman & Guillery, 2004). The evidence that layer 5 inputs determine thalamic receptive field properties (criterion 1) comes from cortical ablation studies. Removal of somatosensory cortex in rats obliterates receptive fields in the higher order relay receiving layer 5 input, the posterior medial nucleus, but not in the first order relay receiving layer 6 input, the ventral posterior nucleus (Diamond et al., 1992); likewise, removal of visual cortex obliterates receptive fields in the higher order pulvinar (Bender, 1983; Chalupa, 1991) but not in the first order lateral geniculate nucleus (Kalil & Chase, 1970; Schmielau & Singer, 1977; Geisert et al., 1981; McClurkin & Marrocco, 1984). Other functional evidence (i.e., criteria 2–3 and 8–9) has been provided largely by Reichova and Sherman (2004).

7.B.3. Lateral Geniculate Input to Cortex as a Driver

Relay cells of the lateral geniculate nucleus and other main sensory thalamic relays have an unusual property that may make them poor exemplars for a general definition of drivers versus modulators. We pointed out earlier that the lateral geniculate relay appears to be the only relay, from retinal receptor to higher cortical visual areas, that produces no significant spatial change in receptive field properties. Geniculate receptive fields are essentially like those of retinal ganglion cells, which makes it particularly easy to identify retinal inputs as the drivers. This is not typical for other relays in the visual pathways, which presumably are also innervated by drivers and modulators. Where new receptive field structures are synthesized, as happens in retina and cortex, we must expect a more complex grouping of convergent driving afferents.

For example, a number of geniculate axons converge to innervate a single cell in layer 4 of striate cortex in the cat. Even here, however, the convergence is relatively small, at roughly 30 (Alonso et al., 2001), compared, say, to the corticogeniculate pathway, at hundreds (see Sherman & Koch, 1986). If the synaptic influences sum linearly, the post-synaptic receptive field will reflect all of the receptive fields of the inputs. This appears to be the case for the geniculocortical pathway (Ferster et al., 1996; Reid & Alonso, 1996; Anderson et al., 2000; Alonso et al., 2001; Kara et al., 2002; reviewed in Ferster, 2004), and the observation that the receptive field of the postsynaptic cell is strongly determined by the input from geniculate axons marks these inputs as drivers. However, action potentials can occur in the postsynaptic cell in relation to action potentials from *any* of its inputs. If the geniculate afferents fired independently of each other, the cross-correlogram based on one of these afferents could still be fairly sharp, but the peak would be smaller and the baseline would be higher and noisier due to firing of the other afferents. A cross-correlogram can identify the driver as long as the number of convergent, independently firing afferents does not prevent the baseline from obscuring the peak that each alone would produce. Indeed, the relatively sharp cross-correlogram seen for geniculocortical synapses (figure 7.1D) marks this as a possible driver identifiable at a synapse in the cortex, which takes our argument beyond the confines of the thalamus.

Clearly, convergence of many independently firing drivers must be limited if a diagnostic, sharp cross-correlogram is to be produced. Large numbers of convergent inputs could produce a sharp cross-correlogram only if their firing were highly correlated. This is well shown in geniculocortical connections: cross-correlograms for geniculate and cortical cells indicate a driver input (figure 7.1D), but they are sharper when the relevant geniculate cells fire in synchrony (see Alonso et al., 1996).

The cross-correlogram for the geniculocortical input (figure 7.1D) further suggests that the synapses must activate mainly ionotropic receptors, because if metabotropic receptors were activated strongly, the result would be a broad peak in the cross-correlogram similar to that seen in figure 7.1B. We can predict, then, that, like the retinogeniculate synapse (a driver), and unlike the corticogeniculate synapse from layer 6 (a modulator), the geniculocortical synapse activates predominantly ionotropic receptors. This hypothesis could be readily tested, but direct evidence is not yet available.

There are other bits of evidence consistent with the role of geniculocortical afferents as drivers based on the criteria outlined in table 7.1. That is, geniculocortical synapses are found in well-localized, dense arbors (criterion 10; Ferster & LeVay, 1978; Humphrey et al., 1985a); they derive from large terminals contacting proximal dendrites (criterion 4; Ahmed et al., 1994; Latawiec et al., 2000); they are glutamatergic (criterion 8; Sáez et al., 1998); they often derive from large axons (criterion 7; Ferster & LeVay, 1978; Humphrey et al., 1985a); as suggested in the preceding paragraph, they activate primarily if not solely ionotropic receptors (criterion 2); they produce large EPSPs with paired-pulse depression (criteria 3 and 9; Stratford et al., 1996; Swadlow & Gusev, 2001; Chung et al., 2002); and they show relatively little convergence of roughly 30 axons onto their target cells (criterion 6; Alonso et al., 2001). The only criteria for driver status from table 7.1 not met by geniculocortical inputs, other than criteria 11 and 12, which can apply only within thalamus, is criterion 5, for which data are presently lacking.

Thus a strong case can be made that geniculocortical inputs represent the driver for layer 4 cells. As noted earlier, these inputs produce only about 6% of the synapses onto their target cells in layer 4. This implies a remarkable similarity to retinogeniculate inputs in terms of function (i.e., driver input) and relative number of synapses provided.

7.B.4. Driver/Modulator Distinction for Branching Axons

As indicated by criterion 11 of table 7.1, most or all retinogeniculate axons branch to innervate midbrain as well. This is generally true of other drivers to thalamic relays, both first order and higher order (see above and chapter 10 for details). A question that can be raised is: if an axon branches and provides a driver (or modulator) input to one target, does it necessarily provide a driver (or modulator) input to all of its targets? For example, does a retinal axon that drives a geniculate relay cell also drive its postsynaptic target in the superior colliculus?

It is interesting that the one example for which we have some, albeit limited information suggests that a driver to one target is a driver to others. The example is the thalamic relay cell. As noted above, it seems to provide driver input to both its targets in cortex and the thalamic reticular nucleus. Nonetheless, the importance of the question dictates that we need much more data, and from more examples, to address this issue.

7.C. Tonic and Burst Modes in Thalamic Relay Cells

Since geniculate relay cells generally show both tonic and burst firing (see chapters 5 and 8) in varying degrees under conditions like those for which the cross-correlograms of figure 7.1A and C were obtained, it is likely that some of the responses forming the peaks in these cross-correlogram were due to bursts. A question that has not been experimentally asked is: what is the difference in the form of the retinogeniculate cross-correlogram for the burst or tonic response modes of the relay cell? Action potentials in the tonic firing mode result directly from EPSPs, but during bursting, they result from the Ca^{2+} spike and are thus indirectly linked to the EPSP. This would affect the cross-correlograms. During tonic firing, an action potential in the retinal afferent is likely to evoke an action potential in the relay cell with a tight one-to-one coupling, resulting in a cross-correlogram with an extremely narrow peak only 1 msec or so across. During burst firing, an action potential in the retinal afferent may activate a Ca^{2+} spike, and the resultant burst of several action potentials lasts for 20 msec or so. Thus the coupling between input and output action potentials is no longer one-to-one and would produce a broader peak than expected during tonic firing. Nonetheless, one would expect that the peak during burst firing would still be quite sharp compared with that produced by modulators.

7.D. The Sleeping Thalamus

The functioning of the thalamus during wakefulness is very different from its functioning during sleep, a topic that will be briefly considered here in the context of drivers and modulators. The reader is referred to other sources for a fuller account of sleep (Favale et al., 1964; Dagnino et al., 1965, 1966, 1971; Ghelarducci et al., 1970; Marks et al., 1981; Llinás & Pare, 1991). Sleep actually has two very different major components, each of which can be further subdivided. One is slow-wave sleep (or synchronized sleep), which is characterized in electroencephalographic (EEG) recording by low-frequency, high-amplitude oscillations. The other is desynchronized sleep, which is characterized in EEG recording by high-frequency, low-amplitude oscillations. The latter is also sometimes called REM (for rapid eye movement) sleep, because bouts of rapid eye movements occur during this phase of sleep. As one passes from wakefulness to drowsiness to sleep, slow-wave sleep is entered first, and from there, REM sleep can be initiated.

7.D.1. Slow-Wave Sleep

During slow-wave sleep, the cholinergic parabrachial inputs to the thalamus become much less active, and this undoubtedly enhances the propensity of relay cells to fire in burst mode. Indeed, bursting based on low Ca^{2+} threshold spikes is most frequently seen during slow-wave sleep, and when it is seen, it tends to be rhythmic and synchronized among thalamic neurons. As noted in chapter 5, section 5.A, this synchronized, rhythmic bursting depends on interactions among reticular cells and between reticular and relay cells. It is important to note that not all thalamic cells show rhythmic bursting during slow-wave sleep and that such bursting is typically interspersed with periods of tonic firing (McCarley et al., 1983; Ramcharan et al., 2000). The current dogma (Livingstone & Hubel, 1981; McCarley et al., 1983; Steriade & McCarley, 1990; Steriade et al., 1990; Steriade et al., 1993b; Steriade & Contreras, 1995) suggests that rhythmic bursting represents a period during which the thalamic relay of normal driver information is blocked, since the rhythmic bursting does not correspond to the firing pattern of the drivers.

However, it is not clear why rhythmic bursting should interrupt thalamic relays (see also chapter 6). Perhaps the synchronized rhythmic volleys established in the thalamic reticular nucleus come to so dominate thalamic relay cell firing patterns that their normal driver inputs become ineffective (e.g., Sherman & Guillery, 1998). However, recent evidence suggests that rhythmic bursting may not always dominate the responses of all thalamic cells during sleep (Ramcharan et al., 2000), and other evidence suggests that transmission of driver inputs may only be slightly depressed during sleep (Ghelarducci et al., 1970; Dagnino et al., 1971; Meeren et al., 1998). This issue needs further study. We need much better evidence for the status of thalamic relays during the various phases of sleep, and specifically during slow-wave sleep.

If the dogma does prove to be mostly correct, that synchronized, rhythmic bursting indeed reflects a breakdown of relay of normal driver inputs, and we emphasize the "If," then we can suggest the following:

During this synchronized bursting, input from the thalamic reticular nucleus dominates relay cells, and EPSPs generated by driver inputs may be insufficient to break the stranglehold of reticular inputs on thalamic relay cell responses. The relay is interrupted not by silencing relay cells but rather by forcing them to burst rhythmically and independently of normal driver input. Thus, instead of no signal, cortex receives a clear, positive signal that the relay is disrupted. Silence alone would be ambiguous: the absence of a driver-carried message would be indistinguishable from the disruption of an effective relay of such a message. The rhythmic bursting, by signaling the "no-relay" alternative, avoids this ambiguity. However, if this were true, then it is nonetheless puzzling that rhythmic bursting often gives way to simple silence during slow-wave sleep, and as we have pointed out, silence among the relay cells can be ambiguous from the perspective of cortex.

In any case, since reticular input appears to dominate relay cell responses during synchronous, rhythmic bursting, it is interesting to imagine what the cross-correlograms between a reticular cell and its postsynaptic relay cell would look like. We would expect there to be a fairly sharp peak with little baseline in the cross-correlogram during the synchronized, rhythmic bursting. The peak would have a fairly long latency, since the direct synaptic effect of the reticular activity (a burst) would be powerful inhibition, silencing the relay cells for hundreds of milliseconds, and the relay cell would then fire a burst only after it depolarized, partly due to I_h and partly due to cessation of reticular cell firing. Nonetheless, the interval between the reticular firing and the relay cell firing, while hundreds of milliseconds, would be fairly regular, resulting in a peak. This begins to look like one of our major criteria for a driver input. One could argue that the thalamic relay cells are responding to a message sent by the reticular cells. The more general issue of whether an inhibitory input like the reticular input is likely to be a driver is considered below. However, this form of driving by reticular input during slow-wave sleep occurs because of the special relationships that produce the highly correlated firing of the synchronized reticular cells. Without such correlation, there would be no driving. It seems that the action of these afferents has to be distinguished from the action of drivers considered earlier, but that it cannot be regarded as modulation. We suggest that this action be treated as a disrupting action that is distinct from driving and modulation, and that may be special to the thalamic reticular nucleus and its thalamic connections.

7.D.2. REM Sleep

During REM sleep, cholinergic, parabrachial inputs to thalamus become highly active, which makes thalamic cells fire mostly or perhaps even exclusively in tonic mode. Some very limited evidence (Dagnino et al., 1965, 1966; Ghelarducci et al., 1970; Marks et al., 1981) suggests that relay functions are much greater during REM sleep than during slow-wave sleep and may actually be equivalent to the relay seen during the awake state. In fact, there are as yet no clear criteria that distinguish thalamic relay functions during REM sleep and the alert, awake state. A question often asked and not yet answered (e.g., Llinás & Pare, 1991) is: why, if sensory information is effectively relayed through thalamus to cortex during REM sleep, are we generally unaware of it?

7.E. Can GABAergic Inputs to Thalamus Be Drivers?

7.E.1. Extradiencephalic GABAergic Inputs

In the preceding section we considered the role of the input from the thalamic reticular nucleus, which seems clearly to be a modulator under most conditions. However, during slow-wave sleep, these reticular inputs seem to play a different role, something other than driver or modulator, because of the very special condition that they then fire synchronously. We have suggested that this role might be considered as a disruptor. But what of other GABAergic inputs to thalamic relay cells, particularly those of extradiencephalic origin described for some thalamic nuclei (see chapter 3)?

A consideration of basic differences between inhibitory and excitatory inputs suggests that inhibitory afferents are most unlikely to be acting as drivers. It is important to recognize that inhibitory and excitatory afferents to spiking cells are not mirror images of each other functionally. That is, a synapse creating an EPSP or IPSP might convey the same information to a nonspiking postsynaptic cell, as commonly happens in retina, but not to a cell that passes on information based on action potentials activated from a voltage threshold depolarized with respect to rest. This difference between excitatory and inhibitory inputs as possible drivers has been supported by modeling studies (Smith & Sherman, 2002). In the extreme case where the depolarized cell has zero baseline or spontaneous activity, an IPSP will not readily affect the spiking of a cell with no spontaneous activity, and so the message conveyed by an inhibitory afferent is lost,[3] whereas an EPSP can activate an action potential, and so the presynaptic message can be transmitted further. If, however, the postsynaptic cell has enough spontaneous activity, both an EPSP, by elevating the firing rate, and an IPSP, by lowering it, can transmit information through the postsynaptic cell. Nonetheless, for moderate levels of spontaneous activity (i.e., less than roughly 20–50 Hz), the action of EPSPs in creating extra spikes is more likely to be detected in the postsynaptic spike train than is the action of an IPSP in removing occasional spikes. Possibly at very high baseline firing levels the action of IPSPs can influence the firing of the postsynaptic cell strongly and with a high degree of temporal resolution (i.e., the flip side of an EPSP). However, for the IPSP to be effective as a driver, the baseline rate must be high (well over 50 Hz, and the higher the better), because the brief IPSP must have a high likelihood of canceling an action potential and not fall between them, as would often happen with lower firing rates; but such baseline rates are rarely, if ever, observed in thalamic relay cells under normal conditions. For these reasons, we regard inhibitory, GABAergic inputs to thalamus as unlikely candidates to be drivers and suggest they are all modulators. It is interesting in this regard that baseline firing rates of neurons in the deep cerebellar nuclei tend to be fairly high (Gardner & Fuchs, 1975; Armstrong & Edgley, 1988), because these cells are innervated from the cerebellar cortex by GABAergic Purkinje cells.

It is particularly interesting in this context to consider the pathway from the basal ganglia to the thalamus, namely to the ventral anterior

---

3. There is an interesting exception to this argument. If the inhibitory input sustains strong and long enough inhibition in a previously depolarized thalamic relay cell, either by temporal summation of $GABA_A$-mediated IPSPs or by $GABA_B$-mediated IPSPs, this would de-inactivate I_T. When the IPSP(s) ceased, the relay cell would passively depolarize to its previous value, activating I_T and thus a burst of action potentials. Inhibitory input could thereby lead to burst firing. However, burst firing alone would limit the nature of information relayed to cortex (see chapter 6), there would be a long (≥ 50–100 msec) and variable delay before a burst could be activated due to the time needed to de-inactivate I_T, and much temporal information in the input would be lost by a relay limited to burst mode. This, then, would severely limit the information relayed by an inhibitory driver input if it depended on activating burst firing in the relay cell. Nonetheless, Smith and Sherman (2002) showed via modeling that the effectiveness of inhibitory inputs to relay cells as possible drivers was enhanced during burst firing.

and ventral lateral nuclei, because this is a GABAergic, inhibitory input. (In most mammals other than monkeys, the distinction between these nuclei is often difficult to make, so we treat them together for the issues discussed here.) As shown in figure 7.2A, this pathway is conventionally treated as though it were a driver, functionally comparable to the retinal input to the lateral geniculate nucleus or lemniscal input to the ventral posterior nucleus (for, recent articles, see Nakano, 2000; McFarland & Haber, 2002; for representative textbooks, see Purves et al., 1997; Kandel et al., 2000), and yet we have just argued that GABAergic inputs are unlikely to be drivers. We thus offer an alternative model, shown in figure 7.2B, in which the basal ganglia input is a modulator. We have

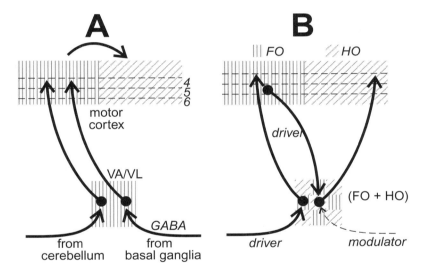

Figure 7.2
Implication of driver/modulator concept for basal ganglia inputs to the ventral lateral and ventral anterior nuclei (VA/VL) of thalamus. *A.* Conventional view. Here, the inputs from the basal ganglia are seen as a route of information, along with parallel information brought by cerebellar inputs, that is relayed through the ventral lateral and ventral anterior nuclei to cortex. In essence, this treats basal ganglia input as if it were a driver. *B.* Alternative view. Because the basal ganglia input to thalamus is carried by GABAergic axons, we argue that it must be a modulator (see text). Furthermore, there is evidence that cerebellar and basal ganglia input to the ventral lateral and ventral anterior nuclei terminates mainly in a patchy nonoverlapping distribution and that there is another driver input to this region from layer 5 of motor cortex. Thus, we argue that the cerebellar input is one driver pathway that is largely independent of the basal ganglia input, which, in turn, acts as a modulator for layer 5 input. See text for details.

argued elsewhere (see chapter 3) that cerebellar inputs to the ventral and lateral anterior nuclei are drivers, and thus the relay cells innervated by this pathway represent a first order relay. Evidence exists in the monkey that, although there is some overlap of the inputs from the cerebellum and from the basal ganglia, these different inputs tend to occupy different territories in a patchy distribution in the ventral anterior and ventral lateral nuclei, with the cerebellar input being denser more rostrally and the basal ganglia denser more caudally (Sakai et al., 1996). Furthermore, there is a projection from layer 5 of motor cortex to both of these thalamic nuclei (McFarland & Haber, 2002), and this defines a zone of higher order relay for the ventral and lateral anterior nuclei. Recent physiological evidence confirms a layer 5 input to this region (Sirota et al., 2005). Note that figure 7.2B shows the first order and higher order thalamic relay as separate, but this is only for illustration; in fact, we do not yet know the relationship of cerebellar and layer 5 inputs. However, on the evidence just cited, that inputs from basal ganglia and cerebellum are largely nonoverlapping, we would expect the regions rich in cerebellar input to be poor in input from the basal ganglia, and vice versa. We thus argue that the input from the basal ganglia serves to modulate mainly the layer 5 input to the higher order portion of ventral and lateral anterior nuclei. This, of course, represents a radically different view of the function of the basal ganglia and its influence on motor cortex.

It should be clearly understood that this conclusion is at best provisional and based on limited and indirect evidence generated mostly by modeling synaptic responses (Smith & Sherman, 2002). We need functional, experimental studies of the extradiencephalic inhibitory inputs to thalamus for a more direct test of the hypothesis that they are all modulators. We also need a better understanding of the different roles played by EPSPs and IPSPs in information processing.

7.E.2. Interneurons

In the preceding section, we described why reticular cells are unlikely to serve as drivers, although we suggest they can be disrupters, and we also pointed out why inhibitory inputs in general are poor candidates for drivers, but interneurons have not specifically been discussed in this framework. In addition to the argument that, by providing an inhibitory input to relay cells, GABAergic interneurons are unlikely drivers, there are other reasons to count them among the modulatory inputs. First, the evidence from dual recording of a retinal afferent and its postsynaptic target in the lateral geniculate nucleus makes clear that such a high percentage of postsynaptic action potentials is accounted for by the retinal input (Cleland et al., 1971; Cleland & Lee, 1985; Mastronarde, 1987b; Usrey et al., 1999) that there is simply no room for other driver inputs. This applies to Y cells as well as to X cells with their triadic input (Cleland et al., 1971; Cleland & Lee, 1985; Mastronarde, 1987b; Usrey et al., 1999) and this means that the dendritic terminals of interneurons cannot be drivers. The axonal terminals of interneurons are also unlikely to be drivers, for the reasons previously noted.

7.F. Implications of the Driver Concept for Cortical Processing

We have argued that the concept of a driver input means that it is theoretically possible to identify the subset of pathways that actually convey information in the brain. The evidence summarized above suggests that although these driver pathways may be numerically quite small, it is important to identify them if one is to make functional sense of complex brain areas with multiple interconnections. For example, in order to understand the pathways that link the 30-odd areas of visual cortex in humans, a starting point must be the identification of the driver pathways. This is essential for understanding what fundamental functional relationships actually exist among the areas. Following the drivers and thus information flow provides a firm basis for establishing functional hierarchies.

We have made the case that geniculocortical afferents are driver inputs to layer 4 cells and that these postsynaptic cells can be regarded as the first stage of cortical processing. It is possible to extrapolate from this and argue that thalamic inputs to middle layers of cortex are always drivers, and that as far as we know, all cortical regions have such input. Whether other driver inputs to cortex exist, for instance from other cortical areas through direct corticocortical connections, remains an open question.

An important issue arises once it is possible to identify the drivers, whether these are thalamocortical or corticocortical. This has to do with the problem of identifying the functional role of a given cortical area. One way to describe such a function is to identify not only the driver input to the area but also its output, because this identifies the information flowing into and out of an area. The difference between these, the input and the output, serves as transfer function that defines the operation of the area. This idea relates to earlier attempts to define the function of cortical areas such as the middle temporal area as subserving motion and V4 as a color area. These functional classifications are based on the general idea that inputs to these areas lack the specificity (for motion or color) first seen in the area. We are suggesting a more formal and formally quite different way to define these functions, first by identifying the driver input to an area, and second by identifying the driver output.

A great difficulty in applying this idea of a transfer function is to identify the nature of the messages being transformed. One possibility is to compare receptive field properties of the input and output drivers, and of course, this approach is akin to the strategy used to study the functional organization of retina (Dowling, 1970, 1987) and visual cortex (Hubel & Wiesel, 1977; Van Essen, 1979, 1985; Van Essen & Maunsell, 1983; Van Essen et al., 1992). However, as noted earlier in a similar discussion of the function of thalamic relays, this approach might work well for sensory areas of cortex, where receptive fields can often be defined, but it is not a useful concept for cortical areas, such as much of prefrontal cortex, where receptive fields are not obvious. Another possibility might be to develop cross-correlograms between the driver input and driver output, but not only is this a difficult technical task, the data generated could be difficult to interpret. Although the idea of defining a transfer function for a cortical area by describing the difference between driver inputs and outputs might be a difficult task in practice, we suggest that it is nonetheless a useful concept for thinking about functional organization.

This view differs from past thinking on this subject on the crucial point of what to define as the driver input and the driver output. The input, we suggest, is to an important extent thalamocortical. For first order pathways from the thalamus it is almost certainly predominantly or entirely thalamocortical; for higher order pathways, the thalamocortical pathway may be equally important, or there may be a significant contribution from corticocortical pathways. Currently we have no evidence on the relative importance of these two pathways. This line of thought differs from the conventional view, which identifies the driver input as exclusively deriving from another cortical area for higher cortical areas (see chapter 8 and Sherman & Guillery, 1998; Guillery & Sherman, 2002a), and it underscores the importance of identifying the driver input(s). Furthermore, we suggest that the driver output travels mainly in the axons of the layer 5 cells, which send motor instructions to brainstem and spinal cord (see chapter 10), and many of which project to thalamus as the first limb in a corticothalamocortical pathway. These layer 5 cells represent the chief *driver* output of a cortical region or column so far as subcortical centers are concerned (again, the extent to which other corticocortical pathways represent driver outputs is currently undefined). It may be possible to distinguish layer 5 cells that project to thalamus from those that project only to extrathalamic subcortical targets, but that requires further study as well, as does the extent to which the thalamic and the extrathalamic pathways convey the same information. One implication, if there are different driver outputs, is that a cortical area can "multiplex" or subserve multiple functions, with different transfer functions for the different driver outputs. This functional understanding differs from the common way to define a cortical area by noting the response properties of cells therein without regard to layer or hierarchical status.

While we are suggesting a specific way to define a cortical area's function that differs in subtle but important ways from the conventional definition, we recognize that our approach offers no easy solution to obtaining this definition. That is, we suggest that one must define the properties of the thalamic input to an area, but often this input arises from a higher order relay that has not yet been much analyzed; and one must also define the properties of the layer 5 corticothalamic cells, which is again a difficult chore. Nonetheless, understanding the logic of the exercise may prove helpful in grasping the overall significance of the need to define and identify drivers.

7.G. Drivers and Labeled Lines

We normally consider a geniculate relay cell as driven by retinal afferents, but there are many other inputs to the cell, including cortical, brainstem, and local GABAergic inputs. Firing in any of these, in addition to or perhaps instead of modulating, can conceivably lead to action potentials in the relay cell. That is, a corticogeniculate or parabrachial input may produce a weak EPSP, but if the membrane potential of the relay cell is sufficiently close to firing threshold, this could produce a postsynaptic action potential. Even an inhibitory input from an interneuron or reticular cell can lead ultimately to relay cell firing, because if the inhibition is strong enough to de-inactivate T channels, passive repolarization of the relay cell following this input can produce a low threshold spike and burst of action potentials.

What does it mean to cortex if relay cell firing is caused not by retinal input but by modulator input? We suggest that cortex must always interpret relay cell firing as if caused by retinal activity and retinal activity alone. This notion is like the idea of "labeled lines" in sensory pathways. For instance, any event that activates a photoreceptor is interpreted as a visual stimulus. Thus, pressure applied to the eyeball that activates photoreceptors is always perceived as a visual stimulus and not as mechanical pressure. Fortunately, it is clear that virtually all geniculate relay cell firing is in response to retinal input and not in response to any nonretinal source (Cleland et al., 1971; Cleland & Lee, 1985; Mastronarde, 1987a; Usrey et al., 1999), so that mistaken signals are rarely a problem for geniculocortical transmission. Nonetheless, the point here is that one implication of identifying a driver input to a neuron is that all activity of that neuron, whether a thalamic relay cell, a cortical layer 4 cell postsynaptic to thalamic input, or any other example of this sort, will be interpreted as evoked by the driver input alone.

7.H. Modulators and Ionotropic Receptors

One of the criteria that distinguish drivers and modulators is the presence of postsynaptic metabotropic receptors. We wish to be clear: our concept is that metabotropic receptors generally signal the identity of a modulator, but ionotropic receptors do not necessarily signal the presence of a driver. Indeed, many modulatory inputs to thalamus, such as the layer 6 corticogeniculate and the brainstem cholinergic inputs, seem to employ both receptor types (although it is not clear if individual axons do), and the possibility certainly exists that some modulatory inputs activate only ionotropic receptors.

Indeed, recent work of Abbott and colleagues (Chance et al., 2002; Abbott, 2005) provides a plausible role for ionotropic receptors in modulation. Thus, both inhibitory and excitatory modulatory inputs could exist that are purely modulatory. This would assume that most other criteria of modulatory function in table 7.1 other than criterion 2 apply. At least two forms of modulation can be imagined. First, if the excitatory and inhibitory modulatory inputs were well balanced, there would be little effect on the target cell's membrane potential or spontaneous activity, but the increase in synaptic conductance would serve to reduce neuronal input resistance. This in turn would render the cell less sensitive to its driver inputs. In this fashion, these modulatory inputs, using just ionotropic receptors, could modulate the gain of the response to driver input. Second, if the excitatory and inhibitory inputs were out of balance, the imbalance would affect spontaneous activity, which is another effect of modulation. Note that an imbalance in the modulatory inputs such that, for instance, modulatory excitation becomes stronger, thereby raising spontaneous activity, does not mean that these modulatory inputs suddenly become drivers. Spontaneous activity levels affect the signal-to-noise ratio and linearity of response of the target cell and are not part of the basic signal to be conveyed through the target cell.

7.I. Summary

The distinction between drivers and modulators (and possibly disrupters) is important for understanding thalamic relays. Perhaps the most important question to answer for any thalamic nucleus is how its inputs are divided among drivers and modulators. Where receptive fields can be defined, as in the main, first order sensory relays, identifying the drivers versus modulators is fairly straightforward, but there is much to learn about drivers and modulators for most of the rest of the thalamus. We have outlined in this chapter some features other than receptive field properties that can be used to help identify drivers versus modulators, and most of these are summarized in table 7.1. Possibly this distinction can be applied much more broadly to cerebral cortex, as suggested by Crick and Koch (1998), and possibly to other cerebral centers as well, and perhaps generally to broad areas of the CNS, such as spinal cord. Within cortex, we think it likely that thalamocortical axons, especially those going to cortical layer 4 and possibly all of them, will prove to be drivers, whether from a sensory relay nucleus such as the lateral geniculate nucleus or a higher order nucleus such as the pulvinar.

It is important in this context to appreciate that the classification of corticocortical pathways is largely untested in terms of the criteria proposed here. The current dogma is that information flow within cortex is carried exclusively, or nearly so, by direct corticocortical connections (see Felleman & Van Essen, 1991; Bullier et al., 1996; Van Essen, 2005), but this seems largely to be an implicit assumption based on the sheer anatomical number of these connections. Indirect corticocortical routes, such as higher order corticothalamocortical ones, have been largely ignored in terms of information flow, perhaps partly because of their relatively small size anatomically, but also because their existence is still widely unrecognized. A reinvestigation of direct and indirect corticocortical pathways could significantly affect the current dogma that all information travels in the direct connections. By analogy with the anatomy of driver and modulator inputs to thalamic nuclei, such as retinogeniculate input, drivers may generally represent a very small input anatomically, while the modulators are the anatomically dominant input. One distinct and intriguing possibility is that the major source of a functional drive for corticocortical communication actually goes through the thalamus and derives from cells in layer 5 of one cortical area, which then provide a driver input to relay cells in a higher order thalamic nucleus such as the pulvinar (as suggested in chapter 8; see figure 8.1). These thalamic cells then, in turn, send their axons as drivers to layer 4 of another cortical area. An extreme corollary might be that most, and perhaps even all, direct corticocortical pathways serve as modulators. This would mean that information flowing from one cortical area to another, by passing through a thalamic relay, would be subject to the same control of information flow as exists for information coming into cortex from subcortical sources. The thalamus thus serves as a gate not only in the control of information to particular cortical areas about sensory events but also in the control of information passed to other cortical areas about the descending outputs emanating from layer 5.

If the categorization of inputs as driver or modulator (or possibly as disrupter) is to have an agreed general significance, or if one is to determine whether disrupters are unique to thalamus or can also be identified in other parts of the brain, then it becomes important that experimental criteria for identifying the class of an input be clearly understood. We have tried to provide an introduction to the problems that need to be addressed if a classification that has wide applicability is to be employed. Possibly it will prove that there are too many problem areas and intermediate positions for the distinction to be of any service outside the thalamus. The observations remain to be made.

7.J. Unresolved Questions

1. Can any afferent to the thalamus act as a driver under some conditions and as a modulator under other conditions?

2. How clear are distinctions between drivers and modulators in other parts of the brain?

3. Are there types of afferent that need to be considered other than drivers and modulators?

4. Do all driver inputs in the brain use glutamate as a transmitter and activate only ionotropic glutamate receptors? For instance, might some be cholinergic, activating nicotinic receptors?

5. Can cross-correlograms generally serve to distinguish drivers from modulators for the thalamus? Can they also do so for other parts of the brain?

6. Does a metabotropic receptor with its concomitant long time course of transmission represent an identifier of a modulator in the thalamus? Does this apply to other parts of the brain? Does this also apply where timing is less critical, as in olfactory or gustatory pathways?

7. Do modulators outnumber drivers in all (most) parts of the brain? Is the discrepancy generally of the same scale as it appears to be in the thalamus?

8. Must branching axons have the same function, in terms of driver or modulator, at each target zone? For that matter, must all synaptic terminals within a single arbor of one axon have the same effect on their target as regards driver or modulator function?

9. What other differences exist between driver and modulator synapses? For instance, do both show the same sorts of plasticity, such as long-term potentiation or depression, do both have similar or different patterns of presynaptic receptors on their terminals, and so on?

10. Since it seems that only a subset of layer 5 corticofugal projections from a cortical area include a thalamic target, what distinguishes those that do from those that do not innervate thalamus?

8 Two Types of Thalamic Relay: First Order and Higher Order

8.A. Basic Categorization of Relays

Earlier chapters introduced the distinction between first and higher order thalamic relays. This distinction represents a new way of looking at thalamic relays and recognizes a large part of the thalamus—indeed, more than half of the thalamic volume in primates—as playing a significant role in corticocortical communication. First order relays, shown by hatching in figure 8.1 (figure 8.1 repeats figure 1.2) receive their driving afferents from ascending pathways and transmit messages, which the cortex has not seen before, to cortex, and these were called first order for that reason (FO in figure 8.2). Higher order relays receive driver messages to the thalamus from layer 5 cortical output cells for transmission from one cortical area to another. These were called higher order relays (HO in figure 8.2), because the thalamus is here relaying messages that have already reached cortex and have been processed in at least one cortical area. Such higher order relays serve to pass a part of the output of one cortical area to another. That is, from the point of view of thalamocortical organization, this is a second (or third or more) run through the thalamocortical circuitry. These relays were not called second order relays because it is reasonable to expect that there will prove to be third and higher order loops going through thalamus and transmitting information from one higher cortical area to others. In this chapter we summarize the evidence that is currently available about these two functionally distinct types of relay, going over some of the material that has appeared briefly in earlier chapters and looking at how the recognition of these two types of thalamic relay relates to our view of the organization of the thalamic relay in general.

The recognition of higher order circuitry not only adds some vital new features to the classical view of the thalamus, it also removes large

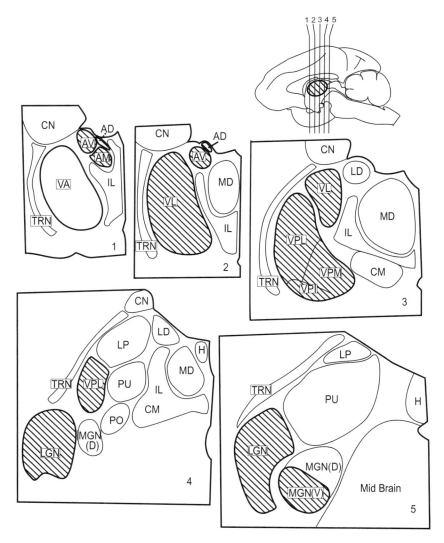

Figure 8.1
This figure, a duplicate of figure 1.2, is a schematic view of five sections through the thalamus of a monkey. The sections are numbered 1 through 5 and were cut in the coronal planes indicated by the arrows in the upper right midsagittal view of the monkey brain from figure 1.1. The major thalamic nuclei in one hemisphere for a generalized primate are shown. The nuclei that are filled by diagonal hatching are described as first order nuclei (see text), and the major functional connections of these, in terms of their afferent (input) and efferent (output) pathways to cortex, are indicated in figure 1.3. Abbreviations: AD, anterior dorsal nucleus; AM, anterior medial nucleus; AV, anterior ventral nucleus; CM, center median nucleus; CN, caudate nucleus (not a part of the thalamus); H, habenular nucleus; IL, intralaminar (and midline) nuclei; LD, lateral dorsal nucleus; LGN, lateral geniculate nucleus; LP, lateral posterior nucleus; MGN, medial geniculate nucleus; PO, posterior nucleus; PU, pulvinar; TRN, thalamic reticular nucleus; VA, ventral anterior nucleus; VL, ventral lateral nucleus; VPI, VPL, and VPM, inferior, lateral, and medial parts of the ventral posterior nucleus or nuclear group.

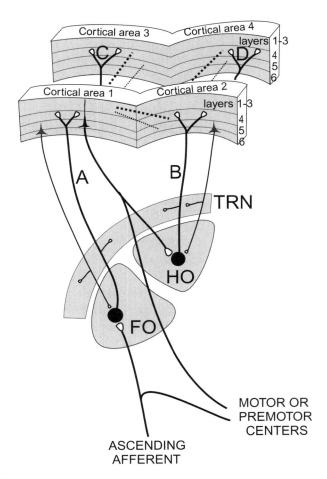

Figure 8.2
Schema to show the thalamocortical, corticothalamic, and corticocortical connections related to first order (FO) and higher order (HO) thalamocortical circuits. The inhibitory connections that go from the thalamic reticular nucleus and from interneurons to the thalamocortical relay cells are not shown. Cortical areas 1–4 show interconnected cortical areas. A, B, C, and D show thalamocortical drivers to 1–4, respectively, although the thalamic course of C and D has not been shown. The dotted arrows show feedforward (thicker arrows) and feedback (thinner arrows) corticocortical connections.

parts of the thalamus from their classical role of "association nuclei" with ill-defined inputs. Further, since many of the layer 5 corticothalamic axons that have been traced to the thalamus have descending branches to motor or premotor centers of the brainstem (discussed in more detail in chapter 10), the new categotization reveals a pattern of corticocortical communication that is sending copies of motor outputs from one cortical area to another, allowing us to see motor instructions as an integral part of perceptual processing (see chapter 10).

In figure 8.1, nuclei that appear to be largely or entirely first order relays are shown in diagonal hatching. They include the ventral posterior nucleus, the ventral part of the medial geniculate nucleus, the lateral geniculate nucleus, the anterior thalamic nuclei, and the ventral lateral nuclei, which receive somatosensory, auditory, visual, mamillary, and cerebellar afferents, respectively.

It is possible to argue that the last two afferent pathways are subject to cortical influences that act on the mamillary bodies from the hippocampus or on the cerebellum via the pons, and that even the first three can also be influenced by cortical pathways that descend to the gracile and cuneate nuclei, the auditory relays or the superior colliculus (which in turn projects to some of the laminae of the lateral geniculate nucleus). We regard the thalamus as serving to relay information from a set of driver afferents to cortex, and from this point of view there is an important difference between driving afferents that may have been influenced by prior corticofugal modifications and driving afferents that themselves come from the cortex. It is this distinction that is important for identifying a particular relay as first or higher order: for a higher order relay, the driver afferents must come from cortex itself.

The GABAergic pathways from the globus pallidus and the substantia nigra to the thalamus were considered in chapter 7, and on the basis of the arguments presented there, namely, that inhibitory pathways are not capable of serving as drivers in relays that do not have extremely high discharge rates, are not regarded as drivers.

An important point already raised in chapter 1 concerns the identification of certain *nuclei* as first or higher order. For each of the nuclei identified as first order by hatching in the figure, all of the driving afferents, or in some of these nuclei all but a small proportion of the driving afferents, are ascending afferents,[1] so that it is appropriate to think of

1. For example, Darian-Smith et al. (1999) show some corticothalamic axons with the characteristics of layer 5 drivers (type II, or R-type axons) in the macaque ventral posterior nucleus.

these as first order relay *nuclei*. However, the identification of higher order nuclei is more problematic, since for most we cannot exclude the possibility that some first order afferents may also have a relay in them. There may well be several of such "mixed" nuclei; possibly, when all the evidence is in, it will turn out that there are no pure higher order nuclei at all, that all contain a mixture of first and higher order relays, and for this reason it is clearer to speak of first and higher order *relays* or *circuits* rather than to identify *nuclei* as being necessarily entirely one or the other.

For example, the evidence, outlined below, that the pulvinar and lateral posterior nuclei receive driving afferents from visual cortex indicates that there are higher order relays in these nuclei. However, there is also a tectal input to the pulvinar and the lateral posterior nucleus, and the interpretation of these axons as driver or modulator afferents has been uncertain. Light and electron microscopic accounts differ as to their appearance (Mathers, 1971; Robson & Hall, 1977a; Ling et al., 1997; Kelly et al., 2003), depending on species and probably also on the particular subdivision of the pulvinar or lateral posterior nucleus that is under study. There are several distinct functionally organized zones in the pulvinar and lateral posterior nuclei (Abramson & Chalupa, 1988; Luppino et al., 1988; Casanova, 2004). Thus, the receptive field properties of some cells in the rabbit's lateral posterior nucleus appear to depend on a collicular input (Casanova & Molotchnikoff, 1990), whereas in the pulvinar of the rabbit, the effect of tectal inactivation produces an augmentation or a diminution of responses, not their abolition (Molotchnikoff et al., 1988). Bender (1988) reported that in the primate brain, "the colliculus contributes rather little to the neuronal response properties in the pulvinar, in contrast to what one would expect if the pulvinar served a major role as a 'relay nucleus.'" That is, much of the pulvinar receives its driving inputs from cortex, but since there may also be some tectal afferents that establish first order relays through parts of the pulvinar or lateral posterior nucleus, there are likely to be parts of these nuclei that probably represent mixed or nonoverlapping but mingled first and higher order regions. However, most parts of the pulvinar and lateral posterior nucleus are likely to be pure higher order relays unless some other, noncortical candidate for a driving input comes to light.

Similarly, there is evidence for mixed inputs to the ventral anterior and ventral lateral nuclei (see figure 7.2 and page 280). In the medial dorsal nucleus, which receives RL terminals from prefrontal cortex

(Schwartz et al., 1991) and from olfactory cortex (Kuroda et al., 1992a) and thus should be regarded as having higher order relays, there may well be first order relays as well, with afferents coming from the amygdala (Aggleton & Mishkin, 1984; Price, 1986; Groenewegen et al., 1990) and from other subcortical sources (Kuroda & Price, 1991). The terminal structures of some of these afferents, which might allow their identification as drivers or modulators, have not yet been sufficiently defined, but their light and electron microscopic appearance as well as their functional relationships to the relay cells of the medial dorsal nucleus clearly become of interest if one is to understand the nature of the relays that pass through this nucleus. For this nucleus it is probable that the larger, lateral parts of the nucleus, characteristic of the primate brain, will prove to be pure higher order relays.

The magnocellular part of the medial geniculate nucleus is a strong candidate for a mixed first and higher order nucleus, with type 2 axons that have large RL terminals coming from cortex but also with a direct, presumably excitatory, afferent component coming in the brachium of the inferior colliculus (Bartlett et al., 2000). The intralaminar nuclei are also very likely to represent a mixture of first and higher order relays. We saw in chapter 3 that injections of horseradish peroxidase into the center median nucleus show that it receives afferents from cortical layer 5 (Royce, 1983), suggesting that there might be some corticothalamic terminals in this nucleus having the character of RL terminals. Since the intralaminar nuclei also receive ascending afferents (Jones, 1985) that may well prove to be to be driving afferents, there is probably also a mixture of first and higher order circuits in these nuclei as well.

On the basis of current evidence, it thus seems likely that there will be several cell groups that represent a mixture of first and higher order circuits. Where such mixed inputs are identified, an important next question will be whether first and higher order relays ever share a thalamic relay cell or whether within one nucleus they are kept as separate parallel pathways going through the nucleus independently, like the X and Y pathways in the A-laminae of the cat (see chapter 3). That is, can there be integrative interactions between first and higher order relays?

8.B. Evidence in Favor of Two Distinct Types of Thalamic Relay

One of the major approaches we have used in this book is to treat the thalamus, including all of its nuclei, as a structure that has a common developmental history and that therefore the morphological features and functional relationships that can be seen in one nucleus will reappear in others. The argument that there are cell groups in the thalamus that receive their major driver afferents from the cerebral cortex has four parts. The evidence for each part has been considered in chapters 3 and 7 but will be summarized here to focus specifically on the distinction between first and higher order circuits.

The first part of the argument is that well-established driver afferents have been identified in the major first order relay nuclei for visual, auditory, and somatosensory afferents, and that these driver afferents have a shared characteristic light and electron microscopic appearance (type II axons with RL terminals, see chapter 3), as well as a common basic pattern of synaptic organization. Generally these axons have no branches to the thalamic reticular nucleus but do have branches going to brainstem or spinal motor or premotor centers (see figure 8.2). We regard axons having these characteristic light and electron microscopic appearances as candidate driver afferents even if they come from pathways whose driver function is not yet established experimentally. It is important to stress that this is a hypothesis, but a testable one about the function of afferent pathways to the thalamus (see chapter 7), and that currently there is no clear counter-evidence showing that any type II axons with RL terminals have only a modulatory and no driver function in any thalamic nucleus. The type II afferents having RL terminals that come from the cerebral cortex, that have no branches going to the thalamic reticular nucleus, but that do have branches going to brainstem motor or premotor centers (see figure 8.2) are therefore reasonably regarded as drivers, determining the nature of the message that is to be passed to another cortical area from the thalamic nucleus in which they terminate.

The second part of the argument is that there are two distinct types of corticothalamic afferent (see figure 8.2) identifiable on the basis of their structure. One, coming from cortical layer 6, appears to provide afferents to all thalamic nuclei, including those that have well-defined ascending, sensory driver afferents. On the basis of their terminal structure and their branches going to the thalamic reticular nucleus, these are type I axons with RS terminals and are quite unlike any known driver afferents. The second type of cortical afferent comes from output pyramidal cells in cortical layer 5, has type II axons with RL thalamic terminals, commonly has descending branches to brainstem, and goes primarily to nuclei that have few, poorly defined or no ascending driver afferents recognizable as type II axons with RL terminals.

The third part of the argument is that there are important differences in the pharmacology and physiology between drivers and modulators. In particular, modulators commonly relate to metabotropic receptors, but drivers, whether corticothalamic or ascending, lack metabotropic receptors. This distinction as well as other differences in synaptic properties and their functional significance, were considered in previous chapters. Here it is relevant to add that recent evidence shows layer 5 corticothalamic axons to have driver properties, whereas layer 6 axons are modulators (see figures 5.2 and 5.3; Li et al., 2003a; Reichova & Sherman, 2004). That is, layer 5 synapses share a number of functional features with retinogeniculate ones, which can be regarded as the prototypical driver, and layer 6 synapses differ in these features. Thus, layer 5 synapses show the properties of paired-pulse depression, a lack of a metabotropic glutamate component, and all-or-none recruitment with increasing electrical activation, a feature that suggests little convergence, whereas layer 6 synapses show paired-pulse facilitation, a metabotropic glutamate component, and graded recruitment, suggesting considerable convergence.

The fourth part of the argument is that in the few situations where it has been possible to test the effects of silencing the candidate corticothalamic driver afferents it has been shown that the basic receptive field properties of the relevant nucleus depend on the cortical input that comes from cortical layer 5 but not on layer 6 input.

We look at the structural evidence supporting the first two parts of the argument first, and then consider the functional evidence.

8.B.1. *Structure and Laminar Origin of the Corticothalamic Axons*

Evidence that corticothalamic afferents can have the same fine structural appearance as afferents coming from the retina or the medial lemniscus has been available for a long time. Mathers (1972) made lesions in the visual cortex of squirrel monkeys and showed that two distinct types of axon terminal in the pulvinar degenerate after such a lesion. One resembled the corticothalamic terminals that had previously been described in the main visual auditory and somatosensory nuclei (RS terminals, see chapter 3), and the other resembled the ascending driver afferents to these nuclei (the RL terminals). This observation was confirmed for the pulvinar of squirrels and primates (Robson & Hall, 1977b; Ogren & Hendrickson, 1979; Feig & Harting, 1998), for the rat lateral posterior nucleus (Vidnyánszky et al., 1996), and for the medial dorsal nucleus in the macaque monkey (Schwartz et al., 1991).

The light microscopic evidence came much more recently than the fine structural evidence. This sequence may seem odd but has a simple explanation: early methods of tracing axons, such as axonal degeneration or axonal labeling with radioactive materials or horseradish peroxidase, did not allow identification of the morphological characteristics of individual terminals, whereas electron microscopy did. Observations made in several species (rat, mouse, cat, monkey) on small groups of axons or single axons that had been filled with an anterograde marker such as biocytin or *Phaseolus* lectin (for these and related methods, see Bolam, 1992) showed the structure of individual axons going from somatosensory cortex to the posterior nucleus (PO; Hoogland et al., 1991; Bourassa et al., 1995), from the auditory cortex to the magnocellular part of the medial geniculate nucleus (Ojima, 1994; Bartlett et al., 2000), and from the visual cortex to the pulvinar or lateral posterior nucleus (Bourassa & Deschênes, 1995; Rockland, 1998; Rouiller & Welker, 2000). It was found, again: there are two characteristic types of axon coming from the cortex, one resembling the type I axons and the other resembling the type II axons described in chapter 3 for the major first order sensory relay nuclei, that is, the layer 6 corticothalamic and the ascending afferents, respectively. It was further shown on the basis of single-cell injections that the former come from layer 6 cells in the cortex, whereas the latter come from layer 5 cells. In addition, in some instances these laminar origins were in accord with earlier experiments that had shown the distribution of retrogradely labeled cortical cells in layer 5 or 6 after injections of horseradish peroxidase into some of the relevant thalamic nuclei (Gilbert & Kelly, 1975; Abramson & Chalupa, 1985).

These experiments, involving injections of one or a few cells, also showed two other potentially important features of the axons that were coming from the cortex. One is that layer 6 cells commonly send branches to the thalamic reticular nucleus, whereas layer 5 cells do so rarely or not at all (see chapter 3). The other is that the layer 5 cells but not the layer 6 cells can often be seen to send long descending branches to more caudal parts of the brainstem (Deschênes et al., 1994; Bourassa & Deschênes, 1995; Bourassa et al., 1995; Rockland, 1998; Guillery et al., 2001). The pattern of some corticothalamic axons as branches of corticotectal axons can also be demonstrated by recording experiments

(Casanova, 1993); it may be that there are some corticothalamic axons that have no descending branches and that other descending axons have no thalamic branches, but resolving these two issues depends on the interpretation of negative results from difficult experiments, so that both questions must be seen as open. Possibly there is a more general statement that can be made about driver afferents to thalamus: no matter whether they come from cortex or from lower centers, they are likely to send branches to brainstem but not the thalamic reticular nucleus, as opposed to the modulator pathways, which, as we have seen, send branches to the thalamic reticular nucleus but not to subthalamic levels of the brainstem.

One line of evidence that is currently available only for the ventral posterior nucleus (Hoogland et al., 1991) and the medial geniculate nucleus (Bartlett et al., 2000) is the demonstration that in higher order nuclei, the type I and type II axons identified light microscopically correspond in fine structural terms to the RS and the RL terminals, respectively. We can feel reasonably secure about the correspondence in first order nuclei such as the lateral geniculate nucleus on the basis of the evidence presented in chapter 3, but for the higher order circuits the evidence is generally less secure and more indirect. On the basis of the terminal sizes, this is a reasonable expectation for most parts of the thalamus, since the small drumstick-like side branches of the type I terminals could hardly form characteristic RL terminals, any more than the large, complex type II terminals coming from layer 5 that have been illustrated and described in the studies cited above could appear as RS terminals in electron microscopic sections. However, the sizes of the terminals of type I and type II cannot be regarded as diagnostic. Although they show no overlap in the A-laminae of the cat's lateral geniculate nucleus (Van Horn et al., 2000), they have not been shown to form distinct populations throughout the thalamus, and it would be reassuring to have a great deal more electron microscopic evidence available about corticothalamic axons that have the light microscopic appearance of type II or type I axons and that can be shown to arise from either cortical layer 5 or 6, respectively.

8.B.2. Functional Evidence for Two Distinct Types of Corticothalamic Afferent

We have proposed, on the basis of evidence from the retinogeniculocortical pathway, that the thalamic relay serves as a modulatory gate, not an integrator. That is, for any one relay cell, the driver afferents are few and generally represent a single function; the function of the relay cell is to pass the driver message to cortex. The message may be passed to cortex in tonic or in burst mode, or it may not be passed to cortex at all, particularly in certain sleep states. There may be slight modifications of the message in the relay, some that yet remain to be defined, but essentially our proposal is that the thalamus will not produce a significant change in the message itself.

The issue of identifying the drivers in any thalamic nucleus and distinguishing them from modulators was considered in the previous chapter, where the problem of making this distinction was also raised in general for any part of the nervous system. We argue that, in the thalamus, drivers can be identified by certain morphological and functional features. Where information about receptive field properties is available, one can use the transmission of receptive field properties for identifying drivers. However, before we look at this functional argument, and explore its use for distinguishing corticothalamic drivers from modulators, it is necessary to recognize two important provisos. One is that for many pathways other than the retinogeniculate pathway, manipulation of cortex can act not only directly on the thalamic relay but also on the driver afferents that innervate this relay. For example, there are pathways that go from somatosensory cortex to the gracile and cuneate nuclei and from auditory cortex to the inferior colliculus, but there is no cortical innervation of the retina. Whereas modifications of activity in visual cortex can have no direct action on the retinogeniculate pathway, the same is not true for the auditory and somatosensory pathways.

The second proviso arises when we extend our argument to nuclei that are not obviously on the route to one of the primary sensory cortical areas. Here, defining the critical properties that characterize the nature of the driver input becomes important, but is as yet largely unexplored. We lack information about the nature of the message that is delivered by the putative driver, either because many of the pathways that pass through the thalamus are not concerned with sensory messages and the concept of a "receptive field" is not applicable, or because for most higher order circuits the nature of the receptive fields has not been defined, even though the circuit is concerned with a particular sensory modality. The distinction between the "nature" of the driver input defined above, which refers to the message that it carries, and the action that the driver has on its postsynaptic cell, which is the contribution that it makes to the discharge of the postsynaptic cell, and which was discussed in the last chapter on drivers and modulators, is of crucial importance. Here we have to recognize that in the past, for all but a few of the thalamic relays, our primary functional clue for identifying an afferent as a driver has been knowledge about the message that it carries and a demonstration that this message is passed on through the relay. Identifying this message is still of vital importance, but other functional and morphological clues considered in the last chapter can now be exploited to identify drivers even where the nature of the message is not clear.

Studies of receptive field properties have provided some useful evidence about the action of corticothalamic axons for first and higher order relays of visual and somatosensory pathways. In the visual pathways, it has been shown that relay cells in the lateral geniculate nucleus, which receive corticothalamic type I (RS) axons but no corticothalamic type II (RL) axons, have receptive fields that survive cortical lesions or cooling in cat or monkey (Kalil & Chase, 1970; Baker & Malpeli, 1977; Schmielau & Singer, 1977; Geisert et al., 1981), whereas receptive field properties in the primate higher order pulvinar, which receives corticothalamic type II axons, are lost after lesions of visual cortex (area 17; Bender, 1983; Chalupa, 1991). Comparably, for the somatosensory pathways of rats, the experiments of Diamond et al. (1992) have shown that the receptive field properties of cells in the ventral posterior nucleus (first order) survive inactivation of the somatosensory cortex, whereas the receptive field properties of cells in the posterior nucleus (POm, higher order) are lost after such cortical inactivation. It should be noted that here we are not discussing subtle changes in receptive field sizes or in the temporal pattern of the thalamic responses (see, e.g., Krupa et al., 1999) but a much more dramatic total loss of the receptive field. That is, these experiments show that the type I axons having RS endings and arising from layer 6, which are the only or the major cortical afferents present in the first order nuclei, can serve to modify the receptive field properties, but that they differ fundamentally from the primary afferents to first order nuclei and the type II axons from layer 5 to higher order nuclei, which on the basis of these experiments should be regarded as the drivers, bringing the impulse traffic that defines the receptive field of the relay.

8.C. Some Differences between First and Higher Order Thalamic Relays

Some intriguing, even puzzling, differences between first and higher order relays have come to light recently, and more may be on the way. One mentioned in chapter 3, section 3.H, relates to relative numbers of driver synapses. While RL terminals, representing the driver afferents, produce about 7% of the synapses in the lateral geniculate nucleus of the cat (Van Horn et al., 2000), these terminals account for only about 2% of the synapses in the cat's pulvinar (Wang et al., 2002a). This difference between the first and higher order visual relays has been extended to the somatosensory relays (Wang et al., 2003) and suggests relatively more modulatory input to higher order relays. A second difference, perhaps related to this relatively heavier modulatory input, is the observation that the zona incerta and anterior pretectal nucleus provide GABAergic inputs to relay cells of higher order relays but provide little or no innervation of first order relays (Barthó et al., 2002; Bokor et al., 2005); similarly, evidence from the monkey suggests that dopaminergic inputs target higher order thalamic relays fairly selectively (Sanchez-Gonzales et al., 2005).

Another curious difference has to do with the cholinergic effects on relay cells, as noted in chapter 5, section 5.B.4. There is evidence that, whereas all relay cells in first order relays are depolarized by acetylcholine acting via an M1 receptor, a subset of relay cells in higher order relays are instead hyperpolarized by acetylcholine via an M2 receptor (Mooney et al., 2004; Varela & Sherman, 2004). Because parabrachial neurons that carry the cholinergic input to relay cells become more active as the animal becomes more awake and alert, it follows that most relay cells in the thalamus, including all in first order relays, would be relatively depolarized during states of arousal, but a subset in higher order relays would be hyperpolarized. These hyperpolarized relay cells would then probably have high levels of I_T de-inactivation, and thus one would predict that these relay cells in higher order relays would exhibit high levels of bursting. The extra GABAergic innervation of higher order relay cells from the zona incerta and anterior pretectal nucleus, mentioned above, would also contribute to more bursting. Preliminary data from behaving monkeys support this prediction, since greater levels of bursting were reported in the higher order thalamic relays, pulvinar, and the medial dorsal nucleus than in the first order lateral geniculate, medial geniculate, and ventral posterior nuclei (Ramcharan et al., 2005).

There may be a pattern here, although the data are still preliminary. Higher order relays seem to have relatively more inputs to relay cells devoted to modulators, especially GABAergic modulators, and they seem to have a subset of cells designed to operate mostly in burst mode during wakefulness, a subset missing from first order relays. If these conclusions remain after more first and higher order relays are compared,

it would suggest that the thalamic relays used for corticothalamocortical processing are under relatively heavy modulatory control and that
bursting, perhaps as a wake up call, is more common for these relays.

8.D. Defining the Functional Nature of Driver Afferents in First and Higher Order Nuclei

There are two distinct ways in which one can think of the functional
nature of a transthalamic pathway. The first is to ask how the thalamic
relay is organized in terms of transmitters, receptors, synaptic junctions,
and membrane properties, so that the messages are passed to cortex
in burst or tonic mode, or for activation of other, currently undefined,
thalamic gating mechanisms. This can be thought of as the *functional
organization* of the relay. The second asks about the particular
function—visual, auditory, somatosensory, head direction, and so on—
that is being relayed in any one part of the thalamus. This can be thought
of as the *functional role* of the relay. The functional organization has
been discussed in earlier chapters, and we have treated it largely as
though it is invariant from one relay to another. The functional role
is characteristic and generally unique for each relay. In this section
we are concerned with this second way of thinking about the functional
nature, that is, the *role*, of the relay.

Identifying the sorts of stimuli that are likely to drive thalamic relay
cells receiving first order visual, auditory, or somatosensory afferents may
seem relatively straightforward, but even that often proves to be a challenge of finding the right stimulus variable for any one particular cell
type. For first order nuclei that are not in receipt of a major sensory
pathway clearly the problem is more difficult, and it becomes increasingly difficult as we move to higher order nuclei. Thus, although there
have been careful studies of the discharge properties of nerve cells in the
deep cerebellar nuclei (Thach et al., 1992; Middleton & Strick, 1997),
it is not yet understood precisely what the nature of the message that
passes through the thalamus is or how it relates to movement control.
Butler et al. (2000) demonstrated in awake monkeys trained to make
wrist movements that manipulated a visual display, with a variable gain
between wrist movement and visual display, that neural activity in the
cerebellothalamic relay was increased when the monkey was adapting to
a new gain level. Their results suggest that the thalamic relay encodes an
error signal, but that in addition other aspects of the movement are also
relayed through the thalamus. Their report provides a good example of

the problems related to the identification of the functional role of a driver. It stresses that for many drivers it is likely to be essential to record from awake animals, and that for any one relay nucleus a variety of different types of signal may well be transmitted.

Another example of a relay with a recently well-defined functional characterization comes from observations of the anterior dorsal thalamic nucleus, which have shown that head orientation in space, "head direction," is a signal that is passed through the tiny lateral mamillary nucleus and the anterior dorsal thalamic nucleus (Taube, 1995; Stackman & Taube, 1998). Since the lateral mamillary nucleus receives afferents from cell groups in the midbrain in receipt of vestibular inputs, and sends bilateral efferents to the anterior dorsal nucleus, which in turn projects to the retrosplenial cortex and thence to the hippocampus, this can be seen as a thalamic relay that transmits a definable message relating to the animal's spatial orientation on to the limbic cortex. However, what the other two, larger, anterior thalamic nuclei, which receive from the medial mamillary nuclei, may be doing remains unknown.

To say for any one thalamic nucleus that the afferents come from the mamillary nucleus, the cerebellum, the tectum, or a particular area of cortex is like identifying a ship by its port of origin, not by its cargo, which is often more important for those waiting to welcome, unload, or consume the cargo. We need to know what aspect of the relevant prethalamic functional organization the messages represent so that we can understand what it is that is being passed on to the cortex. This is a serious and difficult problem for some of the first order nuclei in the thalamus and is largely unresolved for any of the higher order circuits.

8.D.1. Defining the Functional Role of Higher Order Relays

Defining the functional role of a higher order thalamic relay will be difficult. We suggest that all higher order relays serve to pass messages from one area of cortex to another, and that these are messages about the current output to motor or premotor centers from the first cortical area (see figure 8.2). All of these messages must pass through the constraints imposed by the thalamic gate, and we suggest that these constraints are basically similar for all thalamic nuclei. That is, just as sensory information passes through first order nuclei en route to cortex, and there is no direct pathway to cortex, so perhaps most, possibly all, corticocortical *driver* messages must pass through a higher order thalamic relay, with the direct corticocortical pathways performing some other, perhaps modulatory, function (suggested by interrupted arrows in figure 8.2). Another way of looking at this is that any major source of information headed for a cortical area, whether initiated in the periphery or in another cortical area, must first pass through the thalamus. The advantage of information reaching a cortical area by first passing through the thalamus is not yet entirely clear but lies at the heart of understanding the thalamus. It is probable that the thalamic gating functions relating to burst and tonic firing properties of the thalamic relay neurons, discussed in chapter 6, will be equally important for information transmitted via first order and higher order relays. We do not expect a thalamic relay, whether first or higher order, to modify the content of the message or to act as an integrator of two or more messages, but this is an expectation that, although it is in accord with what we know about some first order relays, has not been tested for any higher order relay.

If we now compare first and higher relays, we have to ask whether our proposal that the two are functionally similar is indeed a viable proposal. Are the thalamic relay cells in each type of nucleus simply passing on messages whose characteristics are already established in the ascending afferents or in the afferent cortical layer 5 cells? Or are the higher order nuclei generating new messages either on the basis of their intrinsic, intrathalamic connections or by integrating two or more afferent (driver) pathways? After that, the really interesting and currently unanswered question is about the action of these thalamocortical axons on the cortical areas that they innervate. Are they the effective drivers for the cortical cells that they innervate? Is the laminar distribution of their cortical terminals relevant to determining whether their cortical action is that of driver or modulator? For instance, might corticothalamic inputs to middle layers be drivers, while those to layer 1 are modulators? Do they, like their counterparts from the first order nuclei, dominate the nature of the message that the relevant cortical area processes (see figure 8.2)? Or is there a fundamental difference between cortical cells that receive from first order relays and those that receive from higher order relays? Are the former heavily dominated by their thalamic afferents, as would appear from currently available evidence (e.g., for striate cortex: Hubel & Wiesel, 1977; Reid & Alonso, 1995; Ferster et al., 1996), and are the latter dominated by corticocortical pathways, as would appear from most current speculations about corticocortical connections (Zeki & Shipp, 1988; Van Essen et al., 1992; Salin & Bullier, 1995; Van Essen, 2005)? It is possible, although it seems unlikely to us, that higher cortical areas, which all receive thalamic afferents, generally to layers 3 or 4, depend less or not at all on these thalamic afferents and instead are driven by corticocortical connections. However, it would be more attractive and more in accord with a view of neocortex as having a basic structural pattern for all cortical areas (Mountcastle, 1997) if it could be shown that all areas of cortex resemble the primary visual, auditory, and somatosensory cortical areas in receiving their primary driver input from the thalamus. That is, it would seem reasonable to consider that all of neocortex receives primary driving afferents from the thalamus, and that the corticocortical connections serve modulatory but not driving functions. If this could be demonstrated, then the search for the origin of cortical receptive field properties would be dramatically redirected. At present the question is an open one, waiting for critical experimental evidence to define which axonal pathways are drivers and which are modulators.

Van Essen (2005) has recently argued that the number of connections formed by the thalamocortical pathways from higher order relays like the pulvinar are too low to be serving as drivers for transmitting information from one cortical area to another. The numbers of direct corticocortical pathways are more than an order of magnitude greater, and on this basis Van Essen argues that the direct corticocortical pathways are more suitable for the driver functions necessary for corticocortical communication. We have seen that in the afferents to the thalamus, the modulators greatly exceed the drivers in number, and we know of no reason for thinking that this relationship is likely to be different in the cortex. Estimates of the driver functions and of the number of axons necessary for corticocortical communication from lower to higher order cortical areas are currently based on speculation, not on empirical observations. That is, although a fair amount of information is available about the nature of receptive fields in several interconnected cortical areas, almost nothing is known about the nature of the messages that are passed from one cortical area to another, or indeed about the nature of the messages that might be needed to produce the changes in receptive field properties recorded in a series of higher cortical areas. The extent to which any one area of cortex is capable of synthesizing novel receptive field properties from a limited number of driver afferents has been defined to some extent for area 17 but has been barely explored for higher cortical areas. What is needed are direct observations on the nature of the messages passed along corticocortical pathways, either direct or transthalamic. The extent to which receptive field properties recorded in any one higher cortical area depend on the inputs that they are receiving from lower cortical areas, either by direct or by transthalamic connections, needs to be defined by nondestructive methods.

Van Essen (2005), in support of direct corticocortical pathways as drivers and higher order thalamocortical pathways (specifically those from the pulvinar) as modulators, cites evidence that corticocortical axons passing from cortical area V1 to area MT form relatively large endings in MT which resemble driver axons coming from the thalamus in visual or somatosensory cortex. Three points are relevant to this argument. One is that the number of these putative driver axon terminals described by Anderson et al. (1998) is relatively small, and thus not likely to satisfy the numerical needs postulated by Van Essen. A second point is that the morphological evidence by itself is suggestive but not sufficient to establish an axon in cortex as either a driver or modulator. The limited amount of information we have about the varieties of synaptic terminals in cortex, and the number of characteristic features by means of which a particular axon type can be identified *in cortex*, are currently not sufficient to make the morphological features a strong identifier. None of the features that allow identification of thalamic RL terminals as drivers, such as the glomeruli, the serial synapses, and the close relationship to relatively proximal dendritic sectors, can be identified in cortex. Above all, the evidence about the nature of the receptors and the functional properties of the synapses (outlined in chapter 7) is not available for the cortical terminals. A third point is that these large axon terminals are likely to be coming from Meynert cells, which also send axons to the superior colliculus (Fries et al., 1985). The Meynert cells are variously assigned to layers 5 or 6; if their axons go to the superior colliculus, then these cells are in fact like the layer 5 cells we considered earlier that send motor instructions to the colliculus. They would appear to be sending a copy of these instructions from cortical area V1 to area MT. The possibility that these axons also have a thalamic branch going to the pulvinar merits exploration.

If we now consider examples of higher order relays, we can look at the lateral posterior and pulvinar nuclei and can ask what sorts of information may be needed for us to understand the functional role played by these higher order relays. These nuclei send thalamocortical efferents to several different higher cortical visual areas (Abramson & Chalupa, 1985; Niimi et al., 1985; Lysakowski et al., 1988; Dick et al., 1991; Rockland et al., 1999), and also receive cortical afferents from several cortical visual areas (Updyke, 1977; Wall et al., 1982; Abramson & Chalupa, 1985; Yeterian & Pandya, 1997; Guillery et al., 2001). In order to understand how these relays function in sending messages to cortex it is necessary first to define which corticothalamic afferents come from layer 5 and which from layer 6. Then the functional roles of the cortical layer 5 cells that send axons to the pulvinar will need to be defined. In addition, it is likely to be useful to define the functional outcome of the message passed by the brainstem branches of the same layer 5 cells to motor or premotor centers, since it is a copy of these messages that is being passed from one cortical area to another. That is, there may be instances where the actions of the layer 5 terminals in the brainstem will prove more revealing than the actions in the thalamus.

There are not many studies that specifically define the message passed from cortex to the lateral posterior/pulvinar higher order relays. Casanova (1993, 2004) recorded from nerve cells in area 17 that project to the lateral posterior nucleus in the cat. These must have been layer 5 cells, forming RL axon terminals (see above and Feig & Harting, 1998), since there is only a very sparse layer 6 projection from area 17. Casanova tested these cells with drifting sine wave gratings and showed them to be like cortical complex cells: orientation and directionally selective, with a tendency to favor horizontal or vertical gratings, mostly binocularly driven, with some monocular cells innervated from the contralateral eye. He noted that the response characteristics of the thalamic cells were similar to those of corticotectal cells and found that six of 40 corticothalamic cells that were studied were branches of corticotectal axons. This observation can be compared with the anatomical observations of labeled corticothalamic layer 5 cells to the cat's lateral posterior nucleus, for which it was shown that essentially all had branches going to the midbrain (Guillery et al., 2001). Casanova et al. (1997; and see Casanova, 2004) also recorded from cells in the lateral posterior nucleus. The response properties were similar to those of the corticofugal cells. However, cooling or lesioning area 17, while reducing the responses in a proportion of the thalamic cells, left a significant proportion unaffected, indicating that areas other than cortical area 17 were likely to be making a contribution to the response properties of the cells in the lateral posterior nucleus, a conclusion that is in accord with the rich layer 5 projection to the lateral posterior nucleus coming from many extrastriate cortical areas (Abramson & Chalupa, 1985; Guillery et al., 2001).

For any higher order relay, the distribution of the modulatory layer 6 terminals relative to those of the driver layer 5 terminals will be crucial for understanding the basic connectivity patterns in that relay. The evidence currently available (Bourassa & Deschênes, 1995; Bourassa et al., 1995; Rockland, 1996, 1998; Darian-Smith et al., 1999; Guillery et al.,

2001) shows that the layer 5 terminals form small, well-localized arbors that are topographically organized (see next chapter), whereas the layer 6 terminals have a more diffuse terminal distribution (Darian-Smith et al., 1999; Guillery et al., 2001).

A specific example, for the lateral part of the lateral posterior nucleus of the cat and the adjacent lateral geniculate and pulvinar nuclei (Guillery et al., 2001), shows that areas 17 and 18 send well-localized layer 5 terminals to the lateral posterior nucleus but very few layer 6 terminals to that nucleus. The layer 6 projection goes predominantly to the parts of the lateral geniculate nucleus (figure 8.3) that innervate those cortical areas. Area 19 also sends well-localized layer 5 terminals to the lateral posterior nucleus, but in addition it sends layer 5 terminals to the pulvinar, and it also sends layer 6 terminals to both of these nuclei. These layer 6 terminals are far more widely spread in the nuclei than the layer 5 terminals, and this is similar to the pattern in the lateral geniculate nucleus, where the retinal (driver) input forms a smaller terminal zone than does the layer 6 input (Murphy & Sillito, 1996; Murphy et al., 2000); and see chapter 3. Also, in each nucleus the layer 6 terminals from a small cortical column tend to surround the layer 5 terminals from the same column, with minimal overlap (figure 3 of Guillery et al., 2001). That is, whereas the layer 6 modulatory axons from a cortical area tend to go primarily to the thalamic regions innervating that area, forming predominantly reciprocal connections

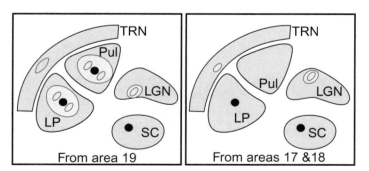

Figure 8.3
Schematic representation of corticothalamic afferents to the thalamic reticular nucleus (TRN), lateral geniculate nucleus (LGN), superior colliculus (SC), lateral posterior nucleus (LP), and pulvinar (Pul) nuclei of the cat. Black circles show layer 5 afferents, pale ovals show layer 6 afferents, with densely populated central zones and sparer periphery in LP, Pul, and LGN. See text for details.

(Van Horn & Sherman, 2004),[2] they do not go to the regions innervated by the drivers from the same small cortical area. In addition to these cortical inputs, the lateral part of the lateral posterior nucleus and the pulvinar also receive afferents from the suprasylvian cortical areas, including both layer 5 and layer 6 afferents (Abramson & Chalupa, 1985).

The above presents a quite preliminary sketch of how higher order relays may be connected to cortex. In summary, it suggests that any one small part of such a relay nucleus can receive driving inputs from several different cortical areas and send its outputs to several different cortical areas. Modulation, relevant for functions such as the control of burst or tonic mode of the outputs, comes (reciprocally) from the latter cortical areas, but it can also come from the cortical areas that are providing the drivers, although here the modulators are not topographically in register with the drivers; their terminals surround the region innervated by the drivers.

This picture of some of the connections of one small zone of a higher order relay has been introduced here to provide a connectional background for considering what it is that any higher order relay may be doing, and how it can be studied. If the drivers to a higher order relay come from several different cortical areas, then it is likely that the relay will represent several different functions. Not only should one expect layer 5 corticothalamic cell functions to differ from one cortical area to another, but one should perhaps also be prepared to find that not all the layer 5 corticothalamic cells in any one cortical area have the same function. That is, one should expect to find that functional properties of the relay cells are nonuniform within the relay. This issue has not been explored experimentally but its implications are considered further in the next chapter.

---

2. The relationship may actually be more complex than this because the lateral part of the lateral posterior nucleus, which receives essentially no layer 6 inputs from areas 17 and 18, does send axons to areas 17 and 18. However, in contrast to the extrastriate areas (19 and suprasylvian), which do send layer 6 axons to this thalamic region, areas 17 and 18 receive afferents primarily in layer 1 of cortex, not in layers 3 and 4 (Abramson & Chalupa, 1985), and it is probably the connection to layers 3 and 4 that represents the thalamocortical limb of the reciprocal link. The point is that, for thalamocortical inputs to middle layers of cortex, the relationship is approximately reciprocal. We know little about thalamocortical inputs to upper layers such as 1, and these may have very different rules.

On the view we have presented here, any one thalamic nucleus has a *functional role* (defined above) that depends entirely on its driver inputs, either ascending or cortical. It also has a *functional organization*, which may vary from one nucleus to another to a limited extent but which essentially represents the gating functions that the thalamus can impose on the relay. The important point is that currently there is no reason to look for anything else in the function of a thalamic relay. That is, we regard it as an error to ascribe a *specific* role to any one thalamic nucleus itself other than the role imposed by the driver inputs. For example, a role in the production of attention has been ascribed to the pulvinar and a role in the production of the symptoms of schizophrenia to the medial dorsal nucleus. A role in attentional mechanisms can depend on the control of burst or tonic modes for any thalamic nucleus, and the nucleus that will best fit the expectations of the experimenter will depend on the modality being studied and on the complexity of the functions tested. That is, the nature of the driver input is the important variable in relation to the function under test. Similarly, to claim a role in the production of schizophrenia for the medial dorsal nucleus is to identify the drivers (presumably the drivers coming from the frontal cortex) as carrying the relevant message. The thalamus transmits the message, it does not create it. If the thalamus itself is to play a role in the production of the symptoms then it must be either through a failure of its relay functions or through an abnormality of the gating functions that act on the messages that are relayed from the frontal cortex. However, the functional *system* that is rendered abnormal is the system that originates in the frontal cortex and that sends copies of its motor outputs through the thalamus from one cortical region to another.

In order to understand a higher order relay it will be necessary not only to understand the messages that the thalamic cells are receiving, and from where, but also to define the cortical areas receiving from these higher order relay cells and the processing that occurs there. That is, one needs to know which of the features that have been defined for the cortical afferents to the thalamic relay cells are the ones that are relevant to the further cortical processing. As pathways are followed further from the first order nuclei we can expect that defining the crucial properties (receptive field or other) will become increasingly more difficult and will depend more on an intuition about what the higher cortical area may be doing than on a clear view of how the first order receiving cortex processes its thalamic afferent messages. The choice of response properties that are to be tested must depend on choices that the experimenter makes as to what are the relevant stimuli to be examined. The assumption that, when there is a response, these are the particular properties that fit the specific functional role of the relay, is one that is not always easy to justify in a sensory system like the visual or somatosensory pathways; it is even more difficult to establish for higher order relays like the medial dorsal or anterior thalamic nuclei where we have very few clues as to the particular properties that are relevant to the functional role of the relay.

A further important point noted above is that whereas anesthetics may have relatively little effect on first order relays and their drivers, such as the lateral geniculate nucleus and retina, the normal functions of many higher order relays and their cortical drivers will depend critically on the absence of anesthesia. The recent report by Guo et al. (2004) of pattern motion in cortical area V1 of unanesthetized but not of anesthetized monkeys highlights the likelihood that complex responses will be missed when anesthetics are used.

This possibility, that the main information route for corticocortical processing uses a thalamic loop involving higher order thalamic relays, runs directly counter to the prevailing assumption that corticocortical pathways convey the main message for corticocortical organization (figure 8.4). The dominant current view is that information initially arrives at cortex after being relayed through first order relays, and once in cortex it remains strictly at the cortical level, being analyzed and communicated among cortical areas strictly along hierarchical, possibly parallel (supposedly "where" or "what') corticocortical pathways, until some instruction is ready to be sent to memory or to lower motor centers. For vision, for example, information first gets to cortex via the geniculostriate pathway and is then analyzed strictly within cortex among the various areas and sent out to centers concerned with producing the necessary responses. The same argument has been made for auditory and somatosensory processing. This view provides no real function for what we call the higher order thalamic relays that represent such a large volume of the thalamus in primates.

In contrast, our very different hypothesis, that corticocortical information transfer is relayed through these higher order thalamic nuclei, invests these relays with a critical function. Not only does it place the thalamus in a key role in corticocortical communication, but it also links that key role to the outputs that the relevant cortical areas are sending to the brainstem and spinal cord. At present we lack the critical data to choose between these competing views, since we know of no experiments

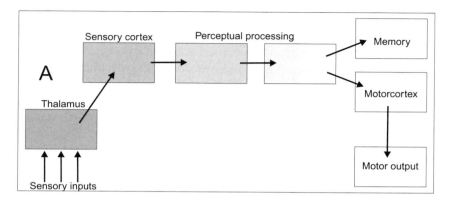

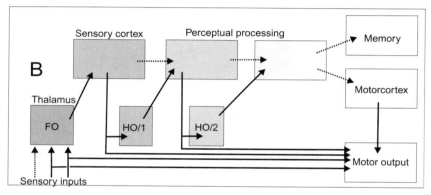

Figure 8.4
Two schematic representations of thalamocortical connections relevant to perceptual processing. *A.* The current conventional view, which sees the thalamic inputs relayed in the thalamus, passed to the cortex for processing, and then passed from higher cortical areas to motor centers or to memory storage sites. *B.* The view of the relevant connections presented here. This includes sensory inputs to first order thalamic relays (FO), transthalamic corticocortical pathways going through higher order thalamic relays (HO), and also includes extensive branches from afferents to the thalamus (ascending and corticothalamic) going directly to motor centers. The branches to the motor centers may be given off by prethalamic relays such as the posterior column nuclei, or by the ascending afferents to the thalamus themselves (see text; not shown in figure). The sensory input, shown as a dotted line at the left of the figure, indicates the (currently unproven) possibility that some ascending afferents may go to the thalamus without sending any branches to lower centers.

that define either the thalamic or the cortical afferents as the drivers for any higher cortical area; however, we do know that the drivers come from thalamus for primary cortical receiving areas, and we have no good reason for thinking that cortical areas differ so dramatically from each other that the component acting as a driver in one cortical area is not likely to do the same for another.

The important question raised at the beginning of this section as to what the functional significance of a higher order relay may be has not been answered in any of the points raised so far. Perhaps the closest we can come to a useful answer is that having a thalamic relay in corticocortical pathways imposes the complex gating functions discussed in earlier chapters on these corticocortical pathways. Of the several possible functions for a thalamic gate the one we understand best is the one that involves the switch from the burst to the tonic mode. We have argued for first order relays that the burst mode may be present when attention is generally reduced, as during drowsiness, or when attention is otherwise directed, to maximize detectability and cortical impact, so that novel stimuli will act as a sort of "wake up call," and that the tonic mode is then initiated to ensure a more faithful relay of the information. It should now be clear that this may happen for messages coming from cortical layer 5 cells and going through the thalamus from one cortical area to another, just as it can for afferent messages on their way to the cortex. For instance, if a corticothalamocortical route has been inactive for a period because of drowsiness or other forms of inattention, the thalamic relay cells may be in burst mode, so that initiation of new activity from the cortical source of the route will wake up the target cortical area, leading then to tonic firing for continued information processing along this route. Just as for the first order relays, the patterns of activity that control the switch between burst and tonic modes can be global or local, and the local controls will depend on the distribution of the layer 6 corticothalamic afferents, considered briefly above, as well as on the connections through the thalamic reticular nucleus (considered in the next chapter).

When we are trying to find the best words with which to express difficult thoughts, our sensory inputs coming through first order relays are barely getting through to cortical levels, perhaps because many relevant thalamic relay cells are in burst mode, but there are active cerebral processes going on, and it would be a reasonable bet to say that to a significant extent, these must involve higher order circuits going through the thalamus and linking cortical areas to each other; when the writing is done and we can relax with some music or conversation, the tonic mode in the first order circuits becomes more important for what we are doing, and the corticothalamic and reticulothalamic afferents will serve to ensure that a new set of thalamocortical pathways is functioning in the tonic mode. Of course, there is also the important possibility of interactions between the first and higher order circuits, which can occur perhaps through type I axons going from higher order cortical areas to first order thalamic relays or through connections in the thalamic reticular nucleus, because it is in this nucleus that one finds the closest relationships between first and higher order circuits for any one modality (see next chapter). Finally, if we next go to sleep, then, if messages from one cortical area to another make an obligatory pass through the thalamus, the rhythmic bursting seen throughout the thalamus during slow-wave sleep would largely disrupt corticocortical communication based on relays through higher order thalamic circuits, and this would be an important aspect of such sleep. It is interesting that dreaming may require this sort of corticocortical integration, and dreaming is not seen in slow-wave sleep but is seen in REM sleep, during which rhythmic bursting in the thalamus is prevented by strong activation of brainstem afferents (Steriade & McCarley, 1990).

The above account could be taken to imply that higher order circuits and the links between first and higher order circuits are significant for abstract thought but that a simple relay through thalamus to cortex is all that is required for simpler processes. There are good reasons for thinking that thalamic pathways to neocortex in all mammals, even in those with relatively simple brains and rather limited amounts of neocortex, always involve first and higher order circuits. This is because all mammals that have been studied from this point of view show a reduplication of cortical areas (Kaas, 1995; Krubitzer, 1998). They have two or more visual, auditory, or somatosensory areas, not just one. It has been shown that even a simple brain like that of the hedgehog has two somatosensory and two visual areas. It looks as though one of the significant advantages that the evolution of thalamocortical pathways offered our ancestors was the opportunity for having a higher order thalamocortical circuit that functioned on the basis of receiving driving afferents that themselves were already the output stage of cortical processing. That is, right from the start, the thalamus could serve as the organ of reflection of cortical activity back upon itself. The reiteration of thalamocortical circuitry may well prove to be one of the special advantages that the evolution of neocortex provided for mammals. This says nothing about the function of multiple cortical areas, but it does address the importance of the way in which they are interconnected, allowing one area to depend for a significant part of its input on the output of another area. One tends to think of the neocortex as sitting on top of the brain and doing all of the really difficult things that need to be done. However, it is worth bearing in mind that thalamus and neocortex have evolved in parallel, and that neither would amount to much without the other. If thalamic circuitry had developed as the deepest cortical layer, we would call it layer 7 and treat it as an integral part of cortex, and it could possibly have developed to do everything that the thalamus and reticular nucleus now do. We don't know why the diencephalic and telencephalic parts of the circuitry evolved as anatomically separate entities, but whatever the reasons, it is likely to be useful to treat the links between the two, particularly the reiterative links formed by higher order circuits, as an essential part of the neocortical mechanisms.

There are two further distinctions between first and higher order thalamic relays that may provide a clue about distinct functional capacities of the higher order relays. One is that in postnatal development of the human brain, the cortical areas receiving from first order relays mature earliest, in terms of myelin formation (Flechsig, 1920; Paus et al., 2001; Gogtay et al., 2002, 2004) and glucose metabolism (Chugani et al., 1987). Brain areas higher in the hierarchy mature later, with temporal and frontal cortex maturing last. The other distinction concerns the presence of a growth-associated protein (GAP-43) in the afferents to the thalamic nuclei. GAP-43 is a protein that is present in growing axons but is generally lost as stable connections are established (Benowitz & Routtenberg, 1997). Further, an increased presence of the protein lowers the threshold for axonal sprouting (Caroni, 1997; Bomze et al., 2001). This protein and its mRNA are present in adult rats in some of the corticothalamic modulators of higher as well as first order relays, and in this respect the two types of relay are similar. The protein is also present in the corticothalamic drivers from layer 5, but is lost at early postnatal stages from the drivers to first order relays (Feig, 2004). Further, the layer 5 corticothalamic cells of primary visual and auditory cortical areas show less of the mRNA for the protein than do the secondary cortical areas. That is, the higher order circuits not only mature later than the first order circuits, they also retain a protein related to axonal growth after it has been lost in first order circuits. This makes sense if one thinks of higher order cortex depending for its inputs on first order circuits as development proceeds. That is, it is probable that the first order circuits have to establish relatively stable circuits before the higher order circuits can take on their mature functions.

8.E. Unresolved Questions

1. Are there any pure higher order thalamic nuclei? Or are all higher order relays mingled with first order pathways?

2. Where the two types of relay, first and higher order, pass through the nucleus, do they do so as parallel, independent pathways, comparable to the X and Y pathways of the cat visual system, or is there an interaction within the thalamic relay?

3. Do the axons that arise in cortex and form RL terminals in the thalamus always arise from layer 5 cells, and are they always (or only sometimes) branches of long descending axons?

4. Can it be demonstrated that the axons considered in question 3 are always the drivers of the relay cells in the nucleus that they innervate? Where this cannot be achieved by the study of receptive fields, can it be done with the methods proposed in the previous chapter?

5. Do higher order relay cells resemble the cells of the lateral geniculate nucleus in passing messages on to cortex without significantly altering the nature of the message, and do they have the same gating functions as first order relay cells?

6. Do higher order cortical areas receive their major driver afferents from higher order thalamic relays or from other cortical areas?

7. Are the actions of thalamocortical axons from higher order nuclei terminating in cortical layers 3 or 4 comparable to the actions of thalamocortical axons from first order nuclei?

8. What is the nature of the message that direct corticocortical pathways transmit from one cortical area to another?

9. Is there a good example in any species of a first order relay that does not have a functionally corresponding or related higher order relay?

9 Maps in the Brain

9.A. Introduction

We have seen in earlier chapters that many of the connections to and from the thalamus are mapped. All of the driver afferents to first order nuclei are mapped, and essentially all of the thalamocortical and corticothalamic pathways, first and higher order, are mapped. In addition, many of the connections of the reticular nucleus are known to be mapped. For some of these pathways we know the functions that are mapped (e.g., visual space, body surface, or frequency), but for many, particularly for higher order relays, we do not know the functions that are mapped. That is, even though we know that there are maps, we have no clear picture of the function that is mapped, and for understanding particular thalamic functions we will need to understand these mapped functions, and also how the several maps for any one function relate to each other. In this chapter we look at some of the early evidence for maps in thalamocortical pathways and consider how maps have been viewed in the past. There have been speculative, theoretical views about the significance of maps, and there have been practical, experimental observations based on altered maps. These perspectives provide some insight into the extent to which maps are an essential part of thalamic function, and also show the extraordinary extent to which detailed maps form an essential part of thalamic organization, linking complex sets of mapped pathways to each other.

For any one sensory function there are multiple, mapped cortical areas; more than 30 have been reported for the macaque monkey's visual system (Felleman & Van Essen, 1991; Van Essen, 2005). Many of these maps, in the thalamus and in cortex, are mirror reversals of each other (Adams et al., 1997), implying extraordinarily complex systems of axonal crossings in their converging and diverging interconnections.

Historically, an early understanding of the basic mapping rules of the geniculocortical pathway was essential for an appreciation of its functional organization. Later, the demonstration of multiple visual cortical maps contributed significantly to our understanding of cortical functions. For many of the thalamic relays whose functions still remain mysterious, particularly the higher order relays, the detailed mapping rules remain undefined or only poorly defined. There can be little doubt that a full appreciation of the mapping rules for any one trans-thalamic pathway will prove essential for understanding its functional organization.

In this chapter we look at the extent to which knowledge about mapping rules can provide insights into the organization of thalamic pathways. In the first part of the chapter we look at what has been learnt in the past about the maps in the retinogeniculocortical pathways in order to demonstrate how experimental observations of normal and abnormal pathways have related to theoretical and speculative views of the role that mapped pathways may play. We look at this evidence in some detail because it demonstrates that the intuitive view of a brain that cannot function without an orderly representation of sensory surfaces does not apply to the thalamus, but does appear to apply to primary visual cortex. In the second part of the chapter we look at two other pathways where the mapping rules are less clearly defined: the thalamic reticular nucleus, and the higher order visual relay through the pulvinar and lateral posterior nucleus. The reticular nucleus has been moved in recent years from a (supposedly) diffusely organized cell group with essentially no topographic rules of connectivity to a topographically well-organized entity with some well-defined, mapped connections. This is one region where careful consideration of the basic mapping rules is proving to have important functional implications. The higher order visual relays represent another part of the thalamus where defining the mapping rules can be expected to lead to a better appreciation of their functional organization.

9.B. The Nature of Thalamic and Cortical Maps

Although it seems intuitively obvious that sensory surfaces, such as those dealing with visual, auditory, or somatosensory inputs, should be mapped, and although this intuition has been significantly exploited in the past, there are no solid theoretical or empirical grounds to support this intuition. The main sensory pathways are indeed mapped within the thalamocortical pathways, but the fact that they are mapped cannot be taken as support for the view that the brain could not function if they were not mapped. For other thalamocortical pathways, such as those from the anterior thalamic nuclei, the medial dorsal nucleus, the lateral dorsal nucleus, or the intralaminar nuclei, there are no intuitive grounds on the basis of which one can make a very good case as to why they should be mapped, nor do we know of any empirical or theoretical evidence that might be relevant. Yet they are mapped, and there appears to be an orderly, topographically organized connection for many, possibly all thalamocortical and corticothalamic pathways (Walker, 1938; Cowan & Powell, 1954; Updyke, 1977, 1981; Goldman-Rakic & Porrino, 1985; see also chapter 2). The simplest explanation for a universal, ordered topographic mapping of thalamus onto cortex would be a developmental one. One might want to argue that if the thalamocortical axons take a relatively orderly course during development, maintaining neighborhood relationships as they go, then the ordered thalamic radiation that would result could provide a neat explanation for the topographic maps (Caviness & Frost, 1983; Hohl-Abrahao & Creutzfeldt, 1991; Dufour et al., 2003). We have already indicated that the pathways from thalamus to cortex do not represent an orderly radiation such as that postulated in the above studies but instead present a very complex network of axonal crossings responsible for a multiplicity of interconnected and often mirror-reversed thalamic and cortical maps. In this chapter we explore the nature of this complex network further and show that the simple developmental view outlined above is not viable. This leads us to see the complex network as requiring a set of separate specified pathways for each mapped projection, producing a possibility for interactions among maps, particularly as they pass through the thalamic reticular nucleus, but it leaves a serious question about the functional variable that is mapped in those thalamocortical pathways in which one cannot see a simple representation of a sensory surface.

If we look at the details of maps, we see that in the thalamus, different aspects of the sensory inputs may map to different parts of the thalamus, so that, for example, the magnocellular and parvocellular pathways map to separate geniculate layers, and the spinothalamic and lemniscal afferents go to separate parts of the ventral posterior nucleus (Krubitzer & Kaas, 1992; Casagrande & Kaas, 1994; see also chapter 3). In the cortex, maps are split up in different ways; for example, connections concerned with orientation selectivity or ocular dominance are mingled within a single map in a regular, interrupted, and repeating pattern (Hubel & Wiesel, 1977). Other afferents are segregated to different cortical areas, a pattern of functional separation that has been strikingly demonstrated in the auditory pathways of bats (Fitzpatrick et al., 1998). It is difficult at present to use this information to formulate a generalization about the basic nature of cortical maps, even though there can be no question that for each major modality, with the exception of olfaction and possibly of taste, the topographic maps of the sensory surfaces play a significant role. That is, although much of what is presented in this chapter deals with the thalamic and cortical representation of sensory, particularly retinal, surfaces, it has to be recognized that, in terms of the detailed distribution of the functional components of the maps, we are not necessarily addressing single continuous representations either of sensory surfaces or of the nerve cells that give origin to the afferents supplying any one map. In the rest of this chapter we are concerned with the overall layout and orientation of maps, and will not deal with the way in which functionally distinct components may be fractionated within a map or distributed over several maps.

9.C. Early Arguments for Maps

The earliest expressions of the view that the brain must receive orderly mapped representations were based, so far as one can tell, on an intuitive evaluation of the capacities of the brain, not on any experimental evidence. The experimental evidence came later. Thus, when Newton in 1704 (cited by Polyak, 1957) argued that there must be a partial decussation at the optic chiasm, of the sort that is now illustrated in any neuroscience textbook and is shown here in figure 9.1C, his argument assumed that the visual pathways had to provide the brain with an orderly representation of the single visual scene transmitted by two pathways, one from each eye, with each image reversed by the lens of the eye. This argument, that the brain needs a single ordered representation, a sort of single internal projection screen of the binocularly viewed visual scene, was not explicitly stated, but Newton's argument could not have been carried to its apparently brilliant and now recognizably correct conclusion if Newton had allowed for the possibility that the brain could have managed with a disrupted, disorderly, or distributed representation of the visual world.

The logic of the argument, however, is not as rigorous as the beautifully correct conclusion might suggest. Descartes had earlier, in 1686 (cited by Polyak, 1957), also recognized the problem presented by a

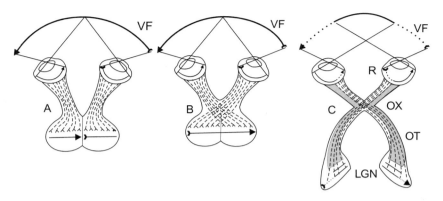

Figure 9.1
A and *B* are based on figures that appear in Cajal's *Histologie* (1911, 1995). *A.*
The visual pathways of an entirely hypothetical "lower" vertebrate, having no
binocular vision and no optic crossing. It is important to stress that there is no
such creature. However, Cajal uses the figure to show the "discrepancy between
the conscious visual image and the object itself" (depicted by the arrows). *B.*
"The benefits" that a complete chiasmatic crossing would produce in such a creature; the arrow is now continuous in the brain. *C.* A heavily modified version of
Cajal's scheme showing what happens in an animal with a significant degree of
binocular overlap. The uncrossed and the crossed pathways are shown, each
going to a different layer of the lateral geniculate nucleus (LGN), where the two
representations of the contralateral visual hemifield are in register. The monocular sectors of the visual field and their central representations are shown by the
interrupted parts of the arrow and its representation. LGN, lateral geniculate
nucleus; OT, optic tract; OX, optic chiasm; R, retina; VF, visual field. *Note:* We
have shown in figure 9.1C, in accord with current evidence (Torrealba et al.,
1982; Guillery et al., 1995), the crossed and the uncrossed axons in the optic
tract intermingling on their way to the lateral geniculate nucleus, and maintaining a rough topographic order. Gross (1999) points out that a schema found in
a Newton manuscript implies just such mixing of the nerve fibers in the optic
tract, and Gross concludes that Newton thought (wrongly, in Gross's view) that
the images from the two eyes fused in the optic tract, rather than in the visual
cortex. Gross bases his view of Newton's supposed error on modern evidence
about neuronal receptive fields: that it is not until the visual inputs reach the
cortex that single binocularly driven nerve cells can first be recorded in the path
from the eye to the cortex. However, the fact that here, too, Newton was
serendipitously correct about the mingling of the two sets of fibers in the pathway
makes one marvel at his capacity to know things that almost 300 years later
Gross still appears to miss. The functional or developmental significance, if any,
of this binocular mingling of axons in the optic tract in rough topographic order,
remains unresolved.

single image transmitted to a single central end-station through two reversing lenses. Descartes's scheme showed each optic nerve going to one hemisphere, so that the image from each eye was represented separately at a first central way station in the brain. Descartes then had fibers from that way station going to the pineal gland, which he proposed as the final receiver of the visual image, through a pathway that involved a partial intrahemispheric crossing. Whereas Descartes had placed the partial crossing in the brain, where we now know that it occurs in a bird like the owl with good binocular vision (Karten et al., 1973), Newton had placed it in the chiasm, where we now know it occurs in mammals. Neither could possibly have had any empirical evidence for his conclusion. Although the junction of the optic nerves at the optic chiasm was known, methods for tissue preservation and study of the fiber systems were not adequate for the type of detail needed to trace the crossed or the uncrossed course of fibers through the optic chiasm, and neither author made an empirical claim. The empirical evidence was not obtained for almost 200 years, a period during which assumptions about localization of functions in the brain were first lost and then regained (Spillane, 1981), all on the basis of arguments that had nothing to do with the rigorous logic applied to the visual system by Descartes and Newton.

Although von Gudden (1874) had been able to demonstrate the partial decussation in the optic chiasm of rabbits experimentally by removing one eye very early in development and showing that the surviving optic nerve split into a large crossed and a smaller uncrossed component, it took Cajal's demonstration of individual axons in Golgi preparations (Cajal, 1911), some crossing in the chiasm, some not crossing, to persuade his contemporaries that there is a partial decussation at the optic chiasm of the mammalian brain. Not only did Cajal show the individual nerve fibers, but he also produced schematic figures (see figure 9.1A and B) based on the same implicit logic that Descartes and Newton had used. With these he explained why there had to be a complete chiasmatic crossing in a vertebrate with laterally placed eyes and no binocular visual field (figure 9.1A and B). The assumption that the brain could not use the broken arrow shown in the brain of figure 9.1A is made explicit by Cajal (1995):

[C]orrect mental perception of visual space can take place only in a brain in which the center responsible for the perception is bilateral, and both halves act in concert so as to render the two images continuous and in the same direction as projected by the right and left halves of the two retinas.

Then he explained why an animal with forward-looking eyes (see figure 9.1C), having a binocular visual field, had to have a partial decussation in the chiasm. Finally, he used these arguments to explain why in the brains of vertebrates, each hemisphere connects to the tactile and other sensory inputs and to motor outputs on the other side of the body. These crossed connections of sensory and motor pathways have not been shown in figure 9.1. The logic that requires them is that, in each hemisphere, visual signals must be related to other sensory and to motor signals from the same side of the body. The implication of Cajal's argument is clear: a disrupted representation, illustrated by a broken arrow in figure 9.1A, could not work to transmit sensory information to the brain.

Although at about the time that Cajal was writing, evidence for orderly, topographic, motor and visual cerebral maps had already been under discussion for some time (Jackson, 1873; Henschen, 1893), he did not refer to this work in his discussion of the chiasm, and for a long time there was no experimental evidence to support the fundamental basis of Cajal's argument, that the brain is unable to function with disrupted maps. It is important to recognize that as sensory messages are traced past the first cortical relay, the accuracy of the maps diminishes, and evidence from other parts of the brain, such as the olfactory pathways and the cerebellum, shows that there are regions of the brain that operate with widely distributed or fractured representations of the input (Welker, 1987; Haberly & Bower, 1989; Hasselmo et al., 1990). The intuitive approach, which assumes that a central "viewing screen" is needed, is not as compelling as perhaps it once seemed. Pattern recognition is possible from distributed, nonmapped systems (Kohonen et al., 1977).

There is a danger, when one is considering the many orderly representations that are found in the thalamocortical pathways, of following the intuitive approach represented in figure 9.1C and not asking what the maps are for. We shall be describing the rich and complex interrelations between numerous cerebral maps in the visual and other pathways, and it will be easy for the reader to forget that the fundamental question of why the brain needs orderly representations of sensory surfaces and also of the motor mechanisms, or better, why the brain uses such maps, and how, remains largely unanswered. There are a few examples, such as visual area V1, where one knows enough about local interactions to argue that without mapped projections such interactions might be very costly in axonal connections, but in general, the significance of maps remains a challenge.

9.D. Clinical and Experimental Evidence for Maps in the Geniculocortical Pathway

9.D.1. Establishing That There Are Maps

The empirical evidence in favor of mapped representations in the visual system came first for the cortex and later for the thalamus. Initially it was shown in human patients that localized lesions of the occipital cortex give rise to localized visual field losses (scotomas; figure 9.2). The history of these studies has a sad link with major international conflicts and with the development of high-speed bullets able to penetrate the skull without killing. These bullets could leave clean entry and exit wounds that allowed quite accurate definition of the cortical damage long before the use of x-rays or modern scanning methods. Studies of visual field losses after damage to the occipital cortex started after the Franco-Prussian war, continued after the Russo-Japanese war, and became highly refined after the 1914–1918, 1939–1945, and subsequent wars (Koerner & Teuber, 1973; Glickstein, 1988).

The fact that local cortical lesions could produce corresponding, well-localized scotomas was evident quite early (figure 9.2; see also figure 2.1). The precise extent of the cortex involved in the production of such scotomas and the precise orientation of the visual field map on the cortical surface were the subject of interesting and quite heated debate for some time, but it is now clear that there is a histologically well-defined area in the occipital lobe, the striate cortex, V1, or area 17, which receives a highly organized, binocular projection of the contralateral visual field. The evidence obtained clinically for the human brain was followed much later by experiments that recorded localized cortical activity in response to visual stimuli delivered to limited parts of the visual field (for monkey: Daniel & Whitteridge, 1961; for cat: Allman and Kaas, 1971; Tusa et al., 1978).

Early knowledge of retinal maps in the thalamus depended on the observations of the cortical lesions and on the rapid and severe retrograde cell losses that these lesions produce in the thalamus (see chapter 2, figure 2.1). When the thalamus was studied in brains with localized lesions it was found that there are correspondingly localized zones of retrograde degeneration in the lateral geniculate nuclei (Minkowski, 1914; Garey & Powell, 1967; Kaas et al., 1972b; see figure 9.2). The fact that each cortical lesion corresponds not only to a particular part of the visual field but also to a particular part of the lateral geniculate nucleus

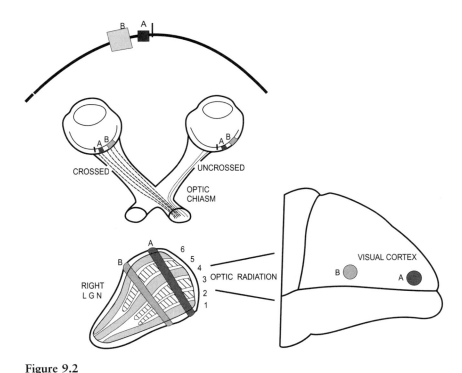

Figure 9.2
In the lower right part of the figure, two localized cortical lesions (A and B) are shown on an outline of a medial view of a right human occipital lobe. The visual field, represented by the arrow at the top of the figure, shows the corresponding visual field losses for the left visual field. There are localized visual losses corresponding to the nasal retina of the left eye and the temporal retina of the right eye. In the lateral geniculate nucleus (shown as a parasagittal section, with posterior to the right) on the side of the lesions in the right hemisphere, each small cortical lesion has produced a localized column of retrograde cell degeneration that goes through all of the geniculate layers, like a toothpick through a club sandwich (see footnote 2). Within the retina one would expect to see degenerative changes in retinal ganglion cells at the points marked A and B, but it should be stressed that the visual losses are a direct result of the cortical damage, not of the retinal damage, which is a secondary, transneuronal retrograde degeneration. Note that due to the magnification factors of mapping retina onto cortex, the visual loss for B is larger than that for A, as is the transneuronal retinal degeneration.

demonstrates that there is a map of the visual field in the nucleus, just as there is in the cortex.

We have seen that the lateral geniculate nucleus is laminated; this lamination has been well studied in carnivores and primates, and figure 9.2 shows that in a primate, each of the six or so laminae receives from either the eye on the same side (shown as hatched layers in figure 9.2) or from that on the other side (shown as white in the figure), but not from both. The relationship of the zones of retrograde degeneration (labeled A and B in the figure), which pass perpendicular to the geniculate layers and through all of them, demonstrates an important point about the way in which the visual field maps onto the lateral geniculate nucleus. The figure shows that all of the layers are receiving inputs from the contralateral visual field but that some layers receive this information through the left eye whereas others receive it through the right eye. Since a localized lesion in the striate cortex produces a scotoma that involves both eyes (a "homonymous visual field loss" involves the same part of the binocular visual field, not of the retina, for each eye), the column of degeneration that passes through the geniculate must correspond to the scotoma for each eye. The astonishing conclusion is that the two maps of the contralateral visual field, one coming from the left eye and the other from the right eye, must be in register through all the laminae of the lateral geniculate nucleus, even though they are largely independent in the lateral geniculate nucleus.[1]

9.D.2 The Alignment of Maps with Each Other

At first sight, this mapping of the visual field in the geniculate layers may not seem as extraordinary as it really is. Figure 9.2 shows that in order to produce such an alignment of visual field representations, small retinal areas of the left and right eye that are both looking at the same part of visual space must project to geniculate cells that are aligned along a single column (A or B in the figure) running through all of the geniculate layers.[2] From a developmental point of view, the two homonymous

1. In the following section we consider the role of corticogeniculate and reticulogeniculate axons (see chapter 3) that pass through several adjacent geniculate layers.

2. Walls (1953) wrote, "The problem of why the lateral geniculate nucleus should ever be stratified has seemed a mystery for half a century. In this time it has been brilliantly shown: first that each LGN embodies an isomorph of one half of the binocular visual field and the adjoining uniocular temporal crescent,

retinal points labeled A have no shared morphological features, nor do those labeled B. They are not symmetrically placed in the head and do not lie in corresponding parts of the two retinas. So far as our current knowledge goes, they are only related because they look at the same point in the visual field. And yet the developing nervous system is able to guide the two sets of retinofugal axons to precisely aligned sites in adjacent geniculate layers. This is a remarkable achievement in itself. It is even more notable because the alignment is completed before eye opening (Shatz, 1996; Crair et al., 1998). We do not know at what developmental stage the projections from the visual cortex and from the thalamic reticular nucleus acquire their mapped order. One can regard the formation of the in-register visual field maps as providing a basis on which the corticogeniculate and the reticulogeniculate axons can pass straight through the nucleus, relating to neurons that receive from just one point in visual space but activated from either the left or the right eye. That is, all of these maps, the retinogeniculate, the corticogeniculate, and the reticulogeniculate, are in matched topographic order in the adult, but the left and the right eye afferents are kept separate (see also chapter 3).

There is one further point, already discussed in chapter 2, that concerns these maps. This is that the retinogeniculate projection is not a single functional or developmental entity. There are functionally distinct retinal ganglion cells (magno, parvo, konio in primates; X, Y, W in cats), which develop at different stages (Walsh & Polley, 1985) and whose axons take distinctly different pathways (Torrealba et al., 1982) to the lateral geniculate nucleus. These all map the geniculate representation of the retina along the same columns (A and B in the figure), although they

---

with each peripheral or central quadrant of each of two hemiretinas projecting to a specific segment of the nucleus; second, that in the strongly binocular carnivores and primates certain laminae receive only from the contralateral retina and others from the ipsilateral; and third, that physiologically correspondent spots in homonymous hemiretinas are scattered along a single 'line' running through all of the gray laminae like one of the toothpicks in a club sandwich. We may marvel at this precision, and we may pardon the old-school localizer for taking refuge in the visual system and crowing a bit. But this knowledge helps us not one jot or tittle to see why the LGN should have lamination per se—not, if no cell in any lamina communicates within the nucleus with any cell in any other lamina. No matter how closely the system may bring binocularly correspondent paths into approximation, if it is not for the purpose of enabling them to 'fuse' in the LGN, then the approximation is senseless; and, the lamination that brings it about continues to seem senseless."

can terminate in different layers, as shown in figure 2.8. That is, we have to recognize that afferents to the thalamus have a capacity for producing accurate matches of several functionally and developmentally distinct, topographically organized projections. This applies not only to ascending afferents but also to corticothalamic connections, which may be heterogeneous, like the retinogeniculate inputs, and which can bring mapped inputs from several cortical areas to a single thalamic nucleus. We will see that it applies to the connections of the thalamic reticular nucleus as well.

One can find many places where two or more maps are brought into precise, or reasonably precise, register with each other. In some instances they are precisely matched within a nucleus or a lamina, in others they form a less rigorous representation, or the matching may be more difficult to demonstrate. For example, in the monkey's ventral posterior nucleus, topographically organized projections to different somatosensory cortical areas come from distinct parts of the nucleus, and these parts interdigitate with each other, so that the functionally distinct representations of the same body part can be seen to lie close to each other (Krubitzer & Kaas, 1992). That is, there is a topographic matching but not the precise alignment seen in the geniculate laminae. The visual system brings out problems of mapping in a particularly striking way because it has to deal with the problem of matching two half-maps from two almost identical inputs, one from each eye, both of them reversed by the lens. However, maps are a common feature of thalamocortical, thalamoreticular, corticoreticular, and corticothalamic pathways, and we can find them in auditory, motor, and somatosensory pathways, where we know something about what it is that is being mapped (Reale & Imig, 1980; Strick, 1988; Beck et al., 1996), as well as in the mamillothalamic pathway (Cowan & Powell, 1954), where the mapped functions are still largely undefined. There is good evidence that activity patterns can play a significant role in some aspects of the development of thalamocortical projections (Shatz, 1996), but the example of the binocular matching across geniculate layers prior to eye opening suggests that other mechanisms are likely to be involved as well, because the patterns of activity coming from the two eyes are not likely to be matched in terms of the visual field alignment that is matched across laminae.

The essential point for us now is that developmental mechanisms have the capacity to produce finely matched maps. Where we fail to see such accuracy it may be that processing is concerned with features other than the precise topography of the afferents. In relays that are not concerned with the location of the stimulus per se, such as taste or smell, or in relays that are a few steps from a sensory surface that is concerned with location, the maps are more difficult to define, presumably because the simple topography of the peripheral map does not play a central role and other features, often more difficult to isolate for study, begin to dominate.[3] This will prove to be a key to understanding many of the "higher" cortical areas and the higher order thalamic nuclei that serve these cortical areas. It may also provide a key to understanding how pathways that carry several cortical and thalamic representations of a single modality, some representations more accurately mapped than others, some perhaps not mapped at all, come to relate to each other as they pass through the thalamic reticular nucleus.

Given that the mammalian visual pathways have achieved such a complex developmental feat of binocular matching in the lateral geniculate nucleus, it is reasonable to ask with Walls (see footnote 2) what it can possibly be for. Although there is some evidence for weak binocular interactions in the lateral geniculate nucleus (Sanderson et al., 1971; Schmielau & Singer, 1977), the problem of why the lateral geniculate nucleus is laminated and why the visual representations in the layers are aligned is not solved. Whereas the lamination clearly serves to separate left eye from right eye inputs, the mapping brings them into register, as though they are meant to interact or to be subjected to a common input. This dual aspect of the functional separation may provide a clue to thalamic organization in general. On the one hand, the thalamus provides a simple, clear relay for sensory pathways on the way to the cortex. For some of the time that is the main relay function of the thalamus; the cortex receives the messages from each eye that come through the one set of geniculate layers; the two inputs are essentially independent and only start to relate to single cells within the visual cortex (Hubel & Wiesel, 1977). On the other hand, we have argued that there is another function for the thalamic relay and that this serves to *modulate* the activity relayed through the thalamus. This modulation can be global or local, and, for the visual pathways, if it is local it would generally need to relate to the binocular visual field, not

---

3. The olfactory system provides an excellent example of how difficult it is to discover the nature of a map in the central nervous system if one does not know what it is that is mapped. In its early stages the system does not map the spatial distribution of odors in the environment, but instead maps distinct groups of molecular structures (Mombaerts et al., 1996; Belluscio et al., 1999).

just to one or the other retina. The two important modulatory inputs considered in chapter 3, one coming from the cerebral cortex, the other coming from the thalamic reticular nucleus (figure 3.7; see also Uhlrich et al., 2003), both have axons that pass through the geniculate laminae like Walls's toothpick (footnote 2). That is, in figure 9.2, corticothalamic afferents coming from the small cortical area indicated by A distribute to the whole of column A of the lateral geniculate nucleus, and correspondingly for the parts labeled B. The experimental evidence for this was illustrated in figure 3.8, and figure 3.10 shows that the same is true for axons that go from the reticular nucleus to the geniculate layers. It appears that these modulatory connections require the alignment of the two maps, so that enhancement or suppression is not limited to a part of the visual field for just one eye but can act on the same visual field representation for each eye. There are rare occasions when modulatory actions may need to be monocular. There is evidence that some modulatory axons from the parabrachial region of the cat innervate a single geniculate layer, thus possibly providing modulation for one eye only (Uhlrich et al., 1988). Possibly there are also some corticogeniculate or reticulogeniculate axons that distribute to left eye or right eye geniculate layers only, but they have not been documented.

Although the arrangement of the binocular inputs to the lateral geniculate nucleus provides a unique relationship that can be found only in the visual pathways, an analysis of how the retinal maps relate to each other helps to illuminate a duality of thalamic functions that is not limited to the visual pathways: transmission of information to cortex and a modulation of that transmission that can be either global or localized. It is worth extending this argument about topographic specificity beyond the most obvious example of local action, with topographic specificity relating to a part of a map, to specificity based on the functional type of relay cell affected, such as geniculate X cell versus Y cell. Although currently we have limited evidence for such connections, it is likely that the differential distribution of some corticogeniculate and reticulogeniculate axons to specific layers of the lateral geniculate nucleus (see chapter 3) relate to such a form of specific functional rather than topographic modulation.

9.E. Multiple Maps in the Thalamocortical Pathways

9.E.1. The Demonstration of Multiple Maps

Evidence that there might be more than one map of the visual field in the cerebral cortex came from electrophysiological recordings (Allman

& Kaas, 1974, 1975; Tusa et al., 1979; Tusa & Palmer, 1980; Van Essen et al., 1992) and from studies of callosal connections between the two hemispheres, which exploited the fact that most of the visually responsive axons in the corpus callosum have receptive fields close to the vertical midline of the visual field, so that a plot of distinct islands of termination of callosal axons could be interpreted as a plot of several representations of the vertical meridian (Zeki, 1969; Cragg, 1969; Olavarria & Montero, 1984, 1989). Studies of cortical responses to other afferents have also shown multiple cortical maps for the somatosensory and auditory pathways (Reale & Imig, 1980; Beck et al., 1996; Kaas et al., 1999), and, similarly, several motor maps have been described (Strick, 1988). Detailed studies of the visually responsive cortex of cats and monkeys now show many distinct, more or less accurately mapped representations of the visual field, over 30 in rhesus monkeys (Van Essen et al., 1992). It is to be stressed that the accuracy of the maps varies from one cortical area to another. Some areas show little or no local sign, others show local sign but appear to represent only a part of the visual field, not all of it.

Many of these cortical areas are thought to represent a different aspect of cortical processing, one, for example, being concerned with color, another with movement (Britten et al., 1993; Zeki, 1993), although for many, no specific functional specialization has yet been recognized. A great deal of attention has been focused in recent years on the way in which these cortical areas are interconnected with each other through corticocortical pathways. Although the functional roles of these corticocortical pathways are almost entirely unexplored in terms of their driver or modulator functions (see chapters 7 and 8; see also Crick & Koch, 1998; Sherman & Guillery, 1998), the interconnections that have been described are complex and have led to complicated schemes of corticocortical communication, the details of which are, fortunately, well beyond the scope of this book.

In addition to this multiplicity of cortical maps, there are also several maps of the visual field in the thalamus itself. These can be displayed by electrophysiological recording (Mason, 1978; Chalupa & Abramson, 1988, 1989; Hutchins & Updyke, 1989) or by studying the connections between the cortical maps and the thalamic maps with neuroanatomical tracers (Updyke, 1977, 1981). A single small, localized injection of an anterograde tracer such as tritiated proline into area 17 or one of the other visual areas produces a number of localized zones, or columns of terminal label, in the thalamus, one in each nucleus or nuclear subdivision. By varying the position of the area 17 injection it can be shown that each zone forms a part of a more or less complete map of the visual field in the thalamus.

The way in which these several thalamic and cortical representations of the visual field are interconnected is likely to be of vital importance to the functioning of the thalamocortical visual system and to our understanding of it, but currently we know relatively little about the precise pattern of the interconnections; we have a far better view of the direct corticocortical connections than we do of those that go through the higher order thalamic relays. Although multiple cortical areas have been defined in rats, mice, cats, and monkeys (Zeki, 1969; Tusa et al., 1979; Tusa & Palmer, 1980; Olavarria & Montero, 1984, 1989; Van Essen et al., 1992), the extent to which cortical areas in different species can be treated as functionally equivalent or developmentally homologous is currently largely unknown, and we have yet to find out whether there is a generalization that can be made across species about the way in which the two-way connections between these several cortical areas and the thalamus are organized. It should perhaps be stressed that the chances of finding true homologies for the many cortical areas in two species that are not closely related will depend on the extent to which the increase in the number of cortical areas has occurred independently in the two species. In view of the dramatic increase in cortical areas that seems to characterize mammalian and particularly primate evolution, it may often be unrealistic to look for close homologies.

9.E.2. *Mirror Reversals of Maps and Pathways*

One important and common feature of thalamocortical pathways that include more than one cortical or thalamic map is that in many of the accounts of multiple maps for a single modality, such as vision or touch, one commonly sees that adjacent maps are mirror reversals of each other. The developmental mechanisms that underlie these many mirror reversals are not understood, nor is it known whether the mirror reversals have any functional significance in the adult. However, from the point of view of the present discussion they demonstrate the capacity of the thalamocortical and corticothalamic pathways to form the complex crossings that are needed within each hemisphere in order to produce orderly connections between a thalamic relay and two or more of such mirror-reversed cortical maps (Adams et al., 1997). It is important to stress that no amount of twisting of axonal pathways can produce the connections that are required. An actual crossing of axons in one dimension of the map is required. In the pathways that link thalamus and cortex, a complex system of crossing axons can be seen in two regions quite early in development. One is immediately beneath the cortex in a region that corresponds to the *subplate* of early development (Allendoerfer & Shatz, 1994), and the other is in the thalamic reticular nucleus and in a region that lies close to it laterally, the *perireticular* nucleus, which lies in the region of the upper thalamic arrow in figure 9.3 (Mitrofanis, 1994; Earle & Mitrofanis, 1996). Both of these cell groups are present as the axons are growing to link thalamus and cortex, but are largely lost due to heavy cell death in later development.

The expected pattern of axons crossing each other is present in the pathways from the lateral geniculate nucleus to the first visual cortical area (area 17) and also in that going from the ventral posterior nucleus to the first somatosensory cortical area (Adams et al., 1997). For the visual pathways the mirror reversal represents a reversal of the horizontal meridian about an axis formed by the vertical meridian. The mirror reversal in the geniculocortical pathway was recognized by Connolly and Van Essen (1984), and the pathway crossing itself was demonstrated experimentally by Nelson and LeVay (1985) for the cat. They showed that the crossing of the thalamocortical fibers occurs in the white matter underlying the visual cortex. In contrast, Lozsádi et al. (1996) showed that the crossing for the corticogeniculate axons in a rat occurs within the thalamic reticular nucleus (as shown schematically in figure 9.3), and also just lateral to this nucleus in the perireticular nucleus. Evidence about where the crossings occur for most of the pathways that link thalamus and cortex is currently unavailable. Possibly the thalamocortical pathways all cross in the subcortical regions that develop from the subplate and the corticothalamic axons all cross in the perireticular nucleus and the thalamic reticular nucleus (see below); that would be a neat arrangement in accord with the fact that the two pathways take quite independent courses. The perireticular nucleus and the subplate are two very similar cell groups. They are present transiently next to cortex and next to the reticular nucleus, they share many immunohistochemical staining properties, and they are most evident at the developmental stages when thalamocortical and corticothalamic axons are growing through these regions (Mitrofanis & Guillery, 1993). They are likely to play a significant role in establishing the complex crossings. In the adult, the region of the thalamic reticular nucleus, where much of the complex pattern of axon crossing occurs, serves as a crucial nexus for thalamocortical and corticothalamic pathways because both sets of axons give

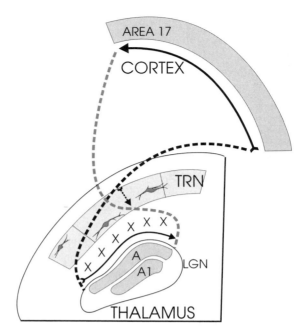

Figure 9.3
Schematic representation of the pathways that connect the visual cortex and lateral geniculate nucleus in a cat. Only two geniculate layers (labeled A and A1) are shown. In order for the two maps, geniculate and cortical, to be topographically interconnected, a pathway crossing is necessary, as shown here for the corticothalamic axons, which are shown crossing in the region of the thalamic reticular nucleus. Three cells of the reticular nucleus are shown with their dendritic arbors stretched out in the plane of the reticular nucleus. The two continuous arrows represent the horizontal meridian of the visual hemifield in the cortex and in the lateral geniculate nucleus. The small interrupted arrow represents representation of the horizontal meridian in the reticular nucleus. TRN, thalamic reticular nucleus; LGN, lateral geniculate nucleus. Xs mark the position of the cells of the perigeniculate nucleus. See text for details.

off collateral branches to the thalamic reticular nucleus as they pass through.

In the thalamic reticular nucleus there is not only the pattern of axon crossing necessitated by the mirror reversals but there is also a significant amount of convergence and divergence in the pathways that link thalamic nuclei and cortical areas. Although in primates, almost all current evidence shows that only a few of the geniculocortical axons go to extrastriate visual cortex (Fries, 1981; Yukie & Iwai, 1981; Sincich et al., 2004), in other species there are projections from the lateral geniculate nucleus to several visual cortical areas. Each of these areas in turn sends axons to the lateral geniculate nucleus and to the pulvinar and lateral posterior nuclei. So far as we know at present, many of these several converging and diverging thalamocortical and corticothalamic pathways send branches to the reticular nucleus and connect to the same portion or sector of the reticular nucleus, described more fully below.

The multiplicity of cortical areas and thalamic nuclei for any one modality produces a combination of crossing pathways, divergent and convergent pathways that link thalamus and cortex (see chapter 1, figure 1.6). Each pathway can give off collateral branches to the same sector of the reticular nucleus, and as several systems pass through the reticular nucleus they can relate several different thalamocortical and corticothalamic pathways concerned with a single modality to the cells of the reticular nucleus.

9.F. Abnormal Maps in the Visual Pathways

Abnormal visual pathways can be produced by naturally occurring mutations or by surgical interference with the developing system. The abnormalities illustrate the extent to which thalamic afferent and efferent connections depend on topographic order and the degree to which the binocular matching across geniculate laminae, discussed earlier, is a necessary part of normal thalamic function. Further, the abnormal pathways demonstrate the extent to which thalamocortical pathways develop in accord with the topographic demands of the sensory inputs rather than with any firmly established intrinsic developmental program. The mutations act like a delicate piece of experimental surgery, causing a particular group of axons, some of the normally uncrossed axons from the temporal retina, to take an abnormal, crossed pathway. The experimental manipulations involve an early postnatal monocular enucleation in hamsters or ferrets. These are both species who have young born at very immature stages, and the enucleation can be done at an early developmental stage, before the thalamocortical pathways are formed. The results are comparable for the mutants and the enucleations. They demonstrate clearly that the input to the thalamus can influence the topography of the map that is passed to the cortex and can produce reversals of the type considered above. The details of the abnormal maps have been worked out more clearly in the mutants.

9.F.1. Abnormal Pathways in Albinos

Much of the work that has attempted to define the developmental basis of the gene action in the mutants or to analyze the functional capacities of the adult visual pathways is beyond the scope of this book. Stent (1978) has written a stimulating analysis, and more recent summaries can be found in Guillery et al. (1995) and Guillery (1996). Here we are concerned to use the mutant systems to look at what happens when the abnormalities produce disrupted maps, as represented by Cajal's broken arrow, or produce nonmatching maps within adjacent geniculate layers, and to compare thalamus and cortex, since there appears to be an important difference in the way that the two structures react to these abnormal connections.

Albino animals, and many other mutants with an abnormal distribution of melanin in the retina early in development, suffer from an abnormal crossing of some of the retinofugal axons. The abnormal pathways have been worked out in most detail for Siamese cats, which are homozygous for an allele of the albino series. In normal cats (left in figure 9.4) the lateral geniculate nucleus receives inputs from the contralateral visual hemifield only. The abnormal pathways (right in figure 9.4) produce a geniculate segment (numbered 9–12 in figure 9.4) that receives from the ipsilateral visual hemifield through the contralateral eye. This abnormal pathway arises in retinal sectors 9–12 and takes a crossed instead of the normally uncrossed route in the chiasm. The misrouted axons go to the appropriate geniculate locus, but on the wrong side. As a result, geniculate segments that normally receive from visual field segments 8, 7, 6, and 5, in mediolateral sequence, now receive from segments 9, 10, 11, and 12, respectively. The retinal axons are terminating on the wrong side and therefore bring a mirror-reversed representation of an abnormally located part of the visual field. Further, in the layer labeled A1 there is a disruption not unlike Cajal's broken arrow, represented by the sequence 9, 10, 11, 12, // 4, 3. Also, whereas normally the numbers match across layers, they match only for sectors 3 and 4.

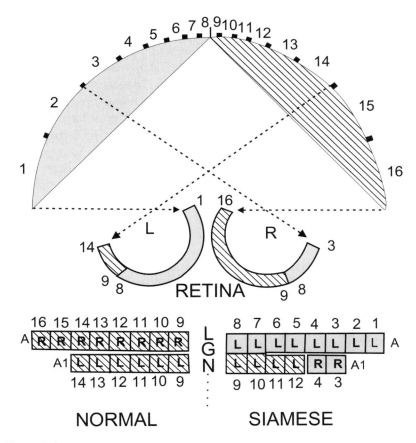

Figure 9.4
Schema to show the layout of the retinogeniculate pathways in normal and Siamese cats. The top half of the figure applies to both types of pathway. It is only the connection from the retina to the lateral geniculate that differs in the two. The normal pattern is shown for the lateral geniculate nucleus on the left side of the figure, and the abnormal, Siamese pattern is shown on the right. R, L, right and left retina and, in the lateral geniculate nucleus, inputs from the right and left retina; LGN, lateral geniculate nucleus.

Electrophysiological recordings in Siamese cats (Hubel & Wiesel, 1971; Kaas & Guillery, 1973) show that all of the geniculate cells, including those in layer A1, respond well to visual stimuli, and the same has been recorded for the superior colliculus (Berman & Cynader, 1972; Lane et al., 1974). That is, contrary to Cajal's suggestion (see figure 9.1), these cell groups can accept a disrupted representation of the visual field.

In the visual cortex the situation is different. Cajal's suggestion seems correct. A broken arrow does not make for a functional connection. Although all geniculate layers send axons to visual cortex, showing the classical retrograde degeneration after cortical lesions (Kaas & Guillery, 1973), the broken arrow representation is not seen in the cortex. Two distinct patterns of visual field representation, neither showing the expected broken arrow, have been defined electrophysiogically and confirmed by retrograde degeneration after small cortical lesions. The two patterns were labeled Boston and Midwestern patterns, to indicate where each was first described. In Midwestern cats (Kaas & Guillery, 1973; see also figure 9.5B), the whole abnormal visual field representation arising from the temporal retina, though present in the lateral geniculate nucleus, is absent in cortex, indicated in figure 9.5B by the struck-out numbers in cortex. Almost all of the cortical cells are driven by inputs from the nasal retina alone. Note that *all* inputs from the temporal retina are lost in the cortex, not just those from the abnormally connected sector of the temporal retina. Confirmation that cortical cells are not responding to inputs from the temporal retina comes from experiments showing that these cats do not respond to stimuli falling on any part of the temporal retina (Elekessy et al., 1973; Guillery & Casagrande, 1977). That is, the parts of the visual fields that do not drive cortical cells also fail to evoke a normal behavioral response.

In Boston cats (figure 9.5C), there is a partial reversal of the geniculocortical projection demonstrable for the abnormally innervated geniculate segment by cortical recording (Hubel & Wiesel, 1971) and by retrograde degeneration (Kaas & Guillery, 1973). The abnormal geniculate segment (9, 10, 11, 12) is now connected to cortex without the normal mirror reversal in the thalamocortical pathway and is inserted next to the 17/18 border. In normal cats this border represents the vertical meridian, but in the Boston pathways it represents about 20° into the ipsilateral visual field. This reversal corrects the disruption, producing an orderly, continuous representation of the normal contralateral visual hemifield and of the adjacent, additional part of the hemifield on the same side (the sequence of large numbers, 1–12, in cortex in figure

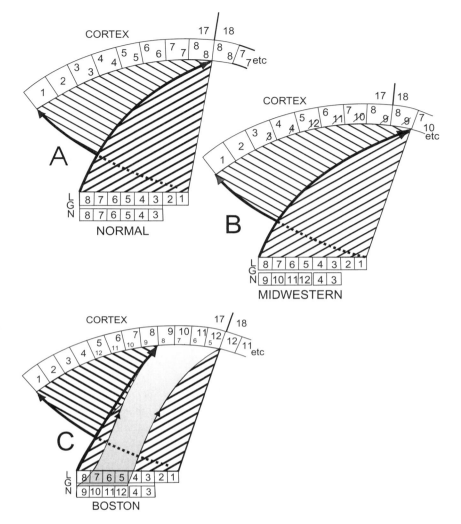

Figure 9.5

A, NORMAL. Schema for a normal cat to show the reversed connections to visual cortex (area 17 or V1) from two geniculate layers in which the visual field representations are in register, as indicated by the numbers. 17/18 shows the boundary between areas 17 and 18; LGN, lateral geniculate nucleus. *B,* MIDWESTERN. Schema using the same conventions as in *A* to show that in the Midwestern geniculocortical pathways of Siamese cats, none of the inputs from the abnormally innervated layer of the lateral geniculate nucleus have effective cortical connections. That is, crossed inputs shown in the figure coming from retinal sectors numbered 9, 10, 11, and 12, and uncrossed inputs numbered 4 and 3, are not received in cortex. Essentially, messages from the temporal retina fail to reach cortex. In contrast, the crossed inputs coming from the nasal retina (sectors 1–8) make normal cortical connections. *C,* BOSTON. Schema to show the correction that occurs in the Boston geniculocortical pathways of Siamese cats. Inputs from nasal and temporal retina provide effective input to cortex; the continuous sequence of visual field representation is recreated by the reversal of a sector of the geniculocortical pathway (9, 10, 11, and 12) to its own cortical area adjacent to the 17/18 boundary. See text for details.

9.5C). Cajal's arrow has been repaired! And the repair involves a mirror reversal of a part of the thalamocortical pathway. Further, these cats respond to visual stimuli for the whole retina, showing that the repaired arrow is functional.[4] The reversal of the abnormal sector in the Boston pathways is of particular interest because it demonstrates that the map in the thalamocortical pathway depends on the map that arrives at the thalamic relay from the driver afferents, and this conclusion is confirmed by the experimental results described in the next section.

Figures 9.5B and C show two strikingly abnormal features of the visual field representation in the geniculate, either one of which might be expected to produce a visual abnormality. One is a "broken arrow" in the abnormally innervated layer, and the other is a mismatch across the layers for just one part of the arrow. Whereas the broken arrow effect can be expected to affect the whole of the relevant geniculate layer (layer A1 in figure 9.5), the mismatch affects only the abnormally innervated segment of layer A1. Since the abnormal cortical and behavioral responses involve the whole of the arrow, it appears that the disruption of the sequence is the relevant feature for the cortical suppression in the Midwestern pathways, not the translaminar mismatch.

This interpretation, that the mismatch across geniculate layers does not produce an abnormal visual response, is confirmed by two lines of evidence. One is that in some cats, in which the normally connected sector of the temporal retina is extremely small (Leventhal & Creel, 1985; Ault et al., 1995), and in albino monkeys, which also have a very small uncrossed component (Guillery et al., 1984), there appears to be no significant loss of responsiveness in the cortex. That is, there is no significant broken arrow effect within the geniculate layer that normally receives the uncrossed afferents (A1). The second is that in Siamese cats in which one eye has been sutured from before eye opening (Guillery & Casagrande, 1977), there is no loss of responsiveness for the normal eye. Figure 9.4 (right side) shows that a right monocular suture would leave the input labeled L in the figure intact, producing no broken arrow, but producing a translaminar mismatch. The mismatched inputs appear not to be in conflict, and the cats react normally to visual stimuli falling on the temporal retina of the normal eye. This behavioral response to visual stimuli on one side can be abolished by a cortical lesion on the other

---

4. Hubel and Wiesel (1971) also described a small number of cortical cells having two receptive fields in mirror position to each other about the vertical meridian. See the smaller figures in the cortex in figure 9.5C.

side, showing that one is dealing with behavioral responses that depend on the cortical mechanisms.

This result may seem odd in view of what we said earlier about the match of visual field maps across layers. If this match is important for the modulatory pathways, then are there subtle abnormalities in such monocularly lid-sutured Siamese cats that remain to be defined? Or has the mismatch been dealt with in some other way? The answer is not known because we do not have appropriate behavioral tests of the function of the modulatory pathways. A partial answer may be in two sets of experiments, one relevant to the Boston, the other to the Midwestern pattern, showing that each has a distinct modification of the corticothalamic pathways, each apparently matching the pattern of the thalamocortical pathway (Montero & Guillery, 1978; Shatz & LeVay, 1979). Perhaps there are corresponding abnormalities of the reticulothalamic and thalamoreticular pathways, but these have not been studied.

The results summarized provide striking evidence that the continuity of Cajal's arrow is important for the development of functional representations of sensory surfaces in the cortex. The Boston animals have also shown that there is a capacity for the developing thalamocortical pathways to produce reversals that serve to recreate a continuous arrow from a discontinuous one. It would seem probable that this capacity reflects a part of the normal developmental repertoire of the thalamocortical system and is not something that the mutant cats have developed de novo in response to the retinofugal abnormalities. This conclusion is confirmed in the next section.

9.F.2. Experimental Modifications of the Thalamocortical Pathway

Evidence that the map formed by the thalamocortical pathways depends on the afferents to the thalamus comes from very early postnatal monocular enucleations in hamsters or ferrets (Trevelyan & Thompson, 1995; Krug et al., 1998). This leaves one lateral geniculate nucleus, the one innervated by the eye on the same side, with an abnormal, partially reversed projection in the retinogeniculate pathway (Schall et al., 1988). By making small injections of different retrograde markers in visual cortex at various stages of development and in the adult, it was shown that there is a mirror reversal of the geniculocortical projection on the side of the enucleation, reminiscent of the Boston abnormality, and that this develops early in postnatal life. These experiments demonstrate clearly that the arrangement of sensory maps that feed into the thalamus plays a significant role in the development and in the functioning of the mapped thalamocortical pathways. That is, the thalamocortical pathways have the capacity to produce modifications and mirror reversals in the early postnatal brain (Krug et al., 1998), and it is probable from the limited evidence we have from Siamese cats that the modulatory pathways that innervate the thalamic relay cells from cortex are correspondingly modified. The important point is that thalamocortical projections are not preprogrammed. The maps that they establish in cortex depend on the maps that they receive from their driver afferents. This is a view that bears serious exploration no matter whether these drivers represent a sensory surface or a higher cortical area, and no matter whether we know or are entirely ignorant about the functional variable that is mapped in the topographically organized pathways that link thalamus and cortex.

9.G. Maps in Higher Order Relays

We have mentioned that thalamocortical pathways in general are topographically ordered, even those that come from higher order relays. Whereas we know what is mapped for many of the first order relays, such as the visual, auditory, or somatosensory relays, we have very little idea about the specific functions that are mapped in higher order relays. We may, for example, be a long way from learning what functions are mapped in the layer 5 projections that go from the frontal cortex to the medial dorsal nucleus, or finding out how those functions are laid out in relation to the morphologically definable maps. The region of the pulvinar and the lateral posterior nucleus provide a relay that is, perhaps, slightly more accessible to such questions, because we know that there are significant parts of these regions concerned with higher visual functions, and because to a significant extent details of the maps are known. This region can serve to illustrate the types of question that are likely to arise as regards the mapped projection to any higher relay, and we use it here to serve as an example.

9.G.1. Maps in the Pulvinar and Lateral Posterior Nuclei

There is good evidence that the pulvinar in primates, and the region that includes the lateral posterior nucleus and the pulvinar in the cat, houses several maps, allowing the identification of several distinct subdivisions (Updyke, 1979, 1981, 1983; Graybiel & Berson, 1980; Hutchins & Updyke, 1989; Adams et al., 2000; Gutierrez et al., 2000; Shipp, 2001,

2003; Lyon et al., 2003; Van Essen, 2005). Subdivisions have been established in different ways: they have been identified as histochemically distinct regions or as regions in receipt of tectal inputs; they have been recorded as distinct representations of the visual field; and they have been identified as distinct representations of one or more cortical areas recorded by transport of marker molecules to the thalamus from visual cortex (areas 17, 18, 19, suprasylvian cortical areas in the cat), or by stimulation of cortex and recording in the thalamus. Whereas there is still significant disagreement about the functionally significant subdivisions in the monkey brain (see Van Essen, 2005), the subdivisions demonstrated by Updyke's studies (1979, 1981, 1983) show that there are several clearly distinguishable maps of cortical areas and of the visual field identifiable in the lateral posterior nucleus and pulvinar of the cat. In general, as would be expected, the maps of the cortex and the maps of the visual fields have shown agreement, although the precision of the maps is not equal to that found in the lateral geniculate nucleus. Demonstrating the maps in the thalamocortical pathways has been more difficult, and the older methods of retrograde degeneration (see chapter 1) were often difficult to interpret in terms of well-defined maps. In the following discussion we focus particularly on the lateral part of the lateral posterior nucleus of the cat, and use this as an example of the questions that can be asked of any higher order relay.

Figure 9.6 shows that it is possible to identify functional columns that run through the lateral posterior nucleus. They have been identified by different terms (Updyke, 1983; Shipp, 2003) but will here be called isocortical columns (Guillery et al., 2001). These columns are comparable with but not identical to the columns that run through the lateral geniculate nucleus (columns A and B in figure 9.2). Unlike the geniculate columns, the isocortical columns receive driver (i.e., layer 5) inputs from several distinct cortical areas, not from the single retinal surface. The modulators, as for the lateral geniculate nucleus, come from several different cortical areas, and the outputs also go to several different cortical areas (Abramson & Chalupa, 1985), but the extent to which the outputs involve axons that send branches to more than one cortical area is only partially defined (Tong & Spear, 1986). The cortical connections are mapped, so that visual field representations in the several cortical areas match visual field maps in the lateral posterior nucleus, and any one column represents a limited part of the visual field. Just as in the lateral geniculate nucleus (see figure 9.2), a plane (or lamina) perpendicular to the columns represents essentially the whole of the contralateral visual field, or a whole of a relevant ipsilateral cortical area. Also, as in

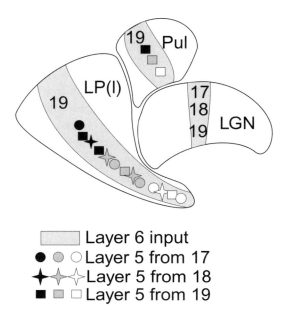

Figure 9.6
Schematic representation of the corticothalamic afferents from areas 17, 18, and 19 to the lateral geniculate nucleus (LGN), the lateral part of the lateral posterior nucleus (LPl), and the pulvinar (Pul) in the cat. Modulatory corticothalamic afferents from layer 6 go to the LGN from all three cortical areas, and to LPl and Pul from area 19 only. Driver afferents from layer 5 do not go to the LGN but do go to LPl from areas 17, 18, and 19, and go to Pul from area 19 only. Note that cortical areas beyond 17, 18, 19, which also have thalamic projections to these nuclei, are not included here. The modulatory afferents from any one small cortical region have a more widespread distribution than do the driver afferents. See text for details. (Based on results in Guillery et al., 2001.)

the geniculate, the pattern of input connections, and probably of output connections (which, however, have not been studied from this point of view), varies along the length of each column.

This comparison of geniculate and lateral posterior organization helps to clarify features that are likely to prove key to understanding the organization of many, possibly all higher order relays, and shows why it has long been so difficult to arrive at any clearly agreed subdivision of the monkey's pulvinar (Van Essen, 2005). Subdivisions made on the basis of architectonic or molecular features may correspond to the whole of the geniculate, to one of the layers of the geniculate, or to a part of the geniculate (e.g., to central versus peripheral representation of the visual field). It is reasonable to suppose that the sensory and cortical maps will provide keys to the subdivisions and that the architectonic and molecular differences can then be understood only in terms of how they relate to these maps.

In the lateral posterior nucleus (lateral part) of the cat, where the columns pass obliquely from anterior (and dorsal) to posterior (and ventral), the posterior and midportions are innervated by cortical areas 17, 18, and 19 (Updyke, 1977; Guillery et al., 2001), receiving well-localized driver terminals from all three cortical areas and very sparse layer 6 inputs from areas 17 and 18, but rich and quite widespread layer 6 inputs from area 19. These layer 6 inputs also extend further anteriorly than do the layer 5 inputs. The posterior parts of the nucleus are innervated by suprasylvian cortex (Updyke, 1981), and the most anterior parts receive from cortical areas 7 and 5 (Heath & Jones, 1971; Robertson & Cunningham, 1981). A further indication of the nonhomogeneity of any one column is seen in the structure of the layer 5 corticothalamic terminals from areas 17, 18, and 19. This structure changes from a relatively open arbor with widely spaced synaptic terminals anteriorly to a more compact structure with tightly packed terminals posteriorly. The former resemble retinal terminals in the geniculate A layers, whereas the latter are more like the terminals in the geniculate C layers (Guillery, 1966; Guillery et al., 2001). That is, the pattern of the cortical innervation varies as any one column is traced from its anterior to its posterior end.

The question arises as to what, if anything, is represented along any one column. In the lateral geniculate nucleus the layers represent different groups of functionally distinct retinal inputs (see chapter 2, figure 2.8) the magno-, parvo-, and koniocellular, or X, Y, and W components. For the magno- and parvocellular portions of the primate geniculate and for the main (A and A1) layers of the cat, these are morphologically identifiable subdivisions of the nucleus. However, in other species, such as the rabbit or rat (Holcombe & Guillery, 1984), in the C layers of the cat, or the koniocellular layers of the primate, there are no morphological, readily identifiable laminar borders to identify the functionally distinct zones. Similarly, in the pulvinar and lateral posterior regions there are no identifiable subdivisons or layers, but this does not imply that there is a functional homogeneity all along any one isocortical column.

Generally the response properties of cells in the lateral posterior nucleus of the cat are described as relatively uniform (Casanova, 2004), resembling those in layer 5 of area 17. However, several points need to be recognized. One is that no one has systematically compared response properties along any one isocortical column. Another is that many of the relevant observations were made with the animals under anesthesia, and a third is that the nature of the response properties that are likely to vary is undefined. The third point can be illustrated from the retinogeniculate pathway: it was not until the distinction between X, Y, and W retinal ganglion cells had been clearly defined that it was possible to show how the response properties in the geniculate A layers in the cat differed from those in the C layers.[5] This is the problem that arises over and over again as one tries to define the functional role (see footnote 2 in chapter 8) of any thalamic relay. This role is not a given; it has to be to be searched for, or it may be found serendipitously (Hubel, 1996).

Finally, as figure 9.6 shows (Guillery et al., 2001), the driver inputs from several different cortical areas can be intermingled within any one segment of an isocortical column, suggesting that there is likely to be a mixture of response types at any one part of a column. That is, in terms of its driver inputs, any one isocortical column represents a mixture of distinct inputs, coming from different cortical areas, and thus distributing distinct functional properties to the column. We know that there is a mingling of cortical inputs within any one part of the column (as represented by the terminals from areas 17, 18, and 19 in figure 9.6) and that there are changes in the pattern of terminals from one end of the column to the other. That is, as indicated above, the comparison with the lateral geniculate nucleus is instructive, because just as the X and the Y inputs in a cat are mingled in one part of a geniculate column (layers A and A1), so cortical driver inputs from several different cortical areas can share one part of an isocortical column. Further, as in the lateral geniculate nucleus, the heterogeneity of the inputs to one end of a column is not the same as the heterogeneity of the inputs to the other end.

On the basis of the above brief view of one higher order relay and the proposed basic similarity of its organization to a first order relay, it makes sense to look at higher order relays generally from this point of view. That is, where a three-dimensional thalamic nucleus maps onto a two-dimensional cortical area, one can expect the map to occupy two dimensions in the thalamus and the third dimension to represent an iso-cortical column. Once the orientation of these columns has been identi-fied, it becomes of interest to consider whether relay functions along any

5. It is worth recalling that Le Gros Clark, knowing of no other relevant variable and finding three pairs of layers, proposed that color was represented in the primate geniculate layers (Walls, 1953).

one column vary or are constant. For this the source of the cortical driver (layer 5) inputs, from one cortical area or several, is important, as is the degree of homogeneity along a column of this input from any one cortical area. Further, since currently the identification of functions for different cortical areas is well ahead of the identification of thalamic functions, the identification of cortical connections may help to establish the functions of higher order thalamic relays.

For this the layer 5 driver inputs may provide some crucial evidence, but it will also be important to define how the corticothalamic layer 6 modulatory input relates to the other connectional patterns. We have argued that a significant part of the layer 6 input to thalamus appears to be a reciprocal feedback connection, although there is evidence that there are layer 6 connections that extend well beyond the boundaries of strict feedback connections (see chapter 3; see also Murphy & Sillito, 1996; Darian-Smith et al., 1999; Murphy et al., 2000; Kakei et al., 2001; Van Horn & Sherman, 2004). The complex relationships between layer 5 and layer 6 inputs are defined for only a few higher order thalamic relays. The distribution of these afferents to different parts of the columns of the lateral posterior nucleus described above and the relationships described in the previous chapter (see chapter 8, figure 8.3) suggest that the relationship between the corticothalamic drivers and modulators, which allows one cortical area to modulate the activity originating in another cortical area, merits comparison with direct corticocortical connections that may have comparable modulatory actions.

As the organization of any one higher order thalamic relay becomes defined and related to drivers for functionally distinct cortical areas, it may prove possible to identify some of the functional properties of that thalamic relay in terms of known cortical functions. It will also be important to understand how the transthalamic corticocortical connections originating in layer 5 cells relate to the direct corticocortical connections. At present there is no clear evidence on this point, although Shipp (2001, 2003) has proposed that there is a "replication principle," with the pattern of corticothalamic interconnections replicating the corticocortical connections. However, the relevant experiments cited by Shipp included some in which no distinction was made between anterograde and retrograde labeling of interconnections between cortex and thalamus, and included none where the layer 5 corticothalamic component was distinguished from the layer 6 component, which, as shown above, establish different patterns of thalamic connections. In order to successfully compare the direct and the transthalamic pathways it will be necessary, as pointed out earlier, to distinguish the drivers from the modulators in each pathway. The rules, if any, by which one can relate corticocortical to corticothalamocortical connections remain to be defined.

9.H. Maps in the Thalamic Reticular Nucleus

The thalamic reticular nucleus is a relatively narrow sheet of cells wrapped around the rostral, lateral, and dorsal aspects of the thalamus (see figure 1.2). Both the thalamocortical and the corticothalamic axons have to pass through this nucleus, and as they do, they give off branches that provide mostly excitatory innervation to the reticular cells (Jones, 1985; Murphy & Sillito, 1996; Cox & Sherman, 1999). The reticular cells in turn provide inhibitory innervation for the thalamic nuclei from which they receive afferents (Ahlsén et al., 1985; Jones, 1985). When the connections of the reticular nucleus were first defined (Rose, 1952; Carman et al., 1964; Jones, 1985), several sectors of the nucleus, each corresponding to a major thalamic nucleus or group of nuclei, were recognized. However, it was thought that each of these sectors received a diffuse, nonmapped input from the thalamus and from the corresponding area of cortex, and the view of the reticular nucleus as essentially a diffusely organized structure has survived long past its sell-by date.[6] The idea that there were no detailed maps within the pathway for any one modality such as the visual, the auditory, or the somatosensory system was reinforced by the observations made some years earlier (Cajal, 1911; Scheibel & Scheibel, 1966) that the individual cells of the reticular nucleus stretched their dendrites in the plane of the reticular sheet, extending over large parts of any one sector, or even between

---

6. Zhang and Jones (2004) claim that "activation of cortical excitatory inputs (within the reticular nucleus) triggers the propagation of inhibitory currents within the RTN and support the view that activation of the RTN from the somatosensory cortex, although focused by the topography of the corticothalamic projection, is capable of disynaptically engaging the whole inhibitory network of the RTN, by local and probably by reentrant GABA(A) receptor-based synapses, thus spreading the corticothalamic influence throughout the RTN." This looks like a curious reintroduction of the older view of the reticular nucleus as a diffusely organized structure, which fails to recognize that the mapped projections are likely to have functional significance per se and that any mapped structure can be incorporated into a diffuse or global response by a few appropriate diffuse connections.

sectors (see figure 9.3). One expected, wrongly as it turned out, that the reticular sheet would correspond to the cortical sheet and that, if there were maps, these would be laid out in the plane of the reticular sheet, as they are in the plane of the cortex, so that the parts of the map would be "smeared out" over the long axis formed by the dendrites of each reticular cell.

During the past two decades it has become clear that there are relatively accurate maps in the thalamic reticular nucleus, but that most of them do not lie in the plane of the reticular nucleus but at right angles to it (Montero et al., 1977; Shosaku et al., 1984; Shosaku, 1985; Crabtree & Killackey, 1989; Cicirata et al., 1990; Cornwall et al., 1990; Conley et al., 1991; Crabtree, 1992a, 1992b; Lozsádi, 1995). The maps have been defined by plotting the terminals of corticoreticular axons, by plotting the terminals of thalamoreticular axons, or by looking at the retrograde labeling of reticular cells after local injections of tracer into the dorsal thalamus. Figure 9.7 shows representations of small cortical areas (A and B) as half-disks in the reticular nucleus. These representations, for the visual pathways, are stacked on top of each other for the horizontal meridian (A, B) of the visual field and next to each other for the vertical meridian. The latter would be represented by B in the section of the reticular nucleus illustrated in figure 9.7 and by a region representing cortical area C, which would lie in a more rostral section that is not shown in the figure. That is, a small cortical injection produces a narrow slab (a whole cheese) of label within a small fraction of the thickness of the reticular sheet, and these slabs extend along the dendrites of the reticular cells (compare figures 9.3 and 9.7), so leading to a reinterpretation of what the spread of reticular dendrites can mean for the capacity of the nucleus to carry reasonably accurate maps.

Not all afferents to the reticular nucleus from cortical areas or thalamic nuclei show this relatively simple mapping. The anterior thalamic nuclei of the rat and cingulate cortex are mapped in a distinctive pattern (Lozsádi, 1995), and the medial dorsal thalamic nucleus and frontal cortex have reticular connections that are topographically mapped but that do not follow the slablike arrangement illustrated for the major sensory modalities in figure 9.7 (Cornwall et al., 1990).

A reticular sector concerned with one modality can receive inputs from the first and second cortical areas (V1 and V2; S1 and S2; A1 and A2) and from the first and higher order thalamic relays concerned with that modality. Separate inputs related to first and higher order circuits have been shown for the visual pathways of rabbit (Crabtree &

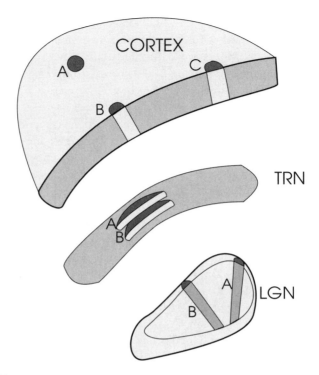

Figure 9.7
The organization of cortical, geniculate, and reticular representations of the visual field in the left hemisphere. The cortex is shown from a medial view, with cortical area C rostral to area B. The thalamic reticular nucleus (TRN) and the lateral geniculate nucleus (LGN) are shown as they would appear in a coronal section, with medial to the right. At the top of the figure, A, B, and C are three small cortical areas; A and B represent small parts of the visual field along the horizontal meridian, B and C represent small parts along the vertical meridian. At the bottom of the figure the lateral geniculate nucleus is shown with the layers not indicated, so that the figure could represent a rat, rabbit, or bush baby. Cortical areas A and B are connected by thalamocortical and corticothalamic axons to columns of cells that run through all of the layers of the lateral geniculate nucleus, as shown for A and B. Cortical area C would be connected to parts of the reticular and geniculate nuclei at more rostral levels, and its representations are not shown.

Killackey, 1989), rat (Coleman & Mitrofanis, 1996), and bush baby (*Galago*; Conley & Diamond, 1990); for the auditory pathways of the cat (Crabtree et al., 1998) and bush baby (Conley et al., 1991); and for the somatosensory pathways of the cat (Crabtree, 1992a) and rat (Pinault & Deschênes, 1998a). Generally but not invariably (Conley et al., 1991; Crabtree, 1998), the higher order thalamic and cortical connections are made with a smaller inner tier of the relevant sector of the reticular nucleus and the first order circuits connect to an outer, larger tier. The higher order connections to the smaller tier generally lack the topographic order seen in the first order tier.

For some cortical areas a single injection of tracer produces not one but two or three slabs running parallel to the plane of the reticular nucleus within the same sector (Cicirata et al., 1990; Conley & Diamond, 1990). The significance of these multiple mappings is not clear and merits further study (Guillery & Harting, 2003).

Several studies have shown that single reticular cells can send two branches of one axon back to different parts of the thalamus (Crabtree, 1992a; Pinault et al., 1995a; Kolmac & Mitrofanis, 1997). Some of these branching axons showed the branches going to modality related first and higher order thalamic relays, suggesting that through the reticular branches of thalamocortical cells, a reticular relay, and the branching reticulothalamic axons, one thalamic nucleus could produce inhibitory actions upon another. Crabtree and Isaac (2002) showed in recordings from slice preparations that there are such inhibitory interactions that can pass from one thalamic relay nucleus to another. The extent to which these may allow interaction between first and higher order relays will prove of particular interest, as will the interactions demonstrated by Crabtree and Isaac for some of the intralaminar and sensory or motor relay nuclei.

One key to understanding what may be happening in the reticular nucleus is to recognize not merely that many of the connections of the reticular nucleus have local sign (that is, they are mapped) but also that the reticular nucleus can provide a site where several different maps related to a single modality may be brought into relation with each other. We indicated that first and second sensory cortical areas connect to the same segment of the reticular nucleus, although to separate tiers, with the second cortical areas providing fewer inputs than the first. At present we know little about the reticular connections of higher cortical areas beyond V2, A2, and S2, and we indicated in chapter 3 that there is some preliminary evidence that higher cortical areas may have sparser inputs than first and second cortical areas. However, if, for example, one considers the higher visual relays, the pulvinar region receives inputs from several higher cortical areas, and also sends efferents to those areas. These connections, together with the two-way connections of the pulvinar and the inner tier of the visual sector of the reticular nucleus, provide an opportunity for the reticular sector to act as a nexus where in one way or another all of the activity relevant to the inputs from one modality can be brought together. That is, in any one sector of the reticular nucleus, several related higher order circuits are brought into close relationship to each other and to the related first order circuit; all innervate the reticular cells within that sector, and the reticular cells serve as a "final common pathway" sending inhibitory afferents to the thalamus, so that these inhibitory pathways can represent all of the thalamoreticular and corticoreticular circuits concerned with the relevant modality.

There is one point about the reticular nucleus that has not been addressed so far. Not only does it receive the thalamocortical and corticothalamic inputs discussed above, it also receives ascending afferents from the brainstem, hypothalamus, and basal forebrain, which were described in chapter 3. So far as we know, most of these afferents lack local sign, and probably act globally within any one reticular sector, and even, for some of the afferents, across all of the sectors. That is, the reticular nucleus can act with local sign, can relate several distinct maps to each other, or can act globally to modify transmission through the thalamus as a whole (see footnote 6).

Three further points need to be stressed about the maps in the reticular nucleus. The first concerns the accuracy of the maps where they have been defined. Even though the slabs extend roughly parallel to the dendritic arbors of the reticular cells, these arbors occupy a fair proportion of the thickness of the reticular nucleus, and the reticular nucleus itself is thin relative to the degree of localization that would be needed if the reticular nucleus were to be able to pass well-localized information back to the thalamus. Although there clearly are maps in the reticular nucleus, the receptive fields of the reticular cells are larger than those of the thalamic or cortical cells (So & Shapley, 1981; Murphy et al., 1994; however, see Shosaku, 1985). It is probable that dendrites of single reticular cells, in accord with the relatively large receptive fields, receive afferents from a quite large sensory area while nonetheless having clear focus within the reticular map. It is important to recognize a distinction between a thalamic relay cell, which signals the presence or absence of a well-localized incoming driving stimulus, and a reticular cell, whose output goes to a thalamic region that is subject to the reticulothalamic modulation.

The second point concerns the surprising orientation of the reticular maps and the relationship of these to the complex axonal crossings in the reticular nucleus. These multiple crossings of axons that link thalamus and cortex, though clearly recognized already more than a century ago by Kölliker (1896), are currently widely ignored. Axons are often represented as passing from thalamus to cortex (or vice versa) in a direct, radiating pattern, where the one set of axons can simply follow the ones going in the opposite direction (Caviness & Frost, 1983; Hohl-Abrahao & Creutzfeldt, 1991; Molnár et al., 1998). If one looks at a preparation in which the axons are well stained, one can recognize that the axons approach the thalamus from the cortex by running roughly parallel to each other. Then, some distance external to the outer or lateral border of the reticular nucleus, the corticothalamic and thalamocortical axons begin the formation of a complex latticework of intertwining axons. This is the site of the embryonic perireticular nucleus, only a few of whose cells survive in the adult. The latticework continues right through to the inner border of the reticular nucleus, where it stops abruptly as the axons continue their course into the substance of the thalamus. As soon as the axons enter the thalamus, they run in strikingly straight, parallel bundles to their final thalamic destination, or origin. In a good preparation these straight, parallel bundles running into the thalamus from the complex intertwining plexus of the perireticular and reticular nuclei look like a rainstorm descending from a cloud (see figure 3 of Mitrofanis & Guillery, 1993). It appears as though the corticothalamic axons, having made the complex traverse of the reticular nucleus, are now directly on the right path, and can proceed without further deviation. The mapped connections to the reticular nucleus, established by branches of corticothalamic and thalamocortical axons passing through the nucleus, form as the several corticothalamic pathways that go through any one sector become lined up (one can think of them as stacked up in register) on their way through the nucleus. This complex latticework is seen not only in the mammalian reticular nucleus but also in the chick and turtle (Adams et al., 1997), demonstrating that it represents a well-established and basic relationship between telencephalon and diencephalon and suggesting that the thalamus and cortex depend on complex interactions with each other. The notion that the thalamus simply serves to provide a supply of afferent messages to cortex, through a neatly ordered thalamic "radiation," is dead.

The third point concerns the perigeniculate nucleus of carnivores. So far we have treated the perigeniculate nucleus as a part of the thalamic reticular nucleus, characteristically found only in cats and other carnivores. It lies between the lateral geniculate nucleus and the reticular nucleus (see figure 9.3). From almost everything we know about the nucleus, including its apparent shared developmental origin with the reticular nucleus (Mitrofanis, 1994), the shape and orientation of its dendritic arbors, its transmitters, receptors, thalamic, cortical, and brainstem connections (Sherman & Guillery, 1996), there appear to be no differences, and the perigeniculate nucleus has long been regarded as simply a part of the reticular nucleus of carnivores that is slightly displaced toward the lateral geniculate nucleus. However, there is one important known difference between, on the one hand, the cat's perigeniculate nucleus, and, on the other hand, the sectors of the reticular nucleus that deal with vision in other species or with somatosensory or auditory pathways in any species, including the cat. This is a difference in the mapping. The cells of the perigeniculate nucleus have receptive fields that are in register with those of the lateral geniculate nucleus (see the lower continuous arrow in figure 9.3; see also Sanderson, 1971), whereas the other maps are oriented perpendicular to this, as shown in figure 9.7.

The difference is not trivial. It is possible to entertain the notion that the perigeniculate nucleus may be developmentally related to the lateral geniculate nucleus and distinct from the reticular nucleus. This can be based on a developmental stage when the perigeniculate nucleus appears to be included with the lateral geniculate nucleus within the terminal field of retinal afferents, which later retreat from the region of the perigeniculate nucleus (Cucchiaro & Guillery, 1984). However, in the rest of this book we have treated the perigeniculate nucleus as a part of the reticular nucleus, in accordance with the developmental account of Mitrofanis (1994), and we interpret the layout of the map as indicative of the fact that where the corticogeniculate fibers reach the perigeniculate nucleus they have completed their crossings and are aligned in accord with their geniculate termination.[7]

9.I. General Conclusions

Perhaps the most important general point to be stressed is that maps are present in most of the thalamocortical and corticothalamic pathways.

---

7. The earlier account (see chapter 3) of geniculate interneurons that may represent "migrated" perigeniculate neurons can perhaps be seen as another indication of a shift during development that brings reticular elements under the influence of developmental forces that are primarily geniculate.

Even where the nature of the function that is mapped is not known, there are topographically organized links between thalamus and cortex, and identifying the functional properties that are mapped in these pathways remains one of the outstanding problems for studies of thalamocortical pathways. Where the issue has been addressed, in the central visual pathways, the maps are not innately determined; they can be reversed (or suppressed) in cortex in response to genetic or experimental challenges. Further, evidence from these pathways indicates that the orderly representation of the afferents may be functionally more important for the cerebral cortex than for the thalamus.

Maps are likely to provide a useful handle for studying thalamocortical pathways. They have helped to define the multiplicity of cortical and thalamic functional subdivisions in the past and one can expect them to serve as a guide to identifying functional distinctions in higher order thalamic nuclei in the future. Further, the confluence of several thalamic and cortical maps within the modality-specific sectors of the thalamic reticular nucleus allows one to see this as a nexus where the several distinct functional thalamocorticothalamic circuits can interact and influence thalamic gating in the related first order thalamic relay nucleus.

9.J. Unresolved Questions

1. Are all driver pathways mapped?

2. Which modulatory pathways are mapped? Which are not mapped?

3. Is the alignment in the lateral geniculate nucleus of visual field representations that come through the left and the right eye related to the local, topographically organized action of modulators, or is there some other way of understanding the functional significance of Walls's toothpick?

4. For each of the pathways that are not concerned with visual, auditory, somatosensory, or motor functions (e.g., pathways to frontal or cingulate cortex), what is the variable, if any, that is mapped? And where the topographic accuracy of sensory or motor maps in higher cortical areas is relatively crude or absent, is there another variable that is mapped?

5. Will it prove possible to define isocortical columns for all higher order thalamic relays?

6. Are the mirror reversals of thalamocortical maps and the consequent crossings of pathways that occur in the thalamic reticular nucleus an essential part of the functional organization of thalamocortical circuitry, characteristic of all major thalamic relays?

7. Are all of the maps in thalamocortical pathways established prenatally?

8. How do first order and higher order circuits relate to each other in the thalamic reticular nucleus? In terms of the maps that can be defined? Or in terms of their synaptic connections to reticular cells?

9. Since first and higher order pathways for any one modality share a reticular sector, should one look for evidence that in the modulation of thalamocortical relays they generally act together, acting in unison, complementing (or perhaps opposing) each other?

10 The Thalamus in Relation to Action and Perception

10.A. Introduction

In earlier chapters we referred to the common pattern seen in afferents to the thalamus, of axons that branch, sending one branch to the thalamus for relay and another branch to a motor or premotor center for some influence on action. In this chapter we explore the evidence for these relationships and look at the functional implications for our view of thalamic function and, more generally, of the relationship between action and perception.

The relationship between perception and action has for a long time been of interest to experimentalists, clinicians, and philosophers. It is not easy to see exactly how action and perception relate to each other in our daily lives, although one can readily appreciate that each is dependent on the other. In previous chapters we have treated the function of the thalamic relay to cortex largely from the point of view of the visual relays, and have been concerned to trace the perceptual process as visual stimuli pass through, in sequence, the first order lateral geniculate nucleus, the primary visual cortex, higher order thalamic relays in the pulvinar, and then cortical areas concerned with higher visual functions.

This approach leads all too readily to a view of perceptual processing as occurring along pathways that pass progressively through cortical connections to motor cortical areas and thence out to action, or to memory storage. Much contemporary analysis of perceptual processing is based on a conceptual structure such as that summarized in figure 10.1A. In this, messages from the outside world are sent through the thalamus to the cerebral cortex, processed in a parallel and hierarchical series of corticocortical connections, and then passed to motor centers for action or to memory centers for storage. This conceptual structure represents perception as a process that records events and seems not to

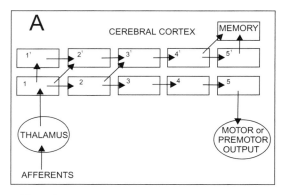

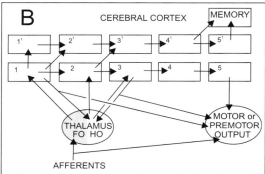

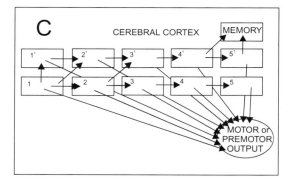

Figure 10.1
Schematic, and simplified, representation of thalamic and cortical connections with motor centers. Only some of the corticocortical links are shown. *A.* A widely used representation of afferent pathways entering through thalamus being processed through a parallel and hierarchical series of cortical connections, and then passed on to motor centers or memory storage. *B.* A representation of the connections described in earlier chapters and in this chapter, showing first order (FO) and higher order (HO) thalamic relays receiving from ascending and corticothalamic afferents, respectively, with each of these afferents sending axonal branches to motor or premotor centers. *C.* A schema to stress that essentially all cortical areas have connections to motor or premotor centers. The extent to which they have branches going to the thalamus remains largely unexplored.

depend on action but primarily acts, eventually, through motor cortical areas to initiate action. A fuller view of such a set of connections for perceptual processing has been provided by Felleman and Van Essen (1991) (figure 10.2), and many proposals for corticocortical communication are implicitly or explicitly based on some such schema (see, e.g., Milner & Goodale, 1993; Romanski et al., 1999; Rizzolatti & Luppino, 2001), essentially focusing on corticocortical communication, but not paying attention either to the close links that inputs to the thalamus have with motor centers (figure 10.1B) or to the many connections that pass from all cortical areas to lower centers (figure 10.1C). Churchland et al. (1994)

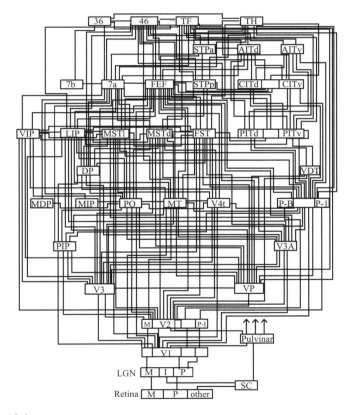

Figure 10.2
Schematic representation of corticocortical pathways for processing of visual information through a proposed system of hierarchical, parallel corticocortical connections. (Redrawn and slightly modified from Felleman and Van Essen, 1991.)

have called the view represented in figure 10.1*A* and 10.2 a "theory of pure vision." It is well represented by Galletti et al. (2001), who summarized the functional position of cortical area V6 as follows:

We suggest that cortical area V6 plays a pivotal role in the dorsal visual stream, by distributing its visual information coming from the occipital lobe to the sensorimotor areas of the parietal cortex. Given the functional characteristics of the cells of this network, we suggest that it could perform the fast form and motion analyses needed for the visual guiding of arm movements as well as their coordination with the eyes and the head,

seeing cortex as an independent executive that can function without reference to lower centers until the need for final action arises.

Such a conceptual separation of the centers concerned with sensation from those concerned with action was recently expressed in an extreme form by Daw and Dayan (2004) with the statement, "Situated in the middle between sensation and action is decision making."

Action, that is, the motor output, is widely seen as the final outcome of a cortical perceptual process, produced as a response that is appropriate to the cortical analysis of external events. Such a view takes no account of the many connections that all cortical areas establish with centers concerned with action (figure 10.1*C*), nor does it recognize the extent to which perception depends on action. For example, vision depends on head and eye movements, the sense of touch depends on finger movements. Many actions and instructions for action precede cortical processing. The extent to which perception depends on action was explored in detail by Helmholtz (Warren & Warren, 1968) and more recently by Churchland et al. (1994) and O'Regan and Noë (2001), among others. In many different ways these authors have explored perceptual and behavioral phenomena that demonstrate the extent to which perception is dependent on action, including evidence from perceptual illusions or the effects of vision through distorting lenses,[1] as well as evidence about the role of movement (e.g., of the eyes or fingers) in visual or tactile perception. In this chapter we will look at some of the pathways that provide links to motor centers on the way into the thalamus, pathways that commit messages for action prior to the perceptual process itself, and we will argue that these messages for action have to be seen as an integral part of the perceptual process.

---

1. Helmholtz even discussed the changed perception obtained when viewing the world upside-down from between the knees.

These pathways for action have not received much attention in past experimental studies of perceptual processing for two main reasons. One is that much of sensory physiology has been obtained from studies of anesthetized animals, where questions about the role of action in perception are made irrelevant. The second is that, where neural responses are studied in awake animals, the nerve cells are almost invariably, and for very good practical reasons, identified in terms of the cortical area they are in, but almost never in terms of their laminar position in the cortex or, more relevantly, their actual connections with other nerve cells. This has created a great deal of fascinating information about what cortical nerve cells can do, without throwing any significant light on the mechanisms by means of which they do it. Commonly, nerve cells are reported in particular cortical areas that can match one or another property of a complex perceptual or motor task performed by a monkey. This is a sort of psychophysical parallelism in which the activity of nerve cells has replaced the mind, perhaps a "neuronophysical parallelism," that convincingly shows that anything a monkey can do can be matched by a corresponding neural activity, but at present, methods that allow an analysis of how the nerve cells do it are largely undeveloped.

The anatomical links that produce a close interdependence of action and perception have not been widely studied and have played virtually no role in experimental studies of neuronal activity in perception. Churchland et al. (1994), writing about vision, summarized some of the pathways that lead from cortex to lower centers concerned with motor outputs, adding, "What is frustrating about this assembly of data, as with neuroanatomy generally, is that we do not know what it all means." However, their conclusion, "The anatomy is consistent with the idea that motor assembly can begin even before sensory signals reach the highest levels," is important. It is based on observations of the output pathways from cortical visual areas to cell groups concerned with the control of movements, such as the striatum, the superior colliculus, or the pons. These pathways demonstrate that even primary *sensory* areas such as area 17 (V1) have significant motor outputs that give these areas access to motor controls independent of any *higher* cortical processing.

We have mentioned in previous chapters that several of the axons that bring inputs to first and higher order thalamic nuclei have branches that innervate cell groups with connections to motor centers (figure 10.1B), but so far we have not explored the implications of these connections. In addition, as indicated by figure 10.1C, most, possibly all, cortical areas have connections with motor or premotor centers. These pathways provide evidence that not only *can* "motor assembly begin before sensory signals reach the highest levels" but that it *must* begin before the sensory signals even reach the thalamus, and that it must accompany corticocortical processing at essentially every stage. The messages that pass along axons to first order relays, and that also pass along branches of the same axons to motor centers, provide a close and essentially unbreakable link between action and perception at the earliest stages of sensory processing, and those that pass along branching axons to higher order relays provide equally secure links between cortical outputs to motor centers and perceptual processing through corticocortical connections. These two sets of pathways, to first order and higher order thalamic nuclei, can be seen as making a significant contribution to, perhaps even forming the major part of, the "sensorimotor contingencies" that O'Regan and Noë (2001) recognize as an essential link between action and perception.

10.B. Evidence for Branching Driver Afferents to First and Higher Order Thalamic Relays

Since this chapter has been added to the chapters that appeared in the first edition of this book, it may seem that it is based on new findings published since the first edition was written. This is only partially so. Evidence that corticothalamic axons from layer 5 cells to higher order thalamic relays commonly send branches to motor centers of the brainstem became available in the 1990s as methods for tracing single axons were developed. The branches were reported for several different corticothalamic pathways in rat, monkey, and cat (Deschênes et al., 1994; Bourassa & Deschênes, 1995; Bourassa et al., 1995; Rockland, 1998; Guillery et al., 2001), and this evidence suggested that most of the layer 5 corticothalamic axons might have brainstem branches. Guillery et al. (2001) traced more than 50 such axons from visual areas 17 and 18 to terminal foci in the thalamus and, although there was some question about the serial tracing of a few of these axons, essentially all of them had branches that continued into the brainstem. Casanova (1993) had earlier reported from electrophysiological observations that some visual corticothalamic axons had collicular branches, but the proportion with demonstrable branches was much smaller.[2]

---

2. The difference is probably the result of the methods used. The problem of negative conclusions about branching axons is discussed later in this section.

These observations of branching axons were, at first consideration, surprising. We had not expected that a driver pathway afferent to the thalamus, and thus concerned with sending information to the cortex, would also be passing information away from the cortex to brainstem centers such as the superior colliculus[3] and pons, which are pathways on the way to motor outputs. It took us a little while to recognize that patterns of branching that connect thalamic driver inputs with motor pathways are not limited to the layer 5 corticothalamic axons. Many of the driver systems that reach the thalamus have branches that pass to motor outputs, and some of the information about these has been available for a long time. This applies to the axons in the posterior column (lemniscal) pathway concerned with touch and position sense, it applies to the anterolateral pathway concerned with pain and temperature, to the cerebellothalamic, to the mamillothalamic pathways, and to the optic tract, just as it does to the layer 5 corticothalamic pathways. It may also apply to the auditory and other pathways, although significant evidence on this last point is not currently available, possibly because it has not been looked for in the past.

Evidence about the branching patterns of afferents to the thalamus has been summarized by Guillery and Sherman (2002b) and more briefly by Guillery (2003, 2005a). Each of the different types of ascending afferent pathway will be considered in the following.

10.B.1. Branching Ascending Driver Afferents to the Thalamus

Patterns of branching that are relevant to understanding the message transmitted to cortex in first order relays indicate that the information being passed to cortex is not simply (or only) about events in the external world represented by visual, auditory, somatosensory, etc., stimuli, or about information from cerebellum or mamillary bodies that needs to be passed to the cortex, but it is also about the current ongoing instructions that are being passed to the motor apparatus.

To understand the nature of the ascending messages that reach the thalamus, it is necessary to recognize that for some pathways, the relevant branching patterns are to be found at early stages, before the cells that innervate the thalamus are reached. That is, for the medial lemnis-

---

3. The position of the superior colliculus in relation to motor centers controlling movements of the head and eyes is discussed in section 10.B.4, Visual Pathways.

cus or the anterolateral pathway, which innervate the ventral posterior nucleus, the inputs to the prethalamic cells in the gracile and cuneate nuclei and in the posterior horn respectively are relevant; one needs to consider not only the branching patterns of the lemniscal and anterolateral axons themselves, but also to know the branching patterns of the axons that innervate the gracile and cuneate nuclei and the posterior horn. Similarly, for the auditory pathways the branching patterns of the axons on the way to the inferior colliculus are as important as the branching patterns of the cells in the inferior colliculus that innervate the medial geniculate nucleus. Given this extra possibility for relevant branching patterns, we now briefly look as several of the major ascending pathways to the thalamus.

10.B.2. Somatosensory Pathways

For the somatosensenory pathways the most striking examples of axons with branches innervating motor centers are to be found in the dorsal roots. Cajal (1911) showed the rich pattern of branching of dorsal root axons as they enter the spinal cord (figure 10.3). These branches have connections with spinal mechanisms at or close to the level of entry, as they innervate the cells of the posterior horn before they ascend toward the gracile and cuneate nuclei or the lateral cervical nucleus (Cajal, 1911; Brown & Fyffe, 1981; Lu & Willis, 1999).

Lu and Willis (1999) stress the difficulty of demonstrating some of these branches or those of ascending axons experimentally. Anatomical methods based on filling single axons anterogradely can fail to show fine branches, just as methods based on labeling single cells with two retrogradely transported markers injected at two different terminal sites can fail. Similarly, methods that use recordings of antidromic action potentials from two branches of an axon can provide false negative results. That is, we know that many of the axons innervating cells that are presynaptic to the anterolateral pathway or medial lemniscus have branches innervating spinal mechanisms (figure 10.4), but the full richness and complexity of this innervation is not yet clearly defined. The same holds for the branching patterns of the axons that form the anterolateral pathways themselves (Lu & Willis, 1999). For the axons that arise in the posterior column nuclei, it is known that most go to the thalamus in the medial lemniscus, but some also pass to the reticular nuclei, the inferior olive, the superior colliculus, or the hypothalamus (see figure 10.4; Berkley, 1975; Berkley et al., 1980; Feldman & Kruger, 1980; Bull &

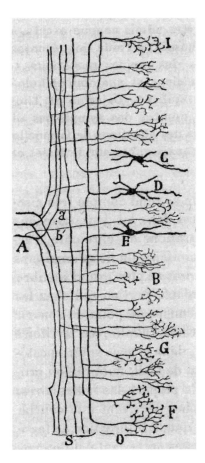

Figure 10.3
Dorsal root axons entering the spinal cord and branching extensively to distribute to spinal neurons at and close to the level of entry. (From Cajal, 1911.)

Berkley, 1984; summarized in Guillery & Sherman, 2002a). Some of these are branching axons, but others appear to arise from distinct cell populations in the posterior column nuclei. Figure 10.4*A* and *B* show the lemniscal and anterolateral pathways as they pass through the spinal cord and brainstem to the thalamus, in *A*, and in *B* show the connections that are established by branching axons at various levels. This indicates the extent to which the message that arrives at the thalamus represents, apart from the activity of the receptors, copies of instructions that are concurrently being widely distributed to other parts of the brain.

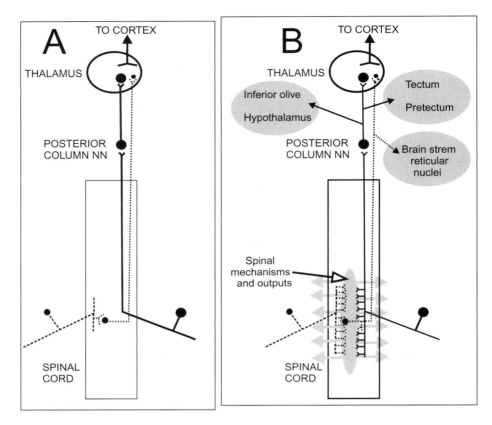

Figure 10.4
A. Schematic representation of the direct lemniscal (continuous lines) and antero-lateral (interrupted lines) pathways to the thalamus. *B.* Additional connections established by branches of the direct pathways. See text for details.

Although the full details of the branching patterns on the pathways from the somatosensory periphery to the thalamus are not completely known, it is clear that the messages reaching the thalamus represent a rich array of copies of messages that are on their way to other centers. These range from autonomic centers in the hypothalamus to cerebellar mechanisms fed by the inferior olive, circuits concerned in the control of head and eye movements in the superior colliculus, and spinal mechanisms. It is important to recognize that the spinal mechanisms can include not only simple segmental reflexes but also more complex multisegmental reflexes and the complex pattern generators of the spinal cord. Information about some of the current inputs to some of these mechanisms will be implicit in the messages that the thalamus sends to cortex, together with the information about activity in the relevant peripheral receptors. This is the information that the cortex must treat as its source for perceptual processing. Each axon reaching the thalamus will carry messages about the condition of one or several receptors and in addition will carry information about the instructions that are already on their way to one or more motor pathways. One should not expect that the cortical analysis will reject or annul this "additional" information simply because it is not a part of what classical physiology has seen as the information carried in sensory pathways. It is reasonable to expect this copy of motor instructions to be an integral part of the perceptual process. It is not surprising that some who have thought seriously about the nature of perceptual processing have been led to a view of sensory processes as "interactive" finding that there is no "pure sensation" (Churchland et al., 1994; on "Pure Vision" above) and that there are complex and often extremely elusive "sensorimotor contingencies" (O'Regan & Noë, 2001). Understanding the nature of these contingencies will likely involve many other connections that do not include the thalamus and are beyond the aims of this chapter, but there can be no doubt that the branching axons that innervate the thalamus represent an absolutely indissoluble link between perception and action, one that is highly complex, involves several different brainstem and spinal circuits, and one that will not be properly understood until we know more about the nature of the action that the nonthalamic branches have at their terminal sites.

It is important to recognize that this rich pattern of connections, which draws many different functional systems into the information brought into the thalamocortical system, represents only the first stage of perceptual processing. The corticothalamic axons that originate in cortical layer 5 and bring the perceptual process to higher cortical areas have branches that provide further potentially widespread involvements of other lower, motor brainstem centers at each stage of the corticothalamocortical cycle.

10.B.3. Mamillothalamic Pathways

The mamillothalamic pathways, which bring afferents to the anterior thalamic nuclei, are an example of a thalamic afferent pathway that is particularly instructive for thinking about the possible functional role of its nonthalamic branches. There is well-documented axonal branching that characterizes the mamillothalamic axons shortly after they leave the mamillary bodies (figure 10.5; see also Kölliker, 1896; Cajal, 1911). The principal mamillary tract leaves the medial and the lateral mamillary nuclei, and then the axons branch to enter the mamillothalamic tract on the way to the anterior thalamic nuclei, or the mamillotegmental tract going to nuclei in the periaqueductal gray and the tegmental parts of the pons at the caudal part of the midbrain. The tiny lateral mamillary nucleus is made up of a few thousand relatively large cells that send their axons bilaterally to the smallest of the anterior thalamic nuclei, the anterior dorsal nucleus. We know more about these two cell groups than we know about the larger medial mamillary nuclei and their recipient thalamic nuclei, the anterior medial and anterior ventral thalamic nuclei, and will therefore focus on these smaller cell groups. In rats, cells in the anterior dorsal thalamic nucleus respond selectively to particular head directions. That is, as a rat explores its environment its head direction

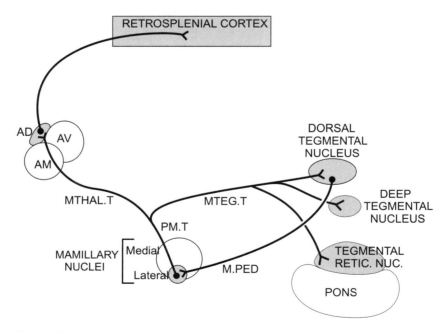

Figure 10.5
Schematic representation of the mamillothalamic and mamillotegmental pathways described in the text. Abbreviations: AD, AM, AV, anterior dorsal, anterior medial, and anterior ventral thalamic nuclei; M.PED, mamillary peduncle; MTEG.T, mamillotegmental tract; MTHAL.T, mamillothalamic tract.

changes, and the different anterior thalamic cells respond selectively to different head directions (Taube, 1995). Cells in the lateral mamillary nucleus show similar response properties (Stackman & Taube, 1998), and the lateral mamillary nucleus in turn receives inputs from a small nucleus at the caudal end of the periaqueductal gray, which in turn receives inputs from the vestibular nuclei (Brown et al., 2002).

These linked nuclei represent an afferent pathway that brings information about head position to the thalamus for subsequent transmittal through the retrosplenial cortex to the hippocampus, contributing to the formation of place maps there (Calton et al., 2003). It might be considered a "pure" sensory system except that we know the lateral mamillary cells send mamillotegmental branches back to the dorsal tegmental nucleus, to a deep tegmental nucleus (which also sends axons to the mamillary bodies), and to the medial and rostral parts of the tegmental reticular nucleus in the pons (Guillery, 1957; Cruce, 1977).

This last cell group does not, so far as is known, send inputs to the mamillary bodies. It lies in the part of the brainstem that is concerned in the control of eye movements (Hess et al., 1989) and that in other species is also concerned with head movements. It is likely to represent a motor output. The precise relationship established between the cells innervated by the mamillotegmental tract and those that play a role in control of eye and head movements remains to be defined, but there is a strong suggestion here that the message going to the thalamus in the mamillothalamic tract also contains a copy of motor instructions that are immediately relevant to the sensory message that is being sent to the thalamus. The centers concerned with the control of eye movements are receiving inputs as the message about head orientation travels to the cortex, and the cortex will be receiving not only the information about head orientation but also the information about instructions to the eye movement centers, which will, presumably, be relevant to the next head position.

10.B.4. Visual Pathways

For the visual pathways, most, possibly all, of the axons that bring messages to the thalamocortical system, the retinogeniculate axons, also send branches to the pretectum and superficial layers of the superior colliculus in the midbrain. For rabbits and rodents there is good evidence that all of the axons that go to the lateral geniculate nucleus also send branches to the midbrain (Chalupa & Thompson, 1980; Vaney et al.,

1981; Linden & Perry, 1983; Dreher et al., 1985; Jhaveri et al., 1991). This evidence, based largely on retrograde labeling of retinal ganglion cells from the terminal stations, demonstrates that all of the information being passed through the lateral geniculate nucleus to cortical area 17 also contains information about the current instructions going to the midbrain. The relevant midbrain centers are the superior colliculus, concerned with control of head and eye movements, and the pretectum, concerned with pupillary control, accommodation and vestibular signals concerning head position.

At one time the retinotectal axons, which terminate in the superficial layers of the superior colliculus, were thought of primarily as providing an alternative, extrageniculate "sensory" route to higher areas of visual cortex through a relay of tectothalamic cells in the pulvinar (Sprague, 1966; Schneider, 1969; Diamond, 1973), because there is a pathway to the pulvinar that arises in the superficial layers of the colliculus (Altman & Carpenter, 1961). However, there have to be serious doubts about the extent to which these tectothalamic (or pretectothalamic) axons can be acting as drivers for cells in the pulvinar. Pulvinar cells lose their characteristic receptive field properties in cats and monkeys after cortical lesions, not after tectal lesions (Bender, 1983; Chalupa, 1991), and a significant number of characteristic corticothalamic driver terminals (see chapter 3) can be identified in the pulvinar of cat and monkey (Rockland, 1996; Guillery et al., 2001). There is some recent evidence that tectopulvinar driver axons in the cat innervate a small part of the pulvinar (Kelly et al., 2003), so perhaps some tectal messages do go to cortex through the pulvinar, but since the superficial layers of the colliculus communicate with the deep layers (Ozen et al., 2000; Schiller & Tehovnik, 2001; Helms et al., 2004) and have the capacity through the deep layers to act on motor centers concerned with the control of head and eye movements, the retinotectal axons must be seen as having ready access to the motor output of the colliculus. That is, no matter what the role of the colliculopulvinar pathway is, whether driver or modulator, the retinal axons that innervate the superior colliculus will be acting through the superficial layers on the deep layers and will be influencing, albeit in a subtle and as yet but poorly understood way, the centers concerned with movement of the head and eyes.

Evidence for the cat shows that the Y pathway and the W pathway both have branching axons that innervate the lateral geniculate nucleus and the superior colliculus (Fukuda & Stone, 1974; Wässle & Illing, 1980; Tamamaki et al., 1994), although it is not known whether all of the W cells branch or only some subgroups of W cells (Guillery & Sherman, 2002a). The X cells were for some time considered as providing a "pure sensory" link through the lateral geniculate nucleus to the cortex, with no branches to midbrain. However, Wässle and Illing (1980) reported that 10% of these cells appeared to project to the superior colliculus, and Koontz et al. (1985) showed that retinal X cells could be retrogradely labeled by injections into the pretectum. Tamamaki et al. (1994) injected individual X cell axons with a small anterogradely transported molecule (biocytin) and reported that six out of six of these axons projected to the pretectum.

In these studies of fine axons, the problem raised by negative evidence, considered for the anterolateral pathway by Lu and Willis (1999; see above), is important. Where only a proportion of a relatively homogeneous cell group appears to show a branch, it is more likely that many branches were missed rather than that the cell group is more heterogeneous than is suggested by observations of other cell properties (see chapter 2 on classification of cells).

The importance of understanding the nature of negative evidence is important for an evaluation of branching patterns of retinofugal axons in the monkey, where Bunt et al. (1975) reported that essentially all retinal ganglion cells were retrogradely labeled by an injection of horseradish peroxidase into the lateral geniculate nucleus, except for the cells in the most central parts of the retina, where the cells are smallest and have the finest axons. Schiller and Malpeli (1977) reported sparse evidence for any parvocellular axons going to the superior colliculus. They found just one. Leventhal et al. (1981) found that whereas all three ganglion cell types could be retrogradely labeled from the lateral geniculate nucleus, all except the parvocellular ganglion cells could be labeled from the superior colliculus or pretectum. Perry and Cowey (1984) reported that although many cells labeled retrogradely after an injection of the superior colliculus had essentially the same size distribution as the parvocellular group labeled after an injection of the lateral geniculate nucleus, their dendritic morphology, where apparent, resembled the koniocellular component, not the parvocellular one. Given the difficulty of finding evidence for the fine branches of X cells reported for the cat, and given that the cat's X cells project to the pretectum, not to the colliculus, the possibility that there is a midbrain branch from parvocellular axons remains open. The alternative would be to see the parvocellular component as representing a "pure vision" component, although one that is closely tied through the magno- and koniocellular components to midbrain mechanisms concerned with movement. That is, even if the primate had no midbrain branches to its parvocellular pathway, information about concurrent instructions going from the magno- and koniocellular groups would almost certainly play a significant role at an early stage of processing within area 17. At present we do not have enough information to know how the midbrain messages that are copied in the geniculocortical pathway relate to the processing that occurs in area 17. So far the question has, to our knowledge, never been raised.

It may be instructive to compare the lemniscal with the visual pathways at this point. Horsley (1909) cited a patient whose motor cortex had been excised and who was asked to identify objects by touch as saying, "If only I could move my hand about I should know what the things were." Although the pathway to the sensory cortex was intact, the perceptual function was lost. The loss of visual perception when the retinal image is stabilized (Riggs et al., 1953) may be comparable to the extent that in each situation, perception depends on movement. However, in the visual example, even when ocular movements are possible, they no longer have any effect on the perceived image if the retinal image has been stabilized by means that compensate for the ocular movements. That is, the two situations are clearly different, but each raises a problem about exactly how perception depends on movement.

10.B.5. Other Afferents to First Order Thalamic Nuclei

These include the auditory afferents, vestibular afferents, taste afferents, and afferents from the cerebellum. For the auditory afferents we know very little about specific branching patterns, because generally they have not been looked for. Brainstem relays of the auditory pathways on the way to the medial geniculate nucleus innervate the reticular nuclei of the brainstem, the periaqueductal gray, and the superior colliculus (Henkel, 1983; Whitley & Henkel, 1984; Harting & Van Lieshout, 2000), and there are several descending pathways from the inferior colliculus (Vetter et al., 1993; Shore & Moore, 1998), but we have no evidence about branching patterns. Brainstem connections that are given off at early stages of the pathway and relate to the startle response or to pinnal movements may be of particular interest. There are groups of neurons, the cochlear root neurons (López et al., 1999), that lie among the axons of the cochlear nerve and that pass to brainstem centers, including the facial nerve nucleus (concerned with pinnal movements) and other brainstem centers. It is not known whether the innervation of these, clearly motor cells, is from axons that also send ascending branches toward the thalamus or whether this is a distinct cochleofacial pathway that is quite independent of other auditory pathways. For these pathways and some others, such as the taste pathways, about which we have no evidence about branching patterns, it may be worth stating a clear hypothesis as a challenge: all pathways that innervate the thalamus have axons that send branches to extrathalamic subcortical centers. As noted above, disproof of the hypothesis may be difficult until better methods for identifying branches are developed, but demonstration of branches that support the hypothesis would in itself be useful, and one day it may be possible to challenge the hypothesis with a method that does not produce false negatives.

For the vestibular pathways there are axons that send branches to the thalamus and to the interstitial nucleus of Cajal and central gray (Matsuo et al., 1994), as well as vestibulothalamic axons that have branches descending to cervical levels of the spinal cord (Isu et al., 1989).

The axons that pass from the deep cerebellar nuclei to the thalamus were shown by Cajal (1911) to have branches going to the red nucleus. More recent evidence supports this conclusion (Tsukahara et al., 1967; Stanton, 1980, 2001; Shinoda et al., 1988) by showing that the brainstem branches innervate rubrospinal axons, as well as other cell groups, including the tegmental reticular nucleus, the pons, and the inferior olive (McCrea et al., 1978).

10.B.6. General Conclusions about Afferents to First Order Thalamic Relays

The main conclusion from this review of afferents to first order nuclei is that there is a great deal of evidence to show that many of these afferents have prethalamic branches that innervate brainstem or spinal centers concerned directly or indirectly with motor control. In general, the importance of these relationships for understanding the nature of the message that the thalamus transmits to the cortex has not been widely recognized, so that the search for the branching patterns of axons in these pathways has been somewhat sporadic. Given the earlier lack of interest in the subject and the experimental difficulties that are often involved in demonstrating finer branches, there is significant evidence that most, possibly even all, of the afferents that reach the first order thalamic relays have motor or premotor branches, or that the inputs to the cells giving rise to these axons have such branches (or both).

The primary and immediate significance of any sensory input, when it first reaches the central nervous system, is the production of an appropriate motor output. This applies whether one is dealing with the first phylogenetic appearance of a newly evolving sensory component or with the immediate outcomes of a well-established sensory input. In contrast to this, the role of perceptual processing is important for memory storage, that is, for comparisons between past and present, for adjustments of responses in the light of current conditions that include very much more than the present sensory input itself. These are longer term goals and must come after the first motor response. In this sense, perceptual processing is secondary to the motor response, which has to have the most direct links to the sensory inputs and which will always be likely to act first, even though there is, of course, a later response that may be produced as the outcome of the perceptual process.

Many of the impulses that travel from the periphery toward first order thalamic relays have important, immediate, subcortical roles to play in the life of the organism. Those subcortical roles are often, by their very nature, not a part of conscious experience. Identification of objects by touch involves finger movements that barely form a part of the perceptual experience of the object touched, and more strikingly eye movements, which are an essential and major part of any visual experience, are not perceived as a part of that experience without a special effort (and possibly not even then). The early motor components are often lost in theoretical or experimental evaluations of perception because they seem to form no part of the perceptual process itself. Even Helmholtz, who was clearly aware of the importance that action played in perception, generally presented the action as a "voluntary" action, made deliberately by an observer (discussed in Guillery, 2003). It is the involuntary and quite unperceived nature of the action that makes it so elusive. Even where the action of the prethalamic branches may be relatively weak, or perhaps even represent an inhibition, insofar as it acts on the receptor organ (its movement, position, ability to respond optimally, etc.) it will be a part of the perceptual process, often not appreciated by the subject and only rarely appreciated by an investigator trying to understand the nature of perception. One finds reports of puzzling relationships between action and perception (see section 10.A), which are puzzling because the action is generally hidden. The anatomical relationships suggest that in order to uncover these hidden actions it will be necessary to study the nature of the actions produced by the prethalamic branches. What are the spinal actions of the axons from the tactile and kinesthetic receptors involved in a tactile exploration of an object? What are the messages that the mamillotegmental tract sends to the pontine tegmental reticular nucleus? How do these act on eye (and head) movements, and how do these actions relate to the head orientation signal that is passed to the thalamus along the mamillothalamic tract? Exactly what changes do particular retinal inputs to pretectal or tectal cell groups produce in terms of retinal position, pupillary size, or accommodative mechanisms?

We need to be aware of these issues before looking at the possible functional role of the brainstem branches given off by corticothalamic drivers from layer 5 to higher order relays. Here, too, we have an early motor or premotor innervation and an action that is every bit as elusive as the actions considered above. Insofar as we know something about the messages arriving along many of the pathways to first order relays, and know almost nothing about the nature of those going to higher order relays, we can expect the role to be that much more elusive, but by the same token, perhaps, that much more intriguing.

10.C. Branching Corticothalamic Axons from Layer 5 Cells

Layer 5 axons that branch to innervate thalamus and brainstem have been demonstrated for visual, somatosensory, or motor pathways in cat, monkey, and rat (Casanova, 1993; Deschênes et al., 1994; Bourassa & Deschênes, 1995; Bourassa et al., 1995; Rockland, 1998; Guillery et al., 2001). The axons that have been traced by axonal fills with axonally transported markers have well-localized terminals in higher order relays in the thalamus and send branches, whose terminals have not been described, or less clearly described, to the superior colliculus, pons, or more caudal centers. In order to understand the functional significance of these branching axons, a number of further studies will be needed. Currently we do not know how many cortical areas have such branching axons, nor do we know whether or not all of the layer 5 afferents to the thalamus have brainstem branches, or only some of them. The evidence for areas 17 and 18 of the cat mentioned above (Guillery et al., 2001) strongly suggests that for those areas, all corticothalamic axons have brainstem branches, and the other published evidence suggests that the same is likely to be true for axons coming from primary sensory and motor cortical areas.

It is important to recognize that, so far as we know, all cortical areas have layer 5 outputs (figure 10.1C), and that many, possibly all, have connections with motor centers in the brainstem. That is, instructions for motor action, which may be driver or modulator, excitatory or inhibitory in their final outcome, emerge from cortical areas early in the stages of perceptual processing, before this process has progressed significantly through the cortical circuitry, and also at later stages. Essentially every stage of perceptual processing produces its particular output to motor centers, so that the motor apparatus is kept in touch, and possibly moved to action as the perceptual process proceeds.

Evidence about the details of the layer 5 outputs from higher cortical areas is not available for most higher cortical areas at present. Many are known to go to the superior colliculus (figure 10.6), others go to the pons, the brainstem reticular nuclei, the inferior olive, or the spinal cord. For the superior colliculus, Harting et al. (1992), using autoradiographic tracing methods, studied corticotectal axons from 25 different, primarily visual, but also auditory, somatosensory, and cingulate cortical areas in the cat (see figure 10.6), and found that all these cortical areas have projections to the superior colliculus. Not one of the cortical areas that they injected lacked a tectal output. Since layer 6 axons have never been seen to project caudal to the thalamus, these are all likely to have been layer 5 axons. All of the areas they studied project to the thalamus, but here again, for most of these cortical areas we do not know whether that projection includes corticothalamic axons from layer 5. Further, where we know that there are corticothalamic projections from layer 5 (Gilbert & Kelly, 1975; Abramson & Chalupa, 1985), there is currently no information about the branching pattern. On the basis of what we know so far one might anticipate that all of the layer 5 axons terminating in the thalamus have extrathalamic branches, but that extrapolation is very insecure at present and needs to be experimentally tested. It is worth noting that the obverse of the above, that all layer 5 axons terminating beyond the thalamus have thalamic branches, is untested and may well be false. However, in spite of our relative ignorance about the details, we know that most, probably all, cortical areas involved in sensory processing have outputs to the brainstem and to the thalamus so that at every stage of cortical processing there is a connection to centers concerned with action. Where branching corticothalamic axons have been demonstrated, it is clear that the higher order thalamic relays that receive these axons are sending, from one cortical area to another, copies of the outputs of the first cortical area.

Figure 10.6 shows that different cortical areas project to a different group of collicular layers. Whereas some (e.g., areas 17 and 18) have

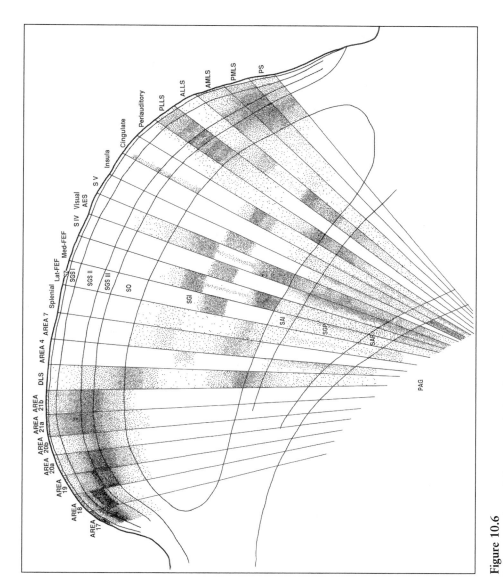

Figure 10.6
Representation of the terminal distribution of corticotectal axons from 22 different cortical areas. (Reproduced from Harting et al., 1992, with permission.)

terminals limited to the most superficial layers, others (e.g., the frontal eye fields) have no terminals in the superficial layers; all of their terminals are in the deeper layers. The superficial layers are to be seen as more "sensory" than the deep layers. That is, although the inputs to the superficial layers have access to the deeper layers which are closely linked to motor outputs for eye and head movements (Ozen et al., 2000; Schiller & Tehovnik, 2001; Tehovnik et al., 2002; Helms et al., 2004), the axons terminating in the deeper layers[4] are more directly linked to the motor outputs. The figure suggests that the cortical areas sending layer 5 outputs to the superior colliculus can be arranged in order, according to the superficial or deep position of their terminals. Area 17 is at one extreme, with terminals limited to the most superficial layers, and areas 18, 19, 20, and 21 follow roughly in sequence, with fewer terminals in the most superficial layers and little or nothing deep to the stratum opticum (SO in figure 10.6). Suprasylvian areas PMLS and PLLS have somewhat more terminals in the deeper layers, together with a rich innervation of the superficial layers, and then there follow a number of cortical areas with few or no terminals superficially and essentially all of their tectal terminals deep. This suggests a rough "hierarchy" along a sensorimotor continuum from area 17 to the frontal eye fields. There may be some problems about the precise position in the hierarchy of some areas, but it becomes of interest to ask how this relates to hierarchies in the direct corticocortical pathways that have been described for the monkey (Van Essen et al., 1992), or how it might relate to hierarchies that can be perhaps be defined for the transthalamic corticocortical pathways once these are known in more detail for monkey or for cat.

10.D. Implications for Corticocortical Processing

In principle, one might expect that the series of corticocortical connections, whether direct or transthalamic, that link the primary cortical receiving area through a chain of higher cortical areas to motor cortical regions such as the frontal eye fields might correspond to the series of superficial to deep terminals in the colliculus. At present, we have information for the colliculus of the cat, and for the direct corticocortical connections in the monkey only. We lack the corresponding information

---

4. The deepest layers are represented by the periventricular gray of the midbrain, which may well be more concerned with autonomic than with oculomotor control mechanisms.

about the colliculus in the monkey and about many of the direct corti-cocortical pathways of the cat. Further, we do not yet have the necessary information about the transthalamic corticocortical pathways in either species. In order to make a comparison we need more information for each species, and we need to recognize that there are some serious questions about the hierarchies that can be identified in the monkey cortex.

One problem is that there is not a single, simple hierarchy but there are some complex side- and cross-connections that make a straightforward interpretation difficult. Further, the proposed hierarchy of direct corticocortical connections is based on a distinction between feedforward and feedback connections that has its experimentally based origins in an analysis of connections between early visual areas (areas V1 and V2; Rockland & Pandya, 1979; Rockland, 1989; Rockland & Virga, 1989; Shipp & Zeki, 1989a, 1989b), which showed that the laminar origin and termination of the connections related closely to the feedforward or feedback nature of the connections in the known functional sequence of cortical processing. This observation was then extrapolated to other areas where the functional sequence is not known (Maunsell & Van Essen, 1983; Felleman & Van Essen, 1991). That is, the functional nature (feedforward or feedback) of the connections for many of the higher cortical areas has not been experimentally defined. In some instances, where specific corticocortical connections have been studied, they do not fit the generalizations that were originally used to distinguish feedforward from feedback connections in terms of laminar origins and terminations (Anderson et al., 1998; Rockland & Knutson, 2000). In terms of the discussion in chapter 7, what one really wants to know is which of the pathways are the drivers and which are the modulators, and on that we have no information at present. Clearly, a rigorous view of the hierarchies will depend on that distinction.

From the point of view of understanding what it is that the thalamus is doing when it transmits messages from one cortical area to another, the descending branches are clearly of great significance. Whereas the direct corticocortical connections, once they are identified as drivers (which so far they are not),[5] can be seen as sending messages from one cortical area to another that represent the ongoing computations within the first cortical area, the transthalamic connections whose corticothalamic axons have descending branches to motor centers have

---

5. For a discussion of the identification of corticocortical axons as drivers or modulators, see chapters 7 and 8.

to be seen, as indicated above, as sending information from one cortical area to another *about the actual output* that the first area is in the process of sending to motor centers. This output represents an involvement in action. The involvement can contribute to an inhibition of action or an initiation of action. The action will generally be in response to a sensory input, but it may be an essential part of the perceptual process, such as finger movements that relate tactile responses to position sense, eye or head movements related to producing a particular head orientation, or eye movements that allow a novel view representing a part of the search that is an essential part of viewing a novel scene; or it may be part of an organism's (final) response to a perceived input. This distinction between a motor instruction that is a part of the perceptual process and one that is a response to a perceptual process may often be a difficult (and somewhat artificial) distinction to make, although one should expect that the former will dominate for the outputs coming from primary and secondary cortical areas, whereas the latter are more likely to dominate for higher cortical areas. On this basis, for example, for the corticotectal descending branches, perhaps one can expect to be able to relate the nature of the motor instructions to the collicular lamina in which the corticotectal branches terminate. These relationships remain to be defined.

Perhaps the most important points about the long descending branches of the layer 5 corticofugal axons are the following: (1) All cortical areas, even the earliest cortical stages like area 17 (V1), have access to subcortical motor outputs. (2) Information about the messages that are passed along these motor outputs plays an important role in the next higher stage of cortical processing. (3) This transfer of information about motor outputs from one stage to the next involves a relay in the thalamus, which implies that this sequence of corticothalamocortical connections is subject to the thalamic gate, able to switch from burst to tonic mode (see chapters 4 and 6). This last point suggests that whereas the descending brainstem branch will be sending an unmodified message to lower motor centers at all times, the transthalamic branch will be sending its messages through the thalamus in either burst or tonic mode, depending on conditions in the relevant thalamic relay. (4) The role of these transthalamic connections, though currently not defined, is not likely to be trivial. The functional significance of thalamic inputs to higher cortical areas should be seen as a challenging area badly in need of study.

An important question that is currently unanswered about the direct and the transthalamic corticocortical pathways is: which of these pathways, or which subsets of these pathways, are likely to be drivers, and which, modulators? One possibility is that only one of the pathways (corticothalamocortical or direct corticocortical) is a driver, the other being modulatory in function. It is worth noting that there is already considerable evidence, summarized in chapter 8, that the cortical input from layer 5 to higher order thalamic relays acts as a driver and all known thalamocortical inputs act as drivers. It is thus probable that corticothalamocortical pathways are mostly or wholly drivers. However, no thalamocortical synapses from higher order relays have yet been tested for this function. There is no evidence to date of the nature, driver or modulator, of any direct corticocortical pathway.

A possibility suggested by the motor relationships of driver inputs to thalamus is of interest. It may be that, as one moves up the cortical hierarchy through the ascending corticothalamocortical chains, the layer 5 descending projections to higher order relays and the target cortical areas of these relays represent increasingly refined motor commands, and it is this continuous updating of motor commands that is transmitted from one cortical area to the next higher cortical area; this process would actually start with the branching driver input to first order relays. Thus, the functional significance of all thalamocortical inputs may be to keep cortex informed about the latest motor commands. In this context, it may be that some subset of direct corticocortical pathways (it remains to be determined which corticocortical pathways are drivers and which are modulators) represents activity of the peripheral receptors, and that this, at each stage of processing, interacts with information related to motor commands. For example, if a command to move the eyes were made, higher areas of cortex need this motor information to distinguish the difference between a stationary visual world and one that is moving.

These speculations emphasize the need for better information about the functional nature, particularly whether driver or modulator, of the various pathways involved in information processing within cortex.

10.E. Relating Action to Perception

Helmholtz (translated by Warren & Warren, 1968) wrote:

If we ask whether there exists some common characteristic distinguishable by direct sensation through which each perception related to objects in space is characterized for us, then we actually find such a characteristic in the circumstance that bodily movement places us in different spatial positions relative to the perceived objects, and in doing so also changes the impressions which these objects make on us. The impulse to movement, however, which we give through the innervation of our motor nerves is something which can be perceived directly. We feel we are doing something when we give such an impulse. But what it is we are doing we do not know directly.

Here a critical point concerns the "impulse to movement," which changes our perceptions. This might be an involuntary act in the first part of the passage, but might appear to be voluntary when "we feel we are doing something" even though we don't know directly "what it is we are doing." In many places Helmholtz writes as though he thinks of the motor component, this "impulse to movement," as voluntary, and in terms of the anatomical pathways, this would suggest a route up to cortex and then down again through the motor centers, possibly in accordance with figure 10.1A. He writes about the infant exploring objects, handling them, and regarding them from different angles, to make judgments about the causes of sensation, and says, "It is only by voluntarily bringing our organs of sense in various relations to objects that we *learn* to be sure as to our judgments of the causes of our sensations" (emphasis added). Here the boundary that would separate a "voluntary" exploration undertaken by an infant from involuntary movements produced at subcortical levels by the many pathways that we have seen linking the relevant somatosensory and visual pathways to midbrain and spinal motor centers is likely to be hard to draw. Perhaps as a first approximation one might draw it by distinguishing subcortical from cortical mechanisms. The branching axons that we have described here would suggest that a large part of the "impulse to movement" will be contributed by subcortical circuits, especially at the earliest stages of a new sensory input. The subcortical circuits will be committed to some particular outputs even before the cortical circuits can be brought into action. That is, much of the action will not be "voluntary."

If we now ask how an appreciation of the motor branches of thalamic afferents should influence current thinking about the relationship between action and perception, it may be worth looking at how the problem is presented in a textbook that looks closely at perceptual processing in relation to action. Churchland (2002) discusses how neuronal activity in the parietal cortex might relate to hand or eye movements toward a target, and shows (her figure 7.17) various sensory (visual, auditory, vestibular, proprioceptive) inputs feeding into posterior parietal cortex. She states, "Normally we reach our hands and move our eyes to a target effortlessly, and the computational resources needed to pull this off are not part of what the brain has conscious access to. The effortlessness makes the task seem easy; but computationally it is anything but simple. The central point is that sensory coordinates have to be transformed into motor coordinates in order to connect to a sensorily specified target." In this situation much depends on how one sees the afferents to parietal cortex. Are they simply the "sensory" inputs that have to be converted to motor coordinates, or are they inputs that relate closely to motor actions and that already implicitly carry messages relevant to the motor coordinates? The messages that parietal cortex is receiving from the thalamus carry information about motor instructions being sent out by other cortical areas to motor centers. The motor coordinates are likely to be there in the inputs, and the "pure sensory" message is an abstraction that we have learned to impose on the world and that philosophers and neuroscientists have imposed on the brain and on their colleagues.

This is not to suggest that the computational problem of converting sensory coordinates to motor coordinates does not exist, but to suggest that it does not have to be solved in the cortex alone. The solution will involve cortical and subcortical centers which establish their connections as an infant learns to relate motor responses to sensory inputs.

In terms of the development of an individual (the infant considered by Helmholtz) who is learning for the first time about the significance of particular perceptual situations, a large part of the impulse to action will also be subcortical. The cortical mechanisms undergo a large part of their development postnatally (figure 10.7). Flechsig (1920) showed that at birth, most of the cortex lacks myelin, and the extent to which its circuitry is capable of connecting adultlike functions to motor centers is questionable. From the point of view of understanding how cortical circuitry develops its connections with subcortical structures, Flechsig's observation that the earliest signs of myelinization appear in primary sensory (auditory, visual, somatosensory) and motor cortical areas is important. Secondary and higher cortical areas develop their myelin later, in sequence, so that the highest cortical areas are generally the last to acquire their adult pattern of myelinization. The extent to which this developmental sequence, characterized by the appearance of cortical myelin, corresponds to a sequence of synaptic development in the cortex is currently not defined, but it is reasonable to expect a close relationship (see chapter 8). Further, one can ask about the extent to which the developmental hierarchy corresponds to other putative hierarchies we have mentioned earlier: the hierarchy of direct corticocortical pathways,

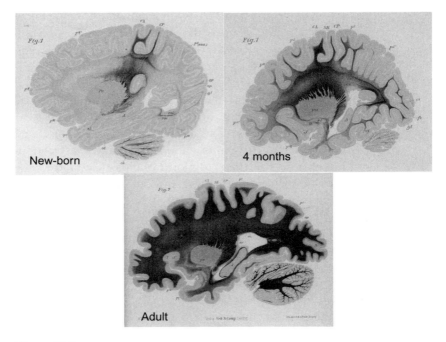

Figure 10.7
Three stages of myelinization of the human cerebral cortex (From Flechsig, 1920.)

the hierarchy of transthalamic corticocortical pathways, or the hierarchy of corticofugal layer 5 terminals in successively more motor regions of the neuraxis, as represented, for example, by the corticotectal terminations in figure 10.6.

Further, the relationship between the developmental sequence demonstrated by Flechsig, and the differential loss of the growth associated protein, GAP-43, mentioned in chapter 8, is of interest. This protein, associated with the growth of axons, is lost from the first order pathways to the thalamus for the innervation of early maturing cortex but is not lost from the higher order pathways that go through the thalamus for the innervation of later maturing cortex (Feig, 2004a), suggesting that there may be different degrees of plasticity that survive in the transthalamic pathways of the adult.

On the basis of Flechsig's sequence of cortical maturation it is possible to see first local—spinal or brainstem—circuits playing a role in the development of perceptual skills,[6] and then, in sequence, a hierarchy of cortical areas becoming involved (figure 10.8). Because our perceptual skills are so natural and generally acquired so early, it is not easy to appreciate the extent to which perceptual tasks that form a natural part of everyday life are learned skills, skills that depend on complex interactions between sensory inputs, on the one hand, and a series of instructions for movement (or inhibition of movement; think of a cat listening for a mouse) on the other. The first and higher order inputs to the thalamus and their brainstem and spinal branches represent a basic essential part of the circuitry that must underlie this learning process. There are, of course, likely to be other higher, largely local cortical circuits involved as well, but the connections we have presented in this chapter must represent the basic building blocks, and present a major opportunity to involve motor systems.

It will be important to learn far more than we know at present about the types of message that are passed along the nonthalamic branches of afferents to first and higher order thalamic relays. At present we know almost nothing about the messages that they are carrying. Consider the ascending axons, for example an axon in the medial lemniscus carrying messages from peripheral receptors in the skin of the arm, that also sends messages to the tectum or pretectum. When impulses from this axon are relayed to the somatosensory cortex (S1), the message received by the cortex will contain information about the specific instruction that this axon has delivered to these midbrain cells. It may be an impulse that prepares for a head or eye movement, probably toward the part of the arm stimulated, or it may be an instruction for the actual production, or inhibition, of a movement. Whatever the message, it is a part of the information that is available for the cortex, and it will be a part of the perceptual process as this progresses through the relevant cortical circuits. Or think about another lemniscal axon, one that perhaps

---

6. The extent to which perception is a *learned* skill is often ignored. Perceptual skills acquired late in life, such as bird watching or wine tasting, are easier to recognize as skills only because they are acquired late. It is easy for microscopists to speak of perceptual "skills," because they have seen students struggle to "perceive," no matter whether it is the image viewed with a light microscope or the photographic image obtained from an electron microscope. In relation to this, the role of movement in perception is strikingly illustrated by someone learning to use the highest powers of a light microscope, where the perceptual outcome depends critically on movements of the fine focus.

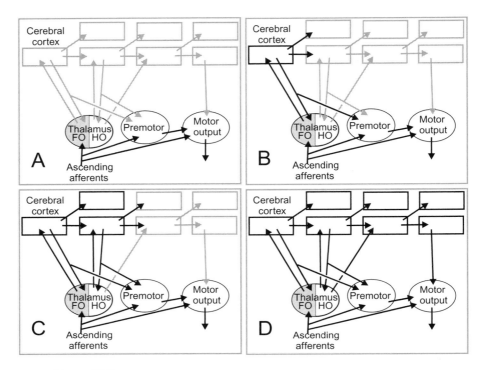

Figure 10.8
Schema to show the chronological sequence of development of the connections illustrated in figure 10.1. Heavy lines indicate the mature connections at each stage (A–D) and gray lines indicate immature ones.

comes from the leg and has a hypothalamic branch. This branch will innervate cells related to specific functions elicited through the hypo-thalamic pathway, such as changes in blood pressure or sweating, or perhaps other reactions related to fear or revulsion. When impulses from these axons are relayed to cortex they will automatically imply not only that skin receptors in the leg have been stimulated (i.e., there is some-thing crawling up my leg), but will also transmit the inseparable impli-cation that a response associated with fear or revulsion is being initiated.

Comparably one can consider axons from the retina that send information about the presence of a large dark object to the geniculate relay and concurrently sends messages to the superficial layers of the col-liculus that change the probability of an ocular movement. When the message from that axon is relayed from the thalamus to cortex, its arrival in cortex implies not only that there is a large object in the visual field, but also that the chances of an eye movement during the next (definable) brief period will be reduced (or enhanced).

Examples can be multiplied, but they must all be hypothetical, because in the past these relationships have not been studied. When it comes to thinking about the function of the branches that the axons of cortical layer 5 cells give off to brainstem centers, the information about their function is no better, and speculation is only worthwhile because it forces thought about the types of functional implication that might be worth investigating. It is possible that a tectal branch of a layer 5 axon from area 17 is simply reinforcing a message that has already been delivered about eye or head movements by the ascending axons, as above. However, it may be a new message that has been generated by the intracortical processing of the visual input, perhaps a directionally selective cortical response that is then related to instructions concerning relevant eye movements. Whatever it is, it will, like the ascending inputs, form an integral part of the information available to the higher cortical areas that are receiving the transthalamic messages from area 17, as well as other areas beyond that. That is, as the perceptual process advances through higher cortical areas it will be not only synthesizing the abstractions about external objects that make up the essential "sensory" side of the perceptual process, it will also be adding information about motor components that are an ongoing part of the response and that will inevitably contribute to the final motor action that is seen by many contemporary studies as coming only at the end of the process when motor cortical regions are reached.

The anatomy of the branched afferents to thalamus is clear. Messages that pass through the thalamus, whether as first or as higher order relays, represent a combination of sensory input and copies of motor instructions, and the effect of the message in thalamus and cortex must include both. The two are inseparable, and perceptual processing inevitably includes both. We should not be asking how perception as a sensory phenomenon relates to action as a motor phenomenon; rather, we should be looking for the intrinsic role of action in perception, wherever a perceptual process is to be studied. We have a system of connections that provides an anatomical skeleton for thinking about how action and perception relate to each other. However, it is only a skeleton. The flesh and the cutaneous cover have yet to be provided by functional studies that recognize this skeleton and show what each part does. Then perhaps will come the time when philosophers can furnish a respectable suit of clothes.

10.F. Unresolved Questions

1. Do all afferents to thalamus have branches innervating motor or premotor centers, or are there some that have no such branches and that might represent a "pure" sensory path?

   a. Specifically, what is the position for the parvocellular component of primates?

   b. Or for the auditory pathways?

2. Are the terminals of layer 5 corticofugal axons that are drivers in the thalamus also drivers at their nonthalamic brainstem synapses? Or are some modulators? More generally, can the nature of the actions that are copied to the thalamocortical pathways be defined for any one system?

3. Are there cortical areas that lack a layer 5 output either to thalamus or to extrathalamic relays in the brainstem? More generally, are there cortical areas whose outputs are confined to cortex, that might participate in perceptual processes but not themselves be involved in action?

4. Do all layer 5 corticothalamic axons have brainstem or spinal branches?

5. Are there layer 5 corticofugal axons to brainstem that lack a thalamic branch?

6. For any one sensory pathway is it possible to define the nonthalamic branches of the thalamic afferents and, more importantly, to understand the functional contribution that they make at their nonthalamic terminal sites?

7. As a specific example of question 6, what are the actions of corticocollicular axons on the motor outputs of the colliculus? How do these vary from one collicular layer to another?

8. Do hierarchies established by direct corticocortical pathways match those of the transthalamic pathways, and how do these match the hierarchies of motor outputs such as those seen in the superior colliculus (see figure 10.6)?

9. Does the developmental sequence seen in the myelinization of cortical areas match any of the hierarchies under question 8? How does this relate to synaptic maturation in the cortex? And how does early learning (perceptual learning or learning more generally) relate to the developmental maturation of the pathways considered in this chapter?

10. Are there rules for the branching corticothalamic axons from layer 5 that relate the terminal sites of the thalamic branch to the terminal sites of the brainstem branch? For example, do axons terminating in the deeper layers of the superior colliculus have branches whose thalamic endings are at sites distinct from the terminal sites of branches coming from axons that terminate in the superficial layers of the colliculus? More generally, is there any tendency for a given extrathalamic target to be associated with a particular thalamic target?

11 Overview

Although it has in the past proved possible to study the cerebral cortex with barely a glance at what might be happening in the thalamus, in the long run a clear understanding of cortical function must depend on knowledge of what it is that the thalamus sends to the cortex. Essentially, the cortex must view the world through the thalamus; that is the only view the cortex has. Understanding how the brain obtains a view of the world must depend to a significant extent on knowing what the thalamus is sending to cortex.

In the past the thalamus has been presented as a gateway to the cortex, sometimes seen as an opening through which information must pass to enter the cortex, at other times as an opening through which the cortex could view the real world. Neither provides a suitable metaphor for understanding thalamocortical relationships. Although today it is generally recognized that the cortex must receive all of its information about lower levels of the nervous system, including the receptors, through the thalamus, contemporary views of cortical function generally allow only a few cortical areas to have a direct view of these lower levels through the thalamus itself. Most cortical areas are presented as receiving their view of lower levels, and thus of the outside world, through other, lower cortical areas, not from the thalamus. That is, the monarch has to rely on reports from courtiers to learn about the realm. In contrast to this view, we have stressed that it is not just primary sensory areas that receive thalamic inputs but that most, probably all, areas of cortex receive afferents from thalamus that are likely to be drivers, and that, further, the thalamic inputs to higher cortical areas represent copies of outputs from lower cortical areas. That is, they represent the actions that the lower levels are currently initiating, so that the higher levels can be informed about the actions likely to occur at lower levels, rather than merely receiving reports about lower levels from intermediaries. The monarch is not just receiving reports from the courtiers but is also kept directly and independently informed about what the courtiers are up to.

We have argued that there are two distinct types of question to ask about any one thalamic relay: (1) What type of information is the relay receiving and passing on to cortex, that is, what is the function of the driver? (2) How do the modulators act on the transfer of information that the driver inputs are bringing to the relay? For these questions, the distinction between the drivers and the modulators is essential.

11.A. The Drivers

Identifying the drivers to the thalamus was initially a question of knowing which pathways carried the critical message for transmission to cortex. Subsequently, drivers were shown to have characteristic features in terms of their structure and synaptic relationships, so that it became possible to identify drivers to thalamic relays even where the particular message being transmitted to cortex was not known. We have suggested other criteria that can serve to identify drivers, including the absence of metabotropic postsynaptic receptors and the nature of cross-correlograms that can be obtained from recording pre- and postsynaptically. Further, we have argued that the relatively slow firing rates of the relay cells make the possibility of a driver function for inhibitory afferents to thalamus unlikely.

It is now possible to recognize three major types of driver input to the thalamus. There are the classical "sensory" afferents—visual, auditory, somatosensory, gustatory—that carry messages from identifiable receptors to the thalamus. The cerebellar and the mamillary afferents are slightly different; we know less about them (except for the small group of lateral mamillary afferents concerned with head direction signals), because it has not been easy to trace the origin of the signal beyond the prethalamic relay (cerebellum, mamillary body) or to identify the precise nature of the message. The corticothalamic layer 5 driver afferents are a third important and relatively newly recognized group of drivers about which we need to learn a great deal more than we know at present. Specifically, we need to understand the nature of the message that they pass to the thalamus. We also need to know how this message compares to any sent via direct corticocortical connections. In relation to this it will be necessary to determine whether all of these layer 5 corticothalamic axons have motor branches to brainstem or spinal cord, and, where such branches are identified, to define the action that the motor branches of these axons have at their brainstem or spinal terminal sites.

The nature of the message that is being sent to the thalamus for transmittal to cortex by any one group of drivers is vital for understanding what any one thalamic relay may actually be sending to cortex. However, when one considers the function of the drivers to the thalamus in these terms, there are two important, currently disappointing, but challenging conclusions to be drawn. One is that we have significant information about the function of relatively few of the drivers. The other is that the information that we do have may be incomplete, and to a certain extent even misleading.

We can provide an account of the function of the visual, somatosensory, auditory, or gustatory drivers to first order relays, but we have only limited knowledge about the function of cerebellar or mamillary drivers, and we know almost nothing about the functions of the layer 5 cortical drivers that innervate higher order relays. However, even the information that we have about the apparently obviously "sensory" inputs to first order relays may be giving us a skewed picture if it leads us to see the thalamus as though it were simply an instrument through which the cortex can view messages coming from the receptors. Yet, these sensory drivers are carrying messages that can be matched to our subjective sensory experiences. They have receptive field properties that correspond to aspects of vision, touch, hearing, and taste, but we have seen that they also represent copies of current motor instructions, and about these we know almost nothing, because the function of the nonthalamic branches has so far not been raised in relation to the relevant thalamocortical pathways, and it is these branches that must produce a significant link between perception and action, establishing some of the basic sensorimotor contingencies of O'Regan and Noë (2001; see chapter 10) that characterize perceptual processing.

The nonthalamic branches of the thalamic driver afferents, both first and higher order, tell us that our view of the world depends on abstractions from (or, perhaps better, on a redirection of) messages that relate to action. We can think about the sensory functions of thalamocortical circuitry as produced by systems that are "listening" to a part of lower level traffic between afferents and efferents, interpreting the copies of the ongoing motor instructions in order to arrive at conclusions about what is happening "out there," about what the world is like. The infant learning about the significance of tactile inputs from the hand learns about them as a part of an ongoing sensorimotor experience of arm and hand movements related to receptor activity. Comparably, the visual inputs will always be closely related to head and eye movements.

This dependence of cortical sensory mechanisms on circuits concerned with action appears to apply to all levels of the thalamic relay. First order relays receiving, for example, lemniscal inputs from branches of axons innervating spinal mechanisms represent the lowest level of this thalamic function, whereas layer 5 corticothalamic axons that are branches of axons innervating midbrain structures represent one of several higher levels, depending on where in a cortical hierarchy these corticothalamocortical pathways take their origin and have their termination. That is, no matter where we look in thalamic relays or in the hierarchy of cortical areas, we find cortex receiving copies of motor instructions, and it is these copies that provide the raw material from which the neuronal activity that can be regarded as representing sensory events is generated. Most, probably all cortical areas, particularly those at the bottom of any proposed hierarchy (i.e., including primary sensory areas), send out a motor signal via their layer 5 efferent projections.

On the view summarized above, the function of a driver to a first order thalamic sensory relay represents information about motor instructions that a particular sensory organ (visual, auditory, etc.) is passing to a particular, definable group of subcortical motor or premotor centers. Understanding the nature of these motor instructions may provide a useful approach to a clearer appreciation of the sensorimotor contingencies. A comparable approach to other branched driver afferents to thalamus may also prove useful. That is, if we want to know more about the type of message that the cerebellum is sending to the cortex through the thalamus, it may be useful to find out about the action of the brainstem branches of the cerebellothalamic drivers. Similarly, it may prove possible to learn more about the function of a higher order relay like the pulvinar by finding out about the action of the brainstem branches of the relevant layer 5 corticothalamic axons.

Learning about the functions of the drivers that are afferent to thalamic relays is important because they are carrying key input messages for transmission to cortex. Not only do we need more information about the function of many of the drivers to thalamic relays, we also need to learn more about the extent to which there are interactions between any two driver afferents to a relay. We have raised the possibility that there may be thalamic relays that have integrative functions, but have argued that until clear evidence of such a relay is available, it is reasonable to treat the lateral geniculate relay of X and Y, on-center and off-center pathways as a model for thalamic organization generally. That is, the relay cells for distinct driver pathways may be intermingled (as in the A layers of the cat's lateral geniculate nucleus), but without any significant interaction at the single-neuron level in the thalamus, and thus there is no real integration of driver pathways through thalamus. Thus, we see the thalamus as not having an integrative function. Interactions among different afferent transthalamic driver pathways occur in the cortex but may never be seen in the thalamus.

From the point of view of understanding how thalamic inputs relate to cortical organization, it is important to understand not only how (and where) several different transthalamic driver pathways interact, in thalamus or in cortex, but also to learn much more than is known at present about how the direct corticocortical pathways interact with the transthalamic corticocortical pathways. The extent to which any particular corticocortical pathway is either a driver or a modulator needs to be experimentally defined, as does the extent to which the laminar origin and termination of a corticocortical pathway can be used as a reliable indicator of its function. Where corticocortical drivers are identified it will become important to understand how the thalamocortical axons, which on the basis of their driver functions for first order relays are also likely to be drivers, interact with the corticocortical drivers. We have argued that a critical unknown currently is the extent to which any one cortical area depends for its major driver afferents on either the thalamus or on other cortical areas, and we have suggested that the functional importance of thalamic afferents to higher order cortical areas may in the past have been seriously underestimated. Arguments about the number of relay cells available to any one pathway (Van Essen, 2005) carry little weight so long as the nature of the information that needs to be transmitted from one cortical area to another remains as poorly defined as it is at present. As noted in chapter 8, the numbers of cells in higher order relays such as the pulvinar seem adequate to the task of retransmitting information from layer 5 drivers.

A further significant point about the drivers is that so far as we know they all show local sign. That is, the driver afferents and the thalamocortical efferent axons are mapped. For some pathways we can see that the maps represent body parts or sensory surfaces, but for others we have no clear idea as to what it is that is mapped other than parts of a thalamic nucleus or cortical area. The significance of the mapping may be revealed at least in part by looking at the modulators, where we find that some are mapped and some are not mapped, and where we can argue that those that are not mapped allow for a global action, whereas those that are mapped allow for a local focus of action, providing for particular, local parts of a sensory or motor system to be modified in accordance with local demands. Such local actions on mapped drivers are perhaps most clearly revealed by looking at the corticothalamic, largely reciprocal inputs that come from layer 6, and at the related afferents from the thalamic reticular nucleus.

11.B. The Modulators

One of the important points about the modulators is that some are mapped and some are not mapped, allowing some to modulate transmission through the thalamus in a remarkably local manner whereas others have a global or relatively widespread action. The largest and possibly most important group of mapped modulators is made up of the corticothalamic axons from layer 6. Although probably every thalamic nucleus receives modulatory (type I) afferents from cortex, there may be important differences that relate to whether these come from just one cortical area or from several different cortical areas. The evidence currently available suggests that a significant part of the layer 6 pathway establishes connections that are reciprocal with the thalamocortical pathways, but there is also evidence for a sparser distribution of nonreciprocal connections. There are rare examples of modulatory corticothalamic axons having a bilateral distribution in the thalamus.

We have presented evidence that the layer 6 cells that give rise to the modulatory corticothalamic afferents are not a functionally uniform population, and neither are their relay cell targets, so that understanding the particular pattern of modulation received by any one thalamic nucleus may well prove important. There is close relationship between the layer 6 corticothalamic afferents and the circuitry of the thalamic reticular nucleus. We have summarized some of the current knowledge about pathways that link the thalamic reticular nucleus and thalamic relay nuclei. At the level of individual thalamic, cortical, and reticular cells, details of connectivity patterns are likely to prove critical to our understanding of what these pathways are doing. At the level of the major reticular segments and their related thalamic nuclei and cortical areas, we need to learn much more about the connections that are established within the reticular nucleus among first and higher order circuits, as well as the mapped (or unmapped) connections that they form. Where the evidence seems to suggest that higher order pathways are not mapped in the reticular nucleus, one has to ask whether the appropriate parameter has been identified for the experiments that appear to show an unmapped (though well-localized) corticoreticular projection. Further, for much of the cortex it is necessary to ascertain the extent to which there are corticothalamic layer 6 axons that lack reticular branches and more generally to determine just how variable the reticular innervation is among distinct groups of these corticothalamic axons.

On the basis of the close connections that it establishes with the thalamic relays, the reticular nucleus is neither entirely intrinsic nor really extrinsic to the thalamic relay. It is an integral part of the links that connect thalamus and cortex. It accommodates many of the complex fiber interchanges that are an essential part of thalamocorticothalamic communication, and although we can anticipate that every thalamic relay has a reticular connection, it is reasonable to expect that the details will not be the same for each relay and may differ, in particular when first order relays are compared to higher order relays. Is the reticular innervation of higher order relays as rich as that to first order relays? Or do higher order relays depend on other inhibitory pathways more than do first order relays?

In relation to this, one finds that there are several distinct extradiencephalic inhibitory afferents, from globus pallidus, substantia nigra, zona incerta, pretectum, which, we have argued, are likely to be modulators. They represent an important difference between thalamic nuclei: although many thalamic nuclei receive these extradiencephalic inhibitory afferents, only a few nuclei receive any one of these inhibitory components, so that the specific function of these afferents may differ from one nucleus to another. However, at present we have no clear picture of the role that these inhibitory afferents play. As the functional role of the several modulatory pathways becomes clear, it will be important to understand how each relates to any one thalamic nucleus, so that the patterns of modulation that can be imposed on that nucleus can be appreciated.

11.C. The Thalamic Nuclei

In the first part of this book we presented the thalamus as it was seen historically: as a group of several different nuclei, each carrying a functionally distinct set of afferents to the cerebral cortex. We have stressed that although this view may be telling us something about the messages that pass to the cortex through some parts of the thalamus, it tells us very little about what these parts of the thalamus actually do, and it tells us nothing about the function of the rest of the thalamus, represented by the nuclei that are entirely or largely higher order relays. Although the concept of a "nucleus" in the thalamus has proved useful in the past, its limitations must be recognized. Any one nucleus or nuclear subdivision can house a variety of intermingled, functionally (and structurally) distinct relay cell types. The mingling of X with Y, parvo with konio cells in a single geniculate layer provides a good example, as does the increasing evidence for mixed first and higher order relays in a single nucleus (see chapter 8), or the mixture of calbindin- and parvalbumin-positive cells (see chapter 3).

In order to explore what it is that the thalamus does, we have used the visual pathways, primarily of cat and primate, to explore some of the functional properties of the thalamic relay in general. This has been a dual approach. On the one hand, it has raised a number of questions about what exactly the thalamus is doing for the visual relay itself, and on the other hand, it asks whether some of the functional properties that can be defined or hypothesized for the visual relay may also apply to other thalamic relays, possibly to all thalamic nuclei. Insofar as our exploration has an expected outcome, it should serve to guide an investigation of the particular thalamic features that can be treated as general properties found in all parts of the thalamus, and of those that are special to one nucleus or to one group of nuclei. It can be argued that it is unlikely, for example, that auditory, cerebellar, visual, and mamillothalamic relays will all show the same thalamic organization in all details. Yet it is clear that in terms of the morphological features seen light and electron microscopically or in terms of membrane properties and transmitter functions, there are many shared features across most, possibly all thalamic nuclei. That is, there is a basic common pattern to thalamic relays. The challenge for future studies is to define exactly what the shared features are and to show where the functional organization of any one thalamic nucleus differs from that of another. That is, although one can reasonably expect to find differences between thalamic nuclei, a systematic search for differences has not been undertaken, and those differences that have been documented represent a small and as yet poorly defined part of our knowledge of the thalamus.

The differences between thalamic nuclei can be treated as either intrinsic or extrinsic. That is, the differences may depend on external connections or on the internal organization of the particular relay. The most important of the extrinsic differences are represented by the origins and the functional properties of the driver afferents to each nucleus, and these are the differences explored by the classical approach, except that this approach did not recognize driver afferents coming from the cortex. Adding the drivers that come from cortex to our analysis of thalamus opens many new doors to the way in which we can look at the functional organization of many previously puzzling thalamic nuclei. However, a key step in such an analysis, defining the nature of the message that is sent by the corticothalamic drivers, must play a crucial role in the future, as must the determination of whether all or only some of these axons are branches of long descending axons going to brainstem or spinal cord. Further, other extrinsic differences include the particular combination of modulator afferents that a nucleus is receiving from, for example, the brainstem cholinergic pathways or from noradrenergic, serotonergic, histaminergic, or other systems, or from the inhibitory pathways from pretectum, zona incerta, or globus pallidus.

A further difference in the extrinsic connections of thalamic nuclei relates to the distribution of their thalamocortical axons. We have seen that there are differences in the cortical layers within which the axons terminate, although there is rather little evidence as to exactly how the differences relate to the actions they have within the receiving cortical area, and there are also differences in the extent to which any one nucleus or relay cell sends its axons to just one cortical area or to more than one cortical area. Possibly, from the point of view of understanding any one cortical area, all one needs to know is where the thalamocortical afferents take origin; but clearly, in terms of understanding overall functional relationships between cortical areas, it will be important to understand where the thalamic afferents to two cortical areas are or are not shared. Finally, in terms of the extrinsic connections that are relevant to understanding differences among thalamic nuclei, there is the difference between thalamic cells that do and those that do not send axonal terminals to the striatum (e.g., Macchi et al., 1984). Does cortical processing of messages that come from afferents having branches to the striatum differ from the cortical processing of messages that go to cortex alone? Clearly, whether the overall action does or does not include the striatum will have major functional significance for the brain as a whole, but exactly what relationship, if any, this has to cortical processing itself remains to be defined.

In terms of the intrinsic organization of thalamic relays there are many significant common features. It appears probable that all thalamic nuclei receive glutamatergic driver afferents as well as local GABAergic inhibitory afferents coming from interneurons, from cells of the thalamic reticular nucleus, or from both. Perhaps more importantly it appears that the capacity to function in either tonic or burst mode is characteristic of all thalamic relay cells, and this has important implications for how information is transmitted to cortex. We have treated this as a key to understanding at least some of the aspects of thalamic gating functions and are inclined to treat it as a general property of thalamus until a group of thalamic relays that fail to show these two modes are demonstrated. We have summarized the several distinct conductances and receptor mechanisms that have been demonstrated for the lateral geniculate nucleus. Only a few have been studied systematically in more than one thalamic nucleus. It remains to be defined exactly how each relates to the relay functions of the thalamus and the extent to which their distribution differs from one thalamic nucleus to another.

The distribution of metabotropic receptors is likely to relate to the distribution of modulator afferents in many, possibly all thalamic relays; it seems unlikely that a driver that is transmitting a message that requires accurate timing could function with metabotropic receptors, but the possibility that there are driver afferents that function on a slower time base remains to be explored for systems such as taste or olfaction and, by implication, for thalamic relays whose functions are currently completely unknown.

Interneurons represent an important component of some but not all thalamic nuclei, and their distribution in relation to different relays, different nuclei, and different species represents perhaps the strongest argument against treating all thalamic relays as precisely equal. We know that there are differences between nuclei that have almost no interneurons and nuclei that have 20% or more thalamic cells serving as interneurons. It is not yet clear exactly what functional difference the presence or absence of interneurons implies for the function of a particular relay. The fact that thalamic somatosensory relays in cat and rat differ markedly in this respect whereas the visual pathways in the two species appear to resemble each other needs to be understood in terms of how each of these relays can affect the messages that are passed on to cortex. However, the difference within the visual pathways of cats, where the X cells appear to be involved in a relay heavily linked to interneuronal connections whereas the Y cells are not, suggests that it may be more appropriate to compare relay cells that are or are not connected to interneurons instead of simply comparing thalamic nuclei. Possibly there are two types of relay characteristic of the thalamus in general, and perhaps they relate to the two types of nerve cell originally described by Kölliker, although on present evidence that is far from an established conclusion. We have seen that the issue of classifying neurons and so distinguishing functionally distinct classes is a difficult one for relay cells and also for interneurons. It is clear that for both of these types of thalamic neuron there are likely to be functionally distinct classes. However, at present we have rather poor criteria for establishing differences and almost no insights into the functional significance of the differences that can be identified.

11.D. Extending the Functional Analysis from the Thalamus to the Cortex

One of the important points we have raised for the thalamus is the distinction between drivers and modulators. It is only when the drivers are identified that it is possible to understand the nature of the message that a thalamic relay is transmitting to cortex. We have indicated that the same distinction will prove important for understanding the messages that pass from one cortical area to another. We need to know whether the transthalamic corticocortical pathways are drivers or modulators, and we need the same information about the direct corticocortical pathways. It is only by identifying the drivers that one can expect to define the nature of the transfer function of any one cortical area. Once we can identify the driver inputs to a cortical area and the driver outputs from that area we can begin to understand the functionally important changes that any one area contributes to the whole perceptual process.

There is a subtle but important difference between this approach and that currently in vogue. Now the general approach is to compare response properties, or more specifically receptive field properties, of cells in two connected areas, for example, by comparing motion sensitivity in V1 and MT or color sensitivity in V1 and V4. However, currently these cells are not identified in terms of laminar position or, more important, in terms of their connections, often because the observations are made in awake animals in which this is not practical. Further, there is no information about the functional role that any particular cell plays in cortical circuitry: driver or modulator. It is worth recalling that the receptive field properties of the modulatory corticogeniculate layer 6 cells are not passed on to geniculate cells; comparably, the origin of particular functional properties in one area of cortex as coming from another cortical area or from the thalamus is currently unresolved in accounts that appear to trace receptive field properties from one cortical area to another. To be specific, we are suggesting that to really home in on the computational properties of a specific cortical area, one should try to define the properties of the driver input and compare them with the properties of the driver output.

Several examples may clarify this point. Suppose, for instance, the only driver to a cortical area derives from thalamus, either the lateral geniculate nucleus for V1 or the pulvinar for MT. To understand the function of MT, then, one needs to define the properties of the pulvinar input and compare those properties with those of the layer 5 output from MT that projects back to the thalamus and to a motor center of the brainstem. Or a cortical area might receive driver input both from thalamus and directly from another cortical area. One can then imagine multiple functions for an area such as MT: one is defined as above by the different properties between the pulvinar input and the layer 5 output, another is defined by the difference between the direct corticocortical input and the direct corticocortical output, and possibly there could be an integrative function with the two inputs combining to produce the layer 5 output. However, there is another important point to make about this latter scenario: even if there are both direct corticothalamocortical and transthalamic information routes, an important difference is that the transthalamic route also has subcortical motor connections, whereas the direct corticocortical route represents information that remains in cortex. Currently, we know nothing about the motor actions of these transthalamic pathways, but, insofar as the corticocortical link carries copies of the motor instructions, knowledge of these actions is likely to provide a new view of the relevance of motor activity for perception. For each thalamocortical relay, first order or higher order, we can ask how the input to cortex differs from the output, and the question can be framed in terms of motor actions or in terms of perceptual processes, with a view to eventually relating action and perception.

11.E. What Does the Thalamus Do?

We are still far from understanding exactly what it is that the thalamus does. Perhaps the most promising leads will come from recognizing the difference, in terms of the information transmitted, between the tonic mode, on the one hand, and the burst mode, either rhythmic or not, on the other. This can provide a clue as to what cortex may be receiving from the thalamus at any one time, provided that we know in turn what it is that the relevant part of the thalamus is receiving from its drivers. Often, as for some first order and most higher order relays, we have all too little information about the nature of the message that the thalamic relay cells are receiving. Defining the functional characteristics of the afferents may prove extremely difficult, and may depend on intuitions about the significant variables as well as on a certain amount of luck. However, knowing what message is carried by the drivers to any one nucleus will prove to be an essential part of understanding that nucleus and the messages that it is sending to cortex. Where a thalamic nucleus receives more than one driver afferent there is a crucial question about how these pathways relate. Is there some integrative interaction in the nucleus, or do the two sets of messages pass through with relatively little or no interaction? If it is a higher order relay, then an important next step will be to define how the messages that are being sent to the cortical receiving area relate to the messages sent to the same area through corticocortical pathways. Which are drivers? Which are modulators? If there is more than one driver reaching cortex, what is the nature of the integration that occurs in the cortex?

We have presented many questions about the thalamus in the course of this book and in the brief overview of this chapter. The reader will almost certainly be able to add others, and may know of some answers that we have missed in our review of the relevant literature. We are inclined to think of the thalamus as central to all cortical functions, and to believe that a better understanding of the thalamus will lead to a fuller appreciation of cortical function. It has become fashionable in journals that deal with neuroscience for authors to introduce their subject, whatever it may be, as "the central problem of neuroscience," or, occasionally, for slightly more modest authors, as "one of the central problems of neuroscience." We are not tempted to make such a claim about the thalamus, although it does occupy a strikingly central position in the brain. However, we suggest that cerebral cortex without thalamus is rather like a great church organ without an organist: fascinating, but useless.

References

Abbott, L. F. (2005). Drivers and modulators from push-pull and balanced synaptic input. *Progress in Brain Research* 149, 147–155.

Abramson, B. P., & Chalupa, L. M. (1985). The laminar distribution of cortical connections with the tecto- and cortico-recipient zones in the cat's lateral posterior nucleus. *Neuroscience* 15, 81–95.

Abramson, B. P., & Chalupa, L. M. (1988). Multiple pathways from the superior colliculus to the extrageniculate visual thalamus of the cat. *Journal of Comparative Neurology* 271, 397–418.

Adams, M. M., Hof, P. R., Gattass, R., Webster, M. J., & Ungerleider, L. G. (2000). Visual cortical projections and chemoarchitecture of macaque monkey pulvinar. *Journal of Comparative Neurology* 419, 377–393.

Adams, N. C., Lozsádi, D. A., & Guillery, R. W. (1997). Complexities in the thalamocortical and corticothalamic pathways. *European Journal of Neuroscience* 9, 204–209.

Adams, P. R. (1982). Voltage-dependent conductances of vertebrate neurones. *Trends in Neurosciences* 5, 116–119.

Adams, P. R., Brown, D. A., & Constanti, A. (1982). Pharmacological inhibition of the M-current. *Journal of Physiology* (*London*) 332, 223–262.

Aggleton, J. P., & Mishkin, M. (1984). Projections of the amygdala to the thalamus in the cynomolgus monkey. *Journal of Comparative Neurology* 222, 56–68.

Ahlsén, G., Lindström, S., & Lo, F.-S. (1984). Inhibition from the brainstem of inhibitory interneurones of the cat's dorsal lateral geniculate nucleus. *Journal of Physiology* (*London*) 347, 593–609.

Ahlsén, G., Lindström, S., & Lo, F.-S. (1985). Interaction between inhibitory pathways to principal cells in the lateral geniculate nucleus of the cat. *Experimental Brain Research* 58, 134–143.

Ahmed, B., Anderson, J. C., Douglas, R. J., Martin, K. A. C., & Nelson, J. C. (1994). Polyneuronal innervation of spiny stellate neurons in cat visual cortex. *Journal of Comparative Neurology* 341, 39–49.

Allendoerfer, K. L., & Shatz, C. J. (1994). The subplate, a transient neocortical structure: its role in the development of connections between thalamus and cortex. *Annual Reviews in Neuroscience* 17, 185–218.

Allman, J. M., & Kaas, J. H. (1971). Representation of the visual field in striate and adjoining cortex of the owl monkey (*Aotus trivirgatus*). *Brain Research* 35, 89–106.

Allman, J. M., & Kaas, J. H. (1974). A crescent-shaped cortical visual area surrounding the middle temporal area (MT) in the owl monkey (*Aotus trivirgatus*). *Brain Research* 81, 199–213.

Allman, J. M., & Kass, J. H. (1975). The dorsomedial cortical visual area: a third tier area in the occipital lobe of the owl monkey (*Aotus trivirgatus*). *Brain Research* 100, 473–487.

Alonso, J. M., Usrey, W. M., & Reid, R. C. (1996). Precisely correlated firing in cells of the lateral geniculate nucleus. *Nature* 383, 815–819.

Alonso, J. M., Usrey, W. M., & Reid, R. C. (2001). Rules of connectivity between geniculate cells and simple cells in cat primary visual cortex. *Journal of Neuroscience* 21, 4002–4015.

Altman, J., & Carpenter, M. B. (1961). Fiber projections of the superior colliculus in the cat. *Journal of Comparative Neurology* 116, 157–177.

Amadeo, A., Ortino, B., & Frassoni, C. (2001). Parvalbumin and GABA in the developing somatosensory thalamus of the rat: an immunocytochemical ultrastructural correlation. *Anatomy and Embryology (Berlin)* 203, 109–119.

Anderson, J. C., Binzegger, T., Martin, K. A. C., & Rockland, K. S. (1998). The connection from cortical area V1 to V5: a light and electron microscopic study. *Journal of Neuroscience* 18, 10525–10540.

Anderson, J. S., Carandini, M., & Ferster, D. (2000). Orientation tuning of input conductance, excitation, and inhibition in cat primary visual cortex. *Journal of Neurophysiology* 84, 909–926.

Angel, A., Magni, F., & Strata, P. (1967). The excitability of optic nerve terminals in the lateral geniculate nucleus after stimulation of visual cortex. *Archives Italiennes de Biologie* 105, 104–117.

Arcelli, P., Frassoni, C., Regondi, M. C., De Biasi, S., & Spreafico, R. (1997). GABAergic neurons in mammalian thalamus: a marker of thalamic complexity? *Brain Research Bulletin* 42, 27–37.

Armstrong, D. M., & Edgley, S. A. (1988). Discharges of interpositus and Purkinje cells of the cat cerebellum during locomotion under different conditions. *Journal of Physiology* 400, 425–445.

Asanuma, C. (1989). Axonal arborizations of a magnocellular basal nucleus input and their relation to the neurons in the thalamic reticular nucleus of rats. *Proceedings of the National Academy of Sciences of the United States of America* 86, 4746–4750.

Asanuma, C. (1992). Noradrenergic innervation of the thalamic reticular nucleus: a light and electron microscopic immunohistochemical study in rats. *Journal of Comparative Neurology* 319, 299–311.

Asanuma, C. (1994). GABAergic and pallidal terminals in the thalamic reticular nucleus of squirrel monkeys. *Experimental Brain Research* 101, 439–451.

Asanuma, C., & Porter, L. I. (1990). Light and electron microscopic evidence for a GABAergic projection from the caudal basal forebrain to the thalamic reticular nucleus in rats. *Journal of Comparative Neurology* 302, 159–172.

Ault, S. J., Leventhal, A. G., Vitek, D. J., & Creel, D. J. (1995). Abnormal ipsilateral visual field representation in areas 17 and 18 of hypopigmented cats. *Journal of Comparative Neurology* 354, 181–192.

Aumann, T. D., Ivanusic, J., & Horne, M. K. (1998). Arborisation and termination of single motor thalamocortical axons in the rat. *Journal of Comparative Neurology* 396, 121–130.

Baas, P. W. (1999). Microtubules and neuronal polarity: lessons from mitosis. *Neuron* 22, 23–31.

Bacci, A., Verderio, C., Pravettoni, E., & Matteoli, M. (1999). The role of glial cells in synaptic function. *Philosophical Transactions of the Royal Society of London, Series B, Biological Sciences* 354, 403–409.

Baker, F. H., & Malpeli, J. G. (1977). Effects of cryogenic blockade of visual cortex on the responses of lateral geniculate neurons in the monkey. *Experimental Brain Research* 29, 433–444.

Bal, T., & McCormick, D. A. (1993). Mechanisms of oscillatory activity in guinea-pig nucleus reticularis thalami in vitro: a mammalian pacemaker. *Journal of Physiology (London)* 468, 669–691.

Bal, T., Von Krosigk, M., & McCormick, D. A. (1995). Synaptic and membrane mechanisms underlying synchronized oscillations in the ferret lateral geniculate nucleus *in vitro*. *Journal of Physiology (London)* 483, 641–663.

Balercia, G., Kultas-Ilinsky, K., Bentivoglio, M., & Ilinsky, I. A. (1996). Neuronal and synaptic organization of the centromedian nucleus of the monkey thalamus: a quantitative ultrastructural study, with tract tracing and immunohistochemical observations. *Journal of Neurocytology* 25, 267–288.

Banke, T. G., & Traynelis, S. F. (2003). Activation of NR1/NR2B NMDA receptors. *Nature Neuroscience* 6, 144–152.

Barthó, P., Freund, T. F., & Acsády, L. (2002). Selective GABAergic innervation of thalamic nuclei from zona incerta. *European Journal of Neuroscience* 16, 999–1014.

Bartlett, E. L., & Smith, P. H. (1999). Anatomic, intrinsic, and synaptic properties of dorsal and ventral division neurons in rat medial geniculate body. *Journal of Neurophysiology* 81, 1999–2016.

Bartlett, E. L., Stark, J. M., Guillery, R. W., & Smith, P. H. (2000). Comparison of the fine structure of cortical and collicular terminals in the rat medial geniculate body. *Neuroscience* 100, 811–828.

Beck, P. D., Pospichal, M. W., & Kaas, J. H. (1996). Topography, architecture, and connections of somatosensory cortex in opossums: evidence for five somatosensory areas. *Journal of Comparative Neurology* 366, 109–133.

Beierlein, M., & Connors, B. W. (2002). Short-term dynamics of thalamocortical and intracortical synapses onto layer 6 neurons in neocortex. *Journal of Neurophysiology* 88, 1924–1932.

Belluscio, L., Koentges, G., Axel, R., & Dulac, C. (1999). A map of pheromone receptor activation in the mammalian brain. *Cell* 97, 209–220.

Bender, D. B. (1983). Visual activation of neurons in the primate pulvinar depends on cortex but not colliculus. *Brain Research* 279, 258–261.

Bender, D. B. (1988). Electrophysiological and behavioral experiments on the primate pulvinar. *Progress in Brain Research 75*, 55–65.

Benjamin, R. M., & Burton, H. (1968). Projection of taste nerve afferents to anterior opercular-insular cortex in squirrel monkey (*Saimiri sciureus*). *Brain Research 7*, 221–231.

Benowitz, L. I., & Routtenberg, A. (1997). GAP-43: an intrinsic determinant of neuronal development and plasticity. *Trends in Neurosciences 20*, 84–91.

Bentivoglio, M., Macchi, G., & Albanese, A. (1981). The cortical projections of the thalamic intralaminar nuclei, as studied in cat and rat with the multiple fluorescent retrograde tracing technique. *Neuroscience Letters 26*, 5–10.

Berardi, N., Pizzorusso, T., Ratto, G. M., & Maffei, L. (2003). Molecular basis of plasticity in the visual cortex. *Trends in Neurosciences 26*, 369–378.

Berendse, H. W., & Groenewegen, H. J. (1991). Restricted cortical termination fields of the midline and intralaminar thalamic nuclei in the rat. *Neuroscience 42*, 73–102.

Berkley, K. J. (1975). Different targets of different neurons in nucleus gracilis of the cat. *Journal of Comparative Neurology 163*, 285–303.

Berkley, K. J., Blomqvist, A., Pelt, A., & Fink, R. (1980). Differences in the collateralization of neural projections from dorsal column nuclei and lateral cervical nucleus to the thalamus and tectum in the cat: an anatomical study using two different double labeling techniques. *Brain Research 202*, 273–290.

Berman, A. L. (1982). *The Thalamus and Basal Telencephalon of the Cat: A Cytoarchitectonic Atlas with Stereotaxic Coordinates.* University of Wisconsin Press, Madison.

Berman, N. E. J., & Cynader, M. S. (1972). Comparison of receptive-field organization of the superior colliculus in Siamese and normal cats. *Journal of Physiology (London) 224*, 363–389.

Bernander, O., Douglas, R. J., Martin, K. A. C., & Koch, C. (1991). Synaptic background activity influences spatiotemporal integration in single pyramidal cells. *Proceedings of the National Academy of Sciences of the United States of America 88*, 11569–11573.

Bickford, M. E., Günlük, A. E., Guido, W., & Sherman, S. M. (1993). Evidence that cholinergic axons from the parabrachial region of the brainstem are the exclusive source of nitric oxide in the lateral geniculate nucleus of the cat. *Journal of Comparative Neurology 334*, 410–430.

Bickford, M. E., Günlük, A. E., Van Horn, S. C., & Sherman, S. M. (1994). GABAergic projection from the basal forebrain to the visual sector of the thalamic reticular nucleus in the cat. *Journal of Comparative Neurology 348*, 481–510.

Bickford, M. E., Carden, W. B., & Patel, N. C. (1999). Two types of interneurons in the cat visual thalamus are distinguished by morphology, synaptic connections, content, and nitric oxide synthase. *Journal of Comparative Neurology 413*, 83–100.

Bielschowsky, M. (1928). Nervengewebe. In *Handbuch der mikroskopischen Anatomie des Menschen. 4 (1) Nervensystem*, ed W. von Möllendorf, pp. 1–142. Springer, Berlin.

Binns, K. E., Turner, J. P., & Salt, T. E. (2003). Kainate receptor (GluR5)-mediated disinhibition of responses in rat ventrobasal thalamus allows a novel sensory processing mechanism. *Journal of Physiology* 551, 525–537.

Birnbacher, D., & Albus, K. (1987). Divergence of single axons in afferent projections to the cat's visual cortical areas 17, 18, and 19: a parametric study. *Journal of Comparative Neurology* 261, 543–561.

Bishop, G. (1959). The relation between nerve fiber size and sensory modality: phylogenetic implications of the afferent innervation of cortex. *Journal of Nervous and Mental Disorders* 128, 89–114.

Bishop, P. O., Jeremy, D., & McLeod, J. G. (1953). Phenomenon of repetitive firing in lateral geniculate of cat. *Journal of Neurophysiology* 16, 437–447.

Black, M. M., & Baas, P. W. (1989). The basis of polarity in neurons. *Trends in Neurosciences* 12, 211–214.

Blasdel, G. G., & Lund, J. S. (1983). Termination of afferent axons in macaque striate cortex. *Journal of Neuroscience* 3, 1389–1413.

Bloomfield, S. A., Hamos, J. E., & Sherman, S. M. (1987). Passive cable properties and morphological correlates of neurones in the lateral geniculate nucleus of the cat. *Journal of Physiology (London)* 383, 653–692.

Bloomfield, S. A., & Sherman, S. M. (1989). Dendritic current flow in relay cells and interneurons of the cat's lateral geniculate nucleus. *Proceedings of the National Academy of Sciences of the United States of America* 86, 3911–3914.

Bodian, D. (1962). The generalized vertebrate neuron. *Science* 137, 323–326.

Boehning, D., & Snyder, S. H. (2003). Novel neural modulators. *Annual Review of Neuroscience* 26, 105–131.

Bokor, H., Frere, S. G. A., Eyre, M. D., Slezia, A., Ulbert, I., Luthi, A., & Acsády, L. (2005). Selective GABAergic control of higher-order thalamic relays. *Neuron* 45, 929–940.

Bolam, J. P. (1992). *Experimental Neuroanatomy: A Practical Approach*. IRL Press, Oxford.

Bomze, H. M., Bulsara, K. R., Iskandar, B. J., Caroni, P., & Skene, J. H. (2001). Spinal axon regeneration evoked by replacing two growth cone proteins in adult neurons. *Nature Neuroscience* 4, 38–43.

Bourassa, J., & Deschênes, M. (1995). Corticothalamic projections from the primary visual cortex in rats: a single fiber study using biocytin as an anterograde tracer. *Neuroscience* 66, 253–263.

Bourassa, J., Pinault, D., & Deschênes, M. (1995). Corticothalamic projections from the cortical barrel field to the somatosensory thalamus in rats: a single-fibre study using biocytin as an anterograde tracer. *European Journal of Neuroscience* 7, 19–30.

Bowling, D. B., & Michael, C. R. (1984). Terminal patterns of single, physiologically characterized optic tract fibers in the cat's lateral geniculate nucleus. *Journal of Neuroscience* 4, 198–216.

Boycott, B. B., & Wässle, H. (1974). The morphological types of ganglion cells of the domestic cat's retina. *Journal of Physiology (London)* 240, 397–419.

Boyd, J. D., & Matsubara, J. A. (1996). Laminar and columnar patterns of geniculocortical projections in the cat: relationship to cytochrome oxidase. *Journal of Comparative Neurology* 365, 659–682.

Britten, K. H., Shadlen, M. N., Newsome, W. T., & Movshon, J. A. (1993). Responses of neurons in macaque MT to stochastic motion signals. *Visual Neuroscience* 10, 1157–1169.

Brodal, A. (1940). Modification of Gudden method for study of cerebral localization. *Archives of Neurology and Psychiatry (Chicago)* 43, 46–58.

Brown, A. G., & Fyffe, R. E. (1981). Direct observations on the contacts made between 1A afferent fibres and alpha motoneurones in the cat's lumbosacral spinal cord. *Journal of Physiology (London)* 313, 121–140.

Brown, D. A., Abogadie, F. C., Allen, T. G., Buckley, N. J., Caulfield, M. P., Delmas, P., Haley, J. E., Lamas, J. A., & Selyanko, A. A. (1997). Muscarinic mechanisms in nerve cells. *Life Sciences* 60, 1137–1144.

Brown, J. E., Yates, B. J., & Taube, J. S. (2002). Does the vestibular system contribute to head direction cell activity in the rat? *Physiology & Behavior* 77, 743–748.

Bull, M. S., & Berkley, K. J. (1984). Differences in the neurones that project from the dorsal column nuclei to the diencephalon, pretectum, and the tectum in the cat. *Somatosensory Research* 1, 281–300.

Bullier, J., & Norton, T. T. (1979). X and Y relay cells in cat lateral geniculate nucleus: quantitative analysis of receptive-field properties and classification. *Journal of Neurophysiology* 42, 243–273.

Bullier, J., Kennedy, H., & Salinger, W. L. (1984). Bifurcation of subcortical afferents to visual areas 17, 18, and 19 in the cat cortex. *Journal of Comparative Neurology* 228, 309–328.

Bullier, J., Schall, J. D., & Morel, A. (1996). Functional streams in occipito-frontal connections in the monkey. *Behavioural Brain Research* 76, 89–97.

Bullock, T. H. (1959). Neuron doctrine and electrophysiology. *Science* 129, 997–1002.

Bunt, A. H., Hendrickson, A. E., Lund, J. S., Lund, R. D., & Fuchs, A. F. (1975). Monkey retinal ganglion cells: morphometric analysis and tracing of axonal projections, with a consideration of the peroxidase technique. *Journal of Comparative Neurology* 164, 265–285.

Butler, E. G., Bourke, D. W., & Horne, M. K. (2000). The activity of primate ventrolateral thalamic neurones during motor adaptation. *Experimental Brain Research* 133, 514–531.

Cajal, S. R. y. (1911). *Histologie du système nerveaux de l'homme et des vertébrés*. Maloine, Paris.

Cajal, S. R. y. (1995). *Histology of the Nervous System of Man and Vertebrates* (translated from the French by N. and L. W. Swanson). Oxford University Press, Oxford.

Callaway, E. M. (2004). Cell types and local circuits in primary visual cortex of the macaque monkey. In *The Visual Neurosciences*, eds. Chalupa, L. M., & Werner, J. S., pp. 680–694. MIT Press, Cambridge, Mass.

Calton, J. L., Stackman, R. W., Goodridge, J. P., Archey, W. B., Dudchenko, P. A., & Taube, J. S. (2003). Hippocampal place cell instability after lesions of the head direction cell network. *Journal of Neuroscience* 23, 9719–9731.

Carden, W. B., & Bickford, M. E. (2002). Synaptic inputs of class III and class V interneurons in the cat pulvinar nucleus: differential integration of RS and RL inputs. *Visual Neuroscience* 19, 51–59.

Carey, R. G., Fitzpatrick, D., & Diamond, I. T. (1979). Layer I of striate cortex of *Tupaia glis* and *Galago senegalensis*: projections from thalamus and claustrum revealed by retrograde transport of horseradish peroxidase. *Journal of Comparative Neurology* 186, 393–438.

Carman, J., Cowan, W. M., & Powell, T. P. S. (1964). Cortical connexions of the thalamic reticular nucleus. *Journal of Anatomy* (*London*) 98, 587–598.

Caroni, P. (1997). Intrinsic neuronal determinants that promote axonal sprouting and elongation. *Bioessays* 19, 767–775.

Carretta, D., Sbriccoli, A., Santarelli, M., Pinto, F., Granato, A., & Minciacchi, D. (1996). Crossed thalamo-cortical and cortico-thalamic projections in adult mice. *Neuroscience Letters* 204, 69–72.

Casagrande, V. A. (1994). A third parallel visual pathway to primate area V1. *Trends in Neurosciences* 17, 305–309.

Casagrande, V. A., & Kaas, J. H. (1994). The afferent, intrinsic, and efferent connections of primary visual cortex in primates. In *Cerbral Cortex*, eds. Peters, A., & Rockland, K. S., pp. 201–259. Plenum, New York.

Casagrande, V. A., & Norton, T. T. (1991). Lateral geniculate nucleus: a review of its physiology and function. In *Vision and Visual Dysfunction*, ed. Leventhal, A. G., pp. 41–84. Macmillan, London.

Casagrande, V. A., & Xu, X. (2004). Parallel visual pathways: a comparative perspective. In *The Visual Neurosciences*, eds. Chalupa, L. M., & Werner, J. S., pp. 494–506. MIT Press, Cambridge, Mass.

Casanova, C. (1993). Response properties of neurons in area 17 projecting to the striate-recipient zone of the cat's lateralis posterior-pulvinar complex: comparison with cortico-tectal cells. *Experimental Brain Research* 96, 247–259.

Casanova, C. (2004). The visual functions of the pulvinar. In *The Visual Neurosciences*, eds. Chalupa, L. M., & Werner, J. S., pp. 592–608. MIT Press, Cambridge, Mass.

Casanova, C., & Molotchnikoff, S. (1990). Influence of the superior colliculus on visual responses of cells in the rabbit's lateral posterior nucleus. *Experimental Brain Research* 80, 387–396.

Casanova, C., Savard, T., & Darveau, S. (1997). Contribution of area 17 to cell responses in the striate-recipient zone of the cat's lateral posterior-pulvinar complex. *European Journal of Neuroscience* 9, 1026–1036.

Castro-Alamancos, M. A. (2002). Properties of primary sensory (lemniscal) synapses in the ventrobasal thalamus and the relay of high-frequency sensory inputs. *Journal of Neurophysiology* 87, 946–953.

Castro-Alamancos, M. A., & Connors, B. W. (1996). Spatiotemporal properties of short-term plasticity in sensorimotor thalamocortical pathways of the rat. *Journal of Neuroscience* 16, 2767–2779.

Castro-Alamancos, M. A., & Oldford, E. (2002). Cortical sensory suppression during arousal is due to the activity-dependent depression of thalamocortical synapses. *Journal of Physiology* 541, 319–331.

Catsman-Berrevoets, C. E., & Kuypers, H. G. (1978). Differential laminar distribution of corticothalamic neurons projecting to the VL and the center median: an HRP study in the cynomolgus monkey. *Brain Research* 154, 359–365.

Caviness, V. S., Jr., & Frost, D. O. (1983). Thalamocortical projections in the reeler mutant mouse. *Journal of Comparative Neurology* 219, 182–202.

Chalupa, L. M. (1991). Visual function of the pulvinar. In *The Neural Basis of Visual Function*, ed. Leventhal, A. G., pp. 140–159. Macmillan, New York.

Chalupa, L. M., & Abramson, B. P. (1988). Receptive-field properties in the tecto- and striate-recipient zones of the cat's lateral posterior nucleus. *Progress in Brain Research* 75, 85–94.

Chalupa, L. M., & Abramson, B. P. (1989). Visual receptive fields in the striate-recipient zone of the lateral posterior-pulvinar complex. *Journal of Neuroscience* 9, 347–357.

Chalupa, L. M., & Thompson, I. D. (1980). Retinal ganglion cell projections to the superior colliculus of the hamster demonstrated by the horseradish peroxidase technique. *Neuroscience Letters* 19, 13–19.

Chance, F. S., Abbott, L. F., & Reyes, A. (2002). Gain modulation from background synaptic input. *Neuron* 35, 773–782.

Cheatwood, J. L., Reep, R. L., & Corwin, J. V. (2003). The associative striatum: cortical and thalamic projections to the dorsocentral striatum in rats. *Brain Research* 968, 1–14.

Chen, C., & Regehr, W. G. (2003). Presynaptic modulation of the retinogeniculate synapse. *Journal of Neuroscience* 23, 3130–3135.

Chugani, H. T., Phelps, M. E., & Mazziotta, J. C. (1987). Positron emission tomography study of human brain functional development. *Annals of Neurology* 22, 487–497.

Chung, S., Li, X., & Nelson, S. B. (2002). Short-term depression at thalamocortical synapses contributes to rapid adaptation of cortical sensory responses in vivo. *Neuron* 34, 437–446.

Churchland, P. S. (2002). *Brain-Wise*. MIT Press, Cambridge, Mass.

Churchland, P. S., Ramachandran, V. S., & Sejnowski, T. J. (1994). A critique of pure vision. In *Large-Scale Neuronal Theories in the Brain*, eds. Koch, C., & Davis, J. L., pp. 23–65. MIT Press, Cambridge, Mass.

Cicirata, F., Angaut, P., Serapide, M. F., & Panto, M. R. (1990). Functional organization of the direct and indirect projection via the reticularis thalami nuclear complex from the motor cortex to the thalamic nucleus ventralis lateralis. *Experimental Brain Research* 79, 325–337.

Cleland, B. G., Dubin, M. W., & Levick, W. R. (1971). Sustained and transient neurones in the cat's retina and lateral geniculate nucleus. *Journal of Physiology (London)* 217, 473–496.

Cleland, B. G., & Lee, B. B. (1985). A comparison of visual responses of cat lateral geniculate nucleus neurones with those of ganglion cells afferent to them. *Journal of Physiology (London)* 369, 249–268.

Colby, C. L. (1988). Corticotectal circuit in the cat: a functional analysis of the lateral geniculate nucleus layers of origin. *Journal of Neurophysiology* 59, 1783–1797.

Coleman, K. A., & Mitrofanis, J. (1996). Organization of the visual reticular thalamic nucleus of the rat. *European Journal of Neuroscience* 8, 388–404.

Collingridge, G. L., & Bliss, T. V. P. (1987). NMDA receptors: their role in long-term potentiation. *Trends in Neurosciences* 10, 288–293.

Colonnier, M. (1968). Synaptic patterns on different cell types in the different laminae of the visual cortex. *Brain Research* 9, 268–287.

Colonnier, M., & Guillery, R. W. (1964). Synaptic organization in the lateral geniculate nucleus of the monkey. *Zeitschrift für Zellforschung* 62, 333–355.

Conley, M., & Diamond, I. T. (1990). Organization of the visual sector of the thalamic reticular nucleus in *Galago*. *European Journal of Neuroscience* 3, 211–226.

Conley, M., Fitzpatrick, D., & Diamond, I. T. (1984). The laminar organization of the lateral geniculate body and the striate cortex in the tree shrew (*Tupaia glis*). *Journal of Neuroscience* 4, 171–197.

Conley, M., Kupersmith, A. C., & Diamond, I. T. (1991). The organization of projections from subdivisions of the auditory cortex and thalamus to the auditory sector of the thalamic reticular nucleus in *Galago*. *European Journal of Neuroscience* 3, 1089–1103.

Conn, P. J. (2003). Physiological roles and therapeutic potential of metabotropic glutamate receptors. *Progress in Neurobiology* 1003, 12–21.

Conn, P. J., & Pin, J. P. (1997). Pharmacology and functions of metabotropic glutamate receptors. *Annual Review of Pharmacology & Toxicology* 37, 205–237.

Connolly, M., & Van Essen, D. C. (1984). The representation of the visual field in parvicellular and magnocellular layers of the lateral geniculate nucleus in the macaque monkey. *Journal of Comparative Neurology* 226, 544–564.

Connor, J. A., & Stevens, C. F. (1971). Prediction of repetitive firing behaviour from voltage clamp data on an isolated neurone soma. *The Journal of Physiology Online* 213, 31–53.

Copenhagen, D. R. (2004). Excitation in the retina: the flow, filtering, and molecules of visual signaling in the glutamatergic pathways from photoreceptors to ganglion cells. In *The Visual Neurosciences*, eds. Chalupa, L. M., & Werner, J. S., pp. 320–333. MIT Press, Cambridge, Mass.

Cornwall, J., Cooper, J. D., & Phillipson, O. T. (1990). Projections to the rostral reticular thalamic nucleus in the rat. *Experimental Brain Research* 80, 157–171.

Cotman, C. W., Monaghan, D. T., & Gamong, A. H. (1988). Excitatory amino acid neurotransmission: NMDA receptors and Hebb-type synaptic plasticity. *Annual Reviews in Neuroscience* 11, 61–80.

Coulter, D. A., Huguenard, J. R., & Prince, D. A. (1989). Calcium currents in rat thalamocortical relay neurones: kinetic properties of the transient, low-threshold current. *Journal of Physiology (London)* 414, 587–604.

Cowan, W. M., & Powell, T. P. S. (1954). An experimental study of the relation between the medial mamillary nucleus and the cingulate cortex. *Proceedings of the Royal Society of London, Series B, Biological Sciences* 143, 114–125.

Cowan, W. M., Sudhof, T. C., & Stevens, C. F. (2002). *Synapses*. Johns Hopkins University Press, Baltimore.

Cox, C. L., Huguenard, J. R., & Prince, D. A. (1996). Heterogeneous axonal arborizations of rat thalamic reticular neurons in the ventrobasal nucleus. *Journal of Comparative Neurology* 366, 416–430.

Cox, C. L., Huguenard, J. R., & Prince, D. A. (1997). Nucleus reticularis neurons mediate diverse inhibitory effects in thalamus. *Proceedings of the National Academy of Sciences of the United States of America* 94, 8854–8859.

Cox, C. L., Zhou, Q., & Sherman, S. M. (1998). Glutamate locally activates dendritic outputs of thalamic interneurons. *Nature* 394, 478–482.

Cox, C. L., & Sherman, S. M. (1999). Glutamate inhibits thalamic reticular neurons. *Journal of Neuroscience* 19, 6694–6699.

Cox, C. L., & Sherman, S. M. (2000). Control of dendritic outputs of inhibitory interneurons in the lateral geniculate nucleus. *Neuron* 27, 597–610.

Cox, C. L., Reichova, I., & Sherman, S. M. (2003). Functional synaptic contacts by intranuclear axon collaterals of thalamic relay neurons. *Journal of Neuroscience* 23, 7642–7646.

Crabtree, J. W. (1992a). The somatotopic organization within the cat's thalamic reticular nucleus. *European Journal of Neuroscience* 4, 1352–1361.

Crabtree, J. W. (1992b). The somatotopic organization within the rabbit's thalamic reticular nucleus. *European Journal of Neuroscience* 4, 1343–1351.

Crabtree, J. W. (1996). Organization in the somatosensory sector of the cat's thalamic reticular nucleus. *Journal of Comparative Neurology* 366, 207–222.

Crabtree, J. W. (1998). Organization in the auditory sector of the cat's thalamic reticular nucleus. *Journal of Comparative Neurology* 390, 167–182.

Crabtree, J. W., Collingridge, G. L., & Isaac, J. T. R. (1998). A new intrathalamic pathway linking modality-related nuclei in the dorsal thalamus. *Nature Neuroscience* 1, 389–394.

Crabtree, J. W., & Isaac, J. T. R. (2002). New intrathalamic pathways allowing modality-related and cross-modality switching in the dorsal thalamus. *Journal of Neuroscience* 22, 8754–8761.

Crabtree, J. W., & Killackey, H. P. (1989). The topographical organization of the axis of projection within the visual sector of the rabbit's thalamic reticular nucleus. *European Journal of Neuroscience* 1, 94–109.

Cragg, B. G. (1969). The topography of the afferent projections in the circumstriate visual cortex of the monkey studied by the Nauta method. *Vision Research* 9, 733–747.

Crair, M. C., Gillespie, D. C., & Stryker, M. P. (1998). The role of visual experience in the development of columns in cat visual cortex. *Science* 279, 566–570.

Crick, F. (1984). Function of the thalamic reticular complex: the searchlight hypothesis. *Proceedings of the National Academy of Sciences of the United States of America* 81, 4586–4590.

Crick, F., & Koch, C. (1998). Constraints on cortical and thalamic projections: The no-strong-loops hypothesis. *Nature* 391, 245–250.

Crowley, J. C., & Katz, L. C. (2002). Ocular dominance development revisited. *Current Opinion in Neurobiology* 12, 104–109.

Cruce, J. A. (1977). An autoradiographic study of the descending connections of the mamillary nuclei of the rat. *Journal of Comparative Neurology* 176, 631–644.

Cucchiaro, J. B., & Guillery, R. W. (1984). The development of the retinogeniculate pathways in normal and albino ferrets. *Proceedings of the Royal Society of London, Series B, Biological Sciences* 223, 141–164.

Cucchiaro, J. B., Uhlrich, D. J., & Sherman, S. M. (1988). Parabrachial innervation of the cat's dorsal lateral geniculate nucleus: an electron microscopic study using the tracer *Phaseolus vulgaris* leucoagglutinin (PHA-L). *Journal of Neuroscience* 8, 4576–4588.

Cucchiaro, J. B., Uhlrich, D. J., & Sherman, S. M. (1991). Electron-microscopic analysis of synaptic input from the perigeniculate nucleus to the A-laminae of the lateral geniculate nucleus in cats. *Journal of Comparative Neurology* 310, 316–336.

Cucchiaro, J. B., Uhlrich, D. J., & Sherman, S. M. (1993). Ultrastructure of synapses from the pretectum in the A-laminae of the cat's lateral geniculate nucleus. *Journal of Comparative Neurology* 334, 618–630.

Cudeiro, J., Rivadulla, C., Rodriguez, R., Martinez-Conde, S., Martinez, L., Grieve, K. L., & Acuña, C. (1996). Further observations on the role of nitric oxide in the feline lateral geniculate nucleus. *European Journal of Neuroscience* 8, 144–152.

Cudeiro, J., & Sillito, A. M. (1996). Spatial frequency tuning of orientation-discontinuity-sensitive corticofugal feedback to the cat lateral geniculate nucleus. *Journal of Physiology* 490, 481–492.

Cusick, C. G., Steindler, D. A., & Kaas, J. H. (1985). Corticocortical and collateral thalamocortical connections of postcentral somatosensory cortical areas in squirrel monkeys: a double-labeling study with radiolabeled wheatgerm agglutinin and wheatgerm agglutinin conjugated to horseradish peroxidase. *Somatosensory Research* 3, 1–31.

Dagnino, N., Favale, E., Loeb, C., & Manfredi, M. (1965). Thalamic transmission changes during the rapid eye movements of deep sleep. *Archives Internationales de Physiologie et de Biochimie* 73, 858–861.

Dagnino, N., Favale, E., Loeb, C., Manfredi, M., & Seitun, A. (1966). Pontine triggering of phasic changes in sensory transmission during deep sleep. *Archives Internationales de Physiologie et de Biochimie* 74, 889–894.

Dagnino, N., Favale, E., Manfredi, M., Seitun, A., & Tartaglione, A. (1971). Tonic changes in excitability of thalamocortical neurons during the sleep-waking cycle. *Brain Research* 29, 354–357.

Daniel, P. M., & Whitteridge, D. (1961). The representation of the visual field on the cerebral cortex in monkeys. *The Journal of Physiology Online* 159, 203–221.

Dankowski, A., & Bickford, M. E. (2003). Inhibitory circuitry involving Y cells and Y retinal terminals in the C laminae of the cat dorsal lateral geniculate nucleus. *Journal of Comparative Neurology* 460, 368–379.

Darian-Smith, C., & Darian-Smith, I. (1993). Thalamic projections to areas 3a, 3b, and 4 in the sensorimotor cortex of the mature and infant macaque monkey. *Journal of Comparative Neurology* 335, 173–199.

Darian-Smith, C., Tan, A., & Edwards, S. (1999). Comparing thalamocortical and corticothalamic microstructure and spatial reciprocity in the macaque ventral posterolateral nucleus (VPLc) and medial pulvinar. *Journal of Comparative Neurology* 410, 211–234.

Datskovskaia, A., Carden, W. B., & Bickford, M. E. (2001). Y retinal terminals contact interneurons in the cat dorsal lateral geniculate nucleus. *Journal of Comparative Neurology* 430, 85–100.

Daw, N. D., & Dayan, P. (2004). Neuroscience. Matchmaking. *Science* 304, 1753–1754.

De Biasi, S., Arcelli, P., & Spreafico, R. (1994). Parvalbumin immunoreactivity in the thalamus of guinea pig: light and electron microscopic correlation with gamma-aminobutyric acid immunoreactivity. *Journal of Comparative Neurology* 348, 556–569.

de Lima, A. D., & Singer, W. (1987a). The serotoninergic fibers in the dorsal lateral geniculate nucleus of the cat: distribution and synaptic connections demonstrated with immunocytochemistry. *Journal of Comparative Neurology* 258, 339–351.

de Lima, A. D., & Singer, W. (1987b). The brainstem projection to the lateral geniculate nucleus in the cat: identification of cholinergic and monoaminergic elements. *Journal of Comparative Neurology* 259, 92–121.

Derrington, A. M., & Lennie, P. (1984). Spatial and temporal contrast sensitivities of neurones in lateral geniculate nucleus of macaque. *Journal of Physiology (London)* 357, 219–240.

Deschênes, M., Paradis, M., Roy, J. P., & Steriade, M. (1984). Electrophysiology of neurons of lateral thalamic nuclei in cat: resting properties and burst discharges. *Journal of Neurophysiology* 51, 1196–1219.

Deschênes, M., Madariaga-Domich, A., & Steriade, M. (1985). Dendrodendritic synapses in the cat reticularis thalami nucleus: a structural basis for thalamic spindle synchronization. *Brain Research* 334, 165–168.

Deschênes, M., Bourassa, J., & Pinault, D. (1994). Corticothalamic projections from layer V cells in rat are collaterals of long-range corticofugal axons. *Brain Research* 664, 215–219.

Deschênes, M., Veinante, P., & Zhang, Z. W. (1998). The organization of corticothalamic projections: reciprocity versus parity. *Brain Research Reviews* 28, 286–308.

Deschênes, M., Timofeeva, E., Lavallée, P., & Dufresne, C. (2005). The vibrissal system as a model of thalamic operations. *Progress in Brain Research* 149, 31–40.

Destexhe, A., & Sejnowski, T. J. (2002). The initiation of bursts in thalamic neurons and the cortical control of thalamic sensitivity. *Philosophical Transactions of the Royal Society of London, Series B, Biological Sciences* 357, 1649–1657.

Destexhe, A., Contreras, D., Steriade, M., Sejnowski, T. J., & Huguenard, J. R. (1996). *In vivo, in vitro*, and computational analysis of dendritic calcium currents in thalamic reticular neurons. *Journal of Neuroscience* 16, 169–185.

Destexhe, A., Contreras, D., & Steriade, M. (1998a). Mechanisms underlying the synchronizing action of corticothalamic feedback through inhibition of thalamic relay cells. *Journal of Neurophysiology* 79, 999–1016.

Destexhe, A., Neubig, M., Ulrich, D., & Huguenard, J. (1998b). Dendritic low-threshold calcium currents in thalamic relay cells. *Journal of Neuroscience* 18, 3574–3588.

Diamond, I. T. (1973). The evolution of the tectal-pulvinar system in mammals: structural and behavioral studies of the visual system. *Symposia of the Zoological Society of London* 33, 205–233.

Diamond, I. T., Conley, M., Itoh, K., & Fitzpatrick, D. (1985). Laminar organization of geniculocortical projections in *Galago senegalensis* and *Aotus trivirgatus*. *Journal of Comparative Neurology* 242, 584–610.

Diamond, I. T., Fitzpatrick, D., & Schmechel, D. (1993). Calcium binding proteins distinguish large and small cells of the ventral posterior and lateral geniculate nuclei of the prosimian galago and the tree shrew (*Tupaia belangeri*). *Proceedings of the National Academy of Sciences of the United States of America* 90, 1425–1429.

Diamond, M. E., Armstrong-James, M., Budway, M. J., & Ebner, F. F. (1992). Somatic sensory responses in the rostral sector of the posterior group (POm) and in the ventral posterior medial nucleus (VPM) of the rat thalamus: dependence on the barrel field cortex. *Journal of Comparative Neurology* 319, 66–84.

Dick, A., Kaske, A., & Creutzfeldt, O. D. (1991). Topographical and topological organization of the thalamocortical projection to the striate and pre-striate cortex in the marmoset (*Callithrix jacchus*). *Experimental Brain Research* 84, 233–253.

Ding, Y., & Casagrande, V. A. (1997). The distribution and morphology of LGN K pathway axons within the layers and CO blobs of owl monkey V1. *Visual Neuroscience* 14, 691–704.

Ding, Y., & Casagrande, V. A. (1998). Synaptic and neurochemical characterization of parallel pathways to the cytochrome oxidase blobs of primate visual cortex. *Journal of Comparative Neurology* 391, 429–443.

Do, K. Q., Benz, B., Binns, K. E., Eaton, S. A., & Salt, T. E. (2004). Release of homocysteic acid from rat thalamus following stimulation of somatosensory afferents in vivo: feasibility of glial participation in synaptic transmission. *Neuroscience* 124, 387–393.

Dowling, J. E. (1970). Organization of vertebrate retinas. *Investigative Ophthalmology* 9, 655–680.

Dowling, J. E. (1987). *The Retina: An Approachable Part of the Brain*. Belknap Press of Harvard University Press, Cambridge, Mass.

Dowling, J. E. (1991). Retina. In *Encyclopedia of Human Biology*, vol. 6, pp. 615–631. Academic Press, New York.

Dreher, B., Sefton, A. J., & Ni, S. Y. (1985). The morphology, number, distribution and central projections of class I retinal ganglion cells in albino and hooded rats. *Brain, Behavior and Evolution* 26, 10–48.

Duffy, K. R., Murphy, K. M., & Jones, D. G. (1998). Analysis of the postnatal growth of visual cortex. *Visual Neuroscience* 15, 831–839.

Dufour, A., Seibt, J., Passante, L., Depaepe, V., Ciossek, T., Frisen, J., Kullander, K., Flanagan, J. G., Polleux, F., & Vanderhaeghen, P. (2003). Area specificity and topography of thalamocortical projections are controlled by ephrin/Eph genes. *Neuron* 39, 453–465.

Dunlap, K., Luebke, J. I., & Turner, T. J. (1995). Exocytotic Ca^{2+} channels in mammalian central neurons. *Trends in Neurosciences* 18, 89–98.

Earle, K. L., & Mitrofanis, J. (1996). Genesis and fate of the perireticular thalamic nucleus during early development. *Journal of Comparative Neurology* 367, 246–263.

Eaton, S. A., & Salt, T. E. (1996). Role of N-methyl-D-aspartate and metabotropic glutamate receptors in corticothalamic excitatory postsynaptic potentials *in vivo*. *Neuroscience* 73, 1–5.

Eccles, J. C., Ito, M., & Szentágothai, J. (1967). *The Cerebellum as a Neuronal Machine*. Springer, New York.

Elekessy, E. I., Campion, J. E., & Henry, G. H. (1973). Differences between the visual fields of Siamese and common cats. *Vision Research* 13, 2533–2543.

Erişir, A., Van Horn, S. C., Bickford, M. E., & Sherman, S. M. (1997a). Immunocytochemistry and distribution of parabrachial terminals in the lateral geniculate nucleus of the cat: a comparison with corticogeniculate terminals. *Journal of Comparative Neurology* 377, 535–549.

Erişir, A., Van Horn, S. C., & Sherman, S. M. (1997b). Relative numbers of cortical and brainstem inputs to the lateral geniculate nucleus. *Proceedings of the National Academy of Sciences of the United States of America* 94, 1517–1520.

Erişir, A., Van Horn, S. C., & Sherman, S. M. (1998). Distribution of synapses in the lateral geniculate nucleus of the cat: differences between laminae A and A1 and between relay cells and interneurons. *Journal of Comparative Neurology* 390, 247–255.

Famiglietti, E. V. J., & Peters, A. (1972). The synaptic glomerulus and the intrinsic neuron in the dorsal lateral geniculate nucleus of the cat. *Journal of Comparative Neurology* 144, 285–334.

Fanselow, E. E., & Nicolelis, M. A. (1999). Behavioral modulation of tactile responses in the rat somatosensory system. *Journal of Neuroscience* 19, 7603–7616.

Fanselow, E. E., Sameshima, K., Baccala, L. A., & Nicolelis, M. A. L. (2001). Thalamic bursting in rats during different awake behavioral states. *Proceedings of the National Academy of Sciences* 98, 15330–15335.

Favale, E., Loeb, C., & Manfredi, M. (1964). Cortical responses evoked by stimulation of the optic pathways during natural sleep and during arousal. *Archives Internationales de Physiologie et de Biochimie* 72, 221–228.

Feig, S. L. (2004). Corticothalamic cells in layers 5 and 6 of primary and secondary sensory cortex express GAP-43 mRNA in the adult rat. *Journal of Comparative Neurology* 468, 96–111.

Feig, S., & Harting, J. K. (1994). Ultrastructural studies of the primate lateral geniculate nucleus: Morphology and spatial relationships of axon terminals arising from the retina, visual cortex (area 17), superior colliculus, parabigeminal nucleus, and pretectum of *Galago crassicaudatus*. *Journal of Comparative Neurology* 343, 17–34.

Feig, S., & Harting, J. K. (1998). Corticocortical communication via the thalamus: ultrastructural studies of corticothalamic projections from area 17 to the lateral posterior nucleus of the cat and inferior pulvinar nucleus of the owl monkey. *Journal of Comparative Neurology* 395, 281–295.

Feig, S. L., & Guillery, R. W. (2000). Corticothalamic axons contact blood vessels as well as nerve cells in the thalamus. *European Journal of Neuroscience* 12, 2195–2198.

Feldman, S. G., & Kruger, L. (1980). An axonal transport study of the ascending projection of medial lemniscal neurons in the rat. *Journal of Comparative Neurology* 192, 427–454.

Felleman, D. J., & Van Essen, D. C. (1991). Distributed hierarchical processing in the primate cerebral cortex. *Cerebral Cortex* 1, 1–47.

Ferster, D. (2004). Assembly of receptive fields in primary visual cortex. In *The Visual Neurosciences*, eds. Chalupa, L. M., & Werner, J. S., pp. 695–703. MIT Press, Cambridge, Mass.

Ferster, D., Chung, S., & Wheat, H. (1996). Orientation selectivity of thalamic input to simple cells of cat visual cortex. *Nature* 380, 249–252.

Ferster, D., & LeVay, S. (1978). The axonal arborizations of lateral geniculate neurons in the striate cortex of the cat. *Journal of Comparative Neurology* 182, 923–944.

Fetz, E. E., Toyama, K., & Smith (1991). Synaptic interactions between cortical neurons. In *Cerebral Cortex*, vol. 9, *Normal and Altered States of Function*, eds. Peters, A., & Jones, E. G., pp. 1–47. Plenum, New York.

Fischer, W. H., Schmidt, M., & Hoffmann, K. P. (1998). Saccade-induced activity of dorsal lateral geniculate nucleus X- and Y-cells during pharmacological inactivation of the cat pretectum. *Visual Neuroscience* 15, 197–210.

Fitzpatrick, D., Conley, M., Luppino, G., Matelli, M., & Diamond, I. T. (1988). Cholinergic projections from the midbrain reticular formation and the parabigeminal nucleus to the lateral geniculate nucleus in the tree shrew. *Journal of Comparative Neurology* 272, 43–67.

Fitzpatrick, D., Diamond, I. T., & Raczkowski, D. (1989). Cholinergic and monoaminergic innervation of the cat's thalamus: comparison of the lateral geniculate nucleus with other principal sensory nuclei. *Journal of Comparative Neurology* 288, 647–675.

Fitzpatrick, D., Usrey, W. M., Schofield, B. R., & Einstein, G. (1994). The sublaminar organization of corticogeniculate neurons in layer 6 of macaque striate cortex. *Visual Neuroscience* 11, 307–315.

Fitzpatrick, D., & Raczkowski, D. (1990). Innervation patterns of single physiologically identified geniculocortical axons in the striate cortex of the tree shrew. *Proceedings of the National Academy of Sciences of the United States of America* 87, 449–453.

Fitzpatrick, D. C., Olsen, J. F., & Suga, N. (1998). Connections among functional areas in the mustached bat auditory cortex. *Journal of Comparative Neurology* 391, 366–396.

Flechsig, P. E. (1920). *Anatomie des menschlichen Gehirn und Rückenmarks, auf myelogenetischer Grundlage.* G. Thieme, Leipzig.

Florence, S. L., & Casagrande, V. A. (1987). Organization of individual afferent axons in layer IV of striate cortex in a primate. *Journal of Neuroscience* 7, 3850–3868.

Francois, C., Percheron, G., Parent, A., Sadikot, A. F., Fenelon, G., & Yelnik, J. (1991). Topography of the projection from the central complex of the thalamus to the sensorimotor striatal territory in monkeys. *Journal of Comparative Neurology* 305, 17–34.

Freeman, R. D. (2004). Binocular interaction in the visual cortex. In *The Visual Neurosciences*, eds. Chalupa, L. M., & Werner, J. S., pp. 765–778. MIT Press, Cambridge, Mass.

Friedlander, M. J., Lin, C.-S., Stanford, L. R., & Sherman, S. M. (1981). Morphology of functionally identified neurons in lateral geniculate nucleus of the cat. *Journal of Neurophysiology* 46, 80–129.

Fries, W. (1981). The projections from the lateral geniculate nucleus to the prestriate cortex of the macaque monkey. *Proceedings of the Royal Society of London, Series B, Biological Sciences* 213, 73–80.

Fries, W., Keizer, K., & Kuypers, H. G. (1985). Large layer VI cells in macaque striate cortex (Meynert cells) project to both superior colliculus and prestriate visual area V5. *Experimental Brain Research* 58, 613–616.

Fukuda, Y., & Stone, J. (1974). Retinal distribution and central projections of Y-, X-, and W-cells of the cat's retina. *Journal of Neurophysiology* 37, 749–772.

Funke, K., & Eysel, U. T. (1995). Possible enhancement of GABAergic inputs to cat dorsal lateral geniculate relay cells by serotonin. *NeuroReport* 6, 474–476.

Galletti, C., Gamberini, M., Kutz, D. F., Fattori, P., Luppino, G., & Matelli, M. (2001). The cortical connections of area V6: an occipito-parietal network processing visual information. *European Journal of Neuroscience* 13, 1572–1588.

Gandia, J. A., De las Heras, S., García, M., & Giménez-Amaya, J. M. (1993). Afferent projections to the reticular thalamic nucleus from the globus pallidus and the substantia nigra in the rat. *Brain Research Bulletin* 32, 351–358.

Gardner, E. P., & Fuchs, A. F. (1975). Single-unit responses to natural vestibular stimuli and eye movements in deep cerebellar nuclei of the alert rhesus monkey. *Journal of Neurophysiology* 38, 627–649.

Garey, L. J., & Powell, T. P. S. (1967). The projection of the lateral geniculate nucleus upon the cortex in the cat. *Proceedings of the Royal Society of London, Series B, Biological Sciences* 169, 107–126.

Geisert, E. E., Jr. (1980). Cortical projections of the lateral geniculate nucleus in the cat. *Journal of Comparative Neurology* 190, 793–812.

Geisert, E. E., Jr., Langsetmo, A., & Spear, P. D. (1981). Influence of the corticogeniculate pathway on reponse properties of cat lateral geniculate neurons. *Brain Research* 208, 409–415.

Geist, F. D. (1933). Chromatolysis of efferent neurons. *Archives of Neurology and Psychiatry (Chicago)* 29, 88–103.

Gentet, L. J., & Ulrich, D. (2003). Strong, reliable and precise synaptic connections between thalamic relay cells and neurones of the nucleus reticularis in juvenile rats. *Journal of Physiology* 546, 801–811.

Gentet, L. J., & Ulrich, D. (2004). Electrophysiological characterization of synaptic connections between layer VI cortical cells and neurons of the nucleus reticularis thalami in juvenile rats. *European Journal of Neuroscience* 19, 625–633.

Gereau, R. W. IV, & Conn, P. J. (1994). A cyclic AMP-dependent form of associative synaptic plasticity induced by coactivation of β-adrenergic receptors and metabotropic glutamate receptors in rat hippocampus. *Journal of Neuroscience* 14, 3310–3318.

Ghelarducci, B., Pisa, M., & Pompeiano, O. (1970). Transformation of somatic afferent volleys across the prethalamic and thalamic components of the lemniscal system during the rapid eye movements of sleep. *Electroencephalography & Clinical Neurophysiology* 29, 348–357.

Gibb, A. J. (2004). NMDA receptor subunit gating—uncovered. *Trends in Neurosciences* 27, 7–10.

Gilbert, C. D., & Kelly, J. P. (1975). The projections of cells in different layers of the cat's visual cortex. *Journal of Physiology (London)* 163, 81–106.

Giménez-Amaya, J. M., McFarland, N. R., Heras, S. D. L., & Haber, S. N. (1995). Organization of thalamic projections to the ventral striatum in the primate. *Journal of Comparative Neurology* 354, 127–149.

Glees, P., & Le Gros Clark, W. E. (1941). The termination of optic fibres in the lateral geniculate body of the monkey. *Journal of Anatomy (London)* 75, 295–308.

Glickstein, M. (1988). The discovery of the visual cortex. *Scientific American* 259, 118–127.

Godwin, D. W., Van Horn, S. C., Erişir, A., Sesma, M., Romano, C., & Sherman, S. M. (1996a). Ultrastructural localization suggests that retinal and cortical inputs access different metabotropic glutamate receptors in the lateral geniculate nucleus. *Journal of Neuroscience* 16, 8181–8192.

Godwin, D. W., Vaughan, J. W., & Sherman, S. M. (1996b). Metabotropic glutamate receptors switch visual response mode of lateral geniculate nucleus cells from burst to tonic. *Journal of Neurophysiology* 76, 1800–1816.

Gogtay, N., Giedd, J., & Rapoport, J. L. (2002). Brain development in healthy, hyperactive, and psychotic children. *Archives of Neurology* 59, 1244–1248.

Gogtay, N., Giedd, J. N., Lusk, L., Hayashi, K. M., Greenstein, D., Vaituzis, A. C., Nugent, T. F. III, Herman, D. H., Clasen, L. S., Toga, A. W., Rapoport, J. L., & Thompson, P. M. (2004). Dynamic mapping of human cortical development during childhood through early adulthood. *Proceedings of the National Academy of Sciences of the United States of America* 101, 8174–8179.

Goldman-Rakic, P. S., & Porrino, L. J. (1985). The primate mediodorsal (MD) nucleus and its projection to the frontal lobe. *Journal of Comparative Neurology* 242, 535–560.

Goldstein, L. S., & Yang, Z. (2000). Microtubule-based transport systems in neurons: the roles of kinesins and dyneins. *Annual Review of Neuroscience* 23, 39–71.

Gomes, A. R., Correia, S. S., Carvalho, A. L., & Duarte, C. B. (2003). Regulation of AMPA receptor activity, synaptic targeting and recycling: role in synaptic plasticity. *Neurochemical Research* 28, 1459–1473.

Gonzalo-Ruiz, A., Lieberman, A. R., & Sanz-Anquela, J. M. (1995). Organization of serotoninergic projections from the raphé nuclei to the anterior thalamic nuclei in the rat: a combined retrograde tracing and 5-HT immunohistochemical study. *Journal of Chemical Neuroanatomy* 8, 103–115.

Goodchild, A. K., & Martin, P. R. (1998). The distribution of calcium-binding proteins in the lateral geniculate nucleus and visual cortex of a New World monkey, the marmoset, *Callithrix jacchus*. *Visual Neuroscience* 15, 625–642.

Govindaiah & Cox, C. L. (2004). Synaptic activation of metabotropic glutamate receptors regulates dendritic outputs of thalamic interneurons. *Neuron* 41, 611–623.

Granseth, B., Ahlstrand, E., & Lindström, S. (2002). Paired pulse facilitation of corticogeniculate EPSCs in the dorsal lateral geniculate nucleus of the rat investigated *in vitro*. *Journal of Physiology* 544, 477–486.

Gray, E. G. (1959). Axo-somatic and axo-dendritic synapses of the cerebral cortex: an electron microscopic study. *Journal of Anatomy (London)* 93, 420–433.

Graybiel, A. M., & Berson, D. M. (1980). Histochemical identification and afferent connections of subdivisions in the lateralis posterior-pulvinar complex and related thalamic nuclei in the cat. *Neuroscience* 5, 1175–1238.

Green, D. M., & Swets, J. A. (1966). *Signal Detection Theory and Psychophysics.* Wiley, New York.

Groenewegen, H. J. (1988). Organization of the afferent connections of the mediodorsal thalamic nucleus in the rat, related to the mediodorsal-prefrontal topography. *Neuroscience* 24, 379–431.

Groenewegen, H. J., Berendse, H. W., Wolters, J. G., & Lohman, A. H. (1990). The anatomical relationship of the prefrontal cortex with the striatopallidal system, the thalamus and the amygdala: evidence for a parallel organization. *Progress in Brain Research* 85, 95–116.

Gross, C. G. (1999). *Brain, Vision, Memory.* MIT Press, Cambridge, Mass.

Guido, W., Lu, S.-M., & Sherman, S. M. (1992). Relative contributions of burst and tonic responses to the receptive field properties of lateral geniculate neurons in the cat. *Journal of Neurophysiology* 68, 2199–2211.

Guido, W., Lu, S.-M., Vaughan, J. W., Godwin, D. W., & Sherman, S. M. (1995). Receiver operating characteristic (ROC) analysis of neurons in the cat's lateral geniculate nucleus during tonic and burst response mode. *Visual Neuroscience* 12, 723–741.

Guido, W., & Weyand, T. (1995). Burst responses in thalamic relay cells of the awake behaving cat. *Journal of Neurophysiology* 74, 1782–1786.

Guillery, R. W. (1957). Degeneration in the hypothalamic connexions of the albino rat. *Journal of Anatomy (London)* 91, 91–115.

Guillery, R. W. (1966). A study of Golgi preparations from the dorsal lateral geniculate nucleus of the adult cat. *Journal of Comparative Neurology* 128, 21–50.

Guillery, R. W. (1967a). A light and electron microscopic study of neurofibrils and neurofilaments at neuro-neuronal junctions in the dorsal lateral geniculate nucleus of the cat. *American Journal of Anatomy* 120, 583–604.

Guillery, R. W. (1967b). Patterns of fiber degeneration in the dorsal lateral geniculate nucleus of the cat following lesions in the visual cortex. *Journal of Comparative Neurology* 130, 197–222.

Guillery, R. W. (1969a). The organization of synaptic interconnections in the laminae of the dorsal lateral geniculate nucleus of the cat. *Zeitschrift für Zellforschung* 96, 1–38.

Guillery, R. W. (1969b). A quantitative study of synaptic interconnections in the dorsal lateral geniculate nucleus of the cat. *Zeitschrift für Zellforschung* 96, 39–48.

Guillery, R. W. (1995). Anatomical evidence concerning the role of the thalamus in corticocortical communication: a brief review. *Journal of Anatomy* 187, 583–592.

Guillery, R. W. (1996). Why do albinos and other hypopigmented mutants lack normal binocular vision, and what else is abnormal in their central visual pathways? *Eye* 10 (Pt. 2), 217–221.

Guillery, R. W. (2003). Branching thalamic afferents link action and perception. *Journal of Neurophysiology* 90, 539–548.

Guillery, R. W. (2005a). Anatomical pathways that link action to perception. *Progress in Brain Research* 149, 235–236.

Guillery, R. W. (2005b). Observations of synaptic structures: origins of the neuron doctrine and its current status. *Philosophical Transactions of the Royal Society of London, Series B, Biological Sciences* 360, 1281–1307.

Guillery, R. W., & August, B. K. (2002). Doubt and certainty in counting. *Progress in Brain Research* 135, 25–42.

Guillery, R. W., & Casagrande, V. A. (1977). Studies of the modifiability of the visual pathways in midwestern siamese cats. *Journal of Comparative Neurology* 174, 15–46.

Guillery, R. W., & Colonnier, M. (1970). Synaptic patterns in the dorsal lateral geniculate nucleus of the monkey. *Zeitschrift für Zellforschung und Mikroskopische Anatomie* 103, 90–108.

Guillery, R. W., & Harting, J. K. (2003). Structure and connections of the thalamic reticular nucleus: advancing views over half a century. *Journal of Comparative Neurology* 463, 360–371.

Guillery, R. W., & Sherman, S. M. (2002a). Thalamic relay functions and their role in corticocortical communication: generalizations from the visual system. *Neuron* 33, 163–175.

Guillery, R. W., & Sherman, S. M. (2002b). The thalamus as a monitor of motor outputs. *Philosophical Transactions of the Royal Society of London, Series B, Biological Sciences* 357, 1809–1821.

Guillery, R. W., Hickey, T. L., Kaas, J. H., Felleman, D. J., DeBruyn, E. J., & Sparks, D. L. (1984). Abnormal central visual pathways in the brain of an albino green monkey (*Cercopithecus aethiops*). *Journal of Comparative Neurology* 226, 165–183.

Guillery, R. W., Mason, C. A., & Taylor, J. S. (1995). Developmental determinants at the mammalian optic chiasm. *Journal of Neuroscience* 15, 4727–4737.

Guillery, R. W., Feig, S. L., & Lozsádi, D. A. (1998). Paying attention to the thalamic reticular nucleus. *Trends in Neurosciences* 21, 28–32.

Guillery, R. W., Feig, S. L., & Van Lieshout, D. P. (2001). Connections of higher order visual relays in the thalamus: a study of corticothalamic pathways in cats. *Journal of Comparative Neurology* 438, 66–85.

Guo, K., Benson, P. J., & Blakemore, C. (2004). Pattern motion is present in V1 of awake but not anaesthetized monkeys. *European Journal of Neuroscience* 19, 1055–1066.

Gutierrez, C., Cola, M. G., Seltzer, B., & Cusick, C. (2000). Neurochemical and connectional organization of the dorsal pulvinar complex in monkeys. *Journal of Comparative Neurology* 419, 61–86.

Gutierrez, C., Cox, C. L., Rinzel, J., & Sherman, S. M. (2001). Dynamics of low-threshold spike activation in relay neurons of the cat lateral geniculate nucleus. *Journal of Neuroscience* 21, 1022–1032.

Haberly, L. B., & Bower, J. M. (1989). Olfactory cortex: model circuit for study of associative memory? *Trends in Neurosciences* 12, 258–264.

Hallanger, A. E., Levey, A. I., Lee, H. J., Rye, D. B., & Wainer, B. H. (1987). The origins of cholinergic and other subcortical afferents to the thalamus in the rat. *Journal of Comparative Neurology* 262, 105–124.

Hallanger, A. E., & Wainer, B. H. (1988). Ultrastructure of ChAT-immunoreactive synaptic terminals in the thalamic reticular nucleus of the rat. *Journal of Comparative Neurology* 278, 486–497.

Hamos, J. E., Van Horn, S. C., Raczkowski, D., Uhlrich, D. J., & Sherman, S. M. (1985). Synaptic connectivity of a local circuit neurone in lateral geniculate nucleus of the cat. *Nature* 317, 618–621.

Hamos, J. E., Van Horn, S. C., & Sherman, S. M. (1986). Synaptic circuitry of an individual retinogeniculate axon from a retinal Y-cell. *Society for Neuroscience* 12, 1037.

Hamos, J. E., Van Horn, S. C., Raczkowski, D., & Sherman, S. M. (1987). Synaptic circuits involving an individual retinogeniculate axon in the cat. *Journal of Comparative Neurology* 259, 165–192.

Harding, B. N. (1973). An ultrastructural study of the termination of afferent fibres within the ventrolateral and centre median nuclei of the monkey thalamus. *Brain Research* 54, 341–346.

Harting, J. K., & Van Lieshout, D. P. (2000). Projections from the rostral pole of the inferior colliculus to the cat superior colliculus. *Brain Research* 881, 244–247.

Harting, J. K., Diamond, I. T., & Hall, W. C. (1973). Anterograde degeneration study of the cortical projections of the lateral geniculate and pulvinar nuclei in the tree shrew. *Journal of Comparative Neurology* 150, 393–440.

Harting, J. K., Hashikawa, T., & Van Lieshout, D. (1986). Laminar distribution of tectal, parabigeminal and pretectal inputs to the primate dorsal lateral geniculate nucleus: connectional studies in *Galago crassicaudatus*. *Brain Research* 366, 358–363.

Harting, J. K., Huerta, M. F., Hashikawa, T., & Van Lieshout, D. P. (1991). Projection of the mammalian superior colliculus upon the dorsal lateral geniculate nucleus: organization of tectogeniculate pathways in nineteen species. *Journal of Comparative Neurology* 305, 275–306.

Harting, J. K., Updyke, B. V., & Van Lieshout, D. P. (1992). Corticotectal projections in the cat: Anterograde transport studies of twenty-five cortical areas. *Journal of Comparative Neurology* 324, 379–414.

Harting, J. K., Updyke, B. V., & Van Lieshout, D. P. (2001). Striatal projections from the cat visual thalamus. *European Journal of Neuroscience* 14, 893–896.

Hartings, J. A., Temereanca, S., & Simons, D. J. (2003). State-dependent processing of sensory stimuli by thalamic reticular neurons. *Journal of Neuroscience* 23, 5264–5271.

Hashikawa, T., Van Lieshout, D., & Harting, J. K. (1986). Projections from the parabigeminal nucleus to the dorsal lateral geniculate nucleus in the tree shrew *Tupaia glis*. *Journal of Comparative Neurology* 246, 382–394.

Hashikawa, T., Rausell, E., Molinari, M., & Jones, E. G. (1991). Parvalbumin- and calbindin-containing neurons in the monkey medial geniculate complex: differential distribution and cortical layer specific projections. *Brain Research* 544, 335–341.

Hashimoto, A., & Oka, T. (1997). Free D-aspartate and D-serine in the mammalian brain and periphery. *Progress in Neurobiology* 52, 325–353.

Hasselmo, M. E., Wilson, M. A., Anderson, B. P., & Bower, J. M. (1990). Associative memory function in piriform (olfactory) cortex: computational modeling and neuropharmacology. *Cold Spring Harbor Symposia in Quantitative Biology* 55, 599–610.

Hassler, R. (1964). Spezifische und unspezifische Systeme des menschlichen Zwischenhirns. *Progress in Brain Research* 5, 1–32.

Havton, L. A., & Ohara, P. T. (1994). Cell body and dendritic tree size of intracellularly labeled thalamocortical projection neurons in the ventrobasal complex of cat. *Brain Research* 651, 76–84.

Haydon, P. G. (2001). Glia: listening and talking to the synapse. *Nature Reviews: Neuroscience* 2, 185–193.

Head, H. (1905). The afferent nervous system from a new aspect. *Brain* 28, 99–116.

Heath, C. J., & Jones, E. G. (1971). An experimental study of ascending connections from the posterior group of thalamic nuclei in the cat. *Journal of Comparative Neurology* 141, 397–426.

Helms, M. C., Ozen, G., & Hall, W. C. (2004). Organization of the intermediate gray layer of the superior colliculus. I. Intrinsic vertical connections. *Journal of Neurophysiology* 91, 1706–1715.

Hendry, S. H., & Calkins, D. J. (1998). Neuronal chemistry and functional organization in the primate visual system. *Trends in Neurosciences* 21, 344–349.

Hendry, S. H., & Reid, R. C. (2000). The koniocellular pathway in primate vision. *Annual Reviews in Neuroscience* 23, 127–153.

Hendry, S. H. C., & Yoshioka, T. (1994). A neurochemically distinct third channel in the macaque dorsal lateral geniculate nucleus. *Science* 264, 575–577.

Henkel, C. K. (1983). Evidence of sub-collicular auditory projections to the medial geniculate nucleus in the cat: an autoradiographic and horseradish peroxidase study. *Brain Research* 259, 21–30.

Henneman, E., & Mendell, L. M. (1981). Functional organization of motoneuron pool and its inputs. In *Handbook of Physiology*. Sect. 1: *The Nervous System*. Vol. II. *Motor Control*, Pt. 1, ed. Brooks, V. B., pp. 423–507. American Physiological Society, Bethesda, Md.

Henschen, S. E. (1893). On the visual path and centre. *Brain* 16, 170–180.

Hernández-Cruz, A., & Pape, H.-C. (1989). Identification of two calcium currents in acutely dissociated neurons from the rat lateral geniculate nucleus. *Journal of Neurophysiology* 61, 1270–1283.

Herrick, C. J. (1948). *The Brain of the Tiger Salamander*. University of Chicago Press, Chicago.

Herron, P., Baskerville, K. A., Chang, H. T., & Doetsch, G. S. (1997). Distribution of neurons immunoreactive for parvalbumin and calbindin in the somatosensory thalamus of the raccoon. *Journal of Comparative Neurology* 388, 120–129.

Hess, B. J., Blanks, R. H., Lannou, J., & Precht, W. (1989). Effects of kainic acid lesions of the nucleus reticularis tegmenti pontis on fast and slow phases of vestibulo-ocular and optokinetic reflexes in the pigmented rat. *Experimental Brain Research* 74, 63–79.

Heynen, A. J., Yoon, B. J., Liu, C. H., Huganir, R. L., & Bear, M. F. (2003). Molecular mechanism for loss of visual cortical responsiveness following brief monocular deprivation. *Nature Neuroscience* 6, 854–862.

Hickey, T. L., & Guillery, R. W. (1979). Variability of laminar patterns in the human lateral geniculate nucleus. *Journal of Comparative Neurology* 183, 221–246.

Hodgkin, A. L., & Huxley, A. F. (1952). Currents carried by sodium and potassium ions through the membrane of the giant axon of *Loligo*. *Journal of Physiology* (*London*) 116, 449–472.

Hoffman, D. A., & Johnston, D. (1998). Downregulation of transient K$^+$ channels in dendrites of hippocampal CA1 pyramidal neurons by activation of PKA and PKC. *Journal of Neuroscience* 18, 3521–3528.

Hohl-Abrahao, J. C., & Creutzfeldt, O. D. (1991). Topographical mapping of the thalamocortical projections in rodents and comparison with that in primates. *Experimental Brain Research* 87, 283–294.

Holcombe, V., & Guillery, R. W. (1984). The organization of retinal maps within the dorsal and ventral lateral geniculate nuclei of the rabbit. *Journal of Comparative Neurology* 225, 469–491.

Holländer, H., & Vanegas, H. (1977). The projection from the lateral geniculate nucleus onto the visual cortex in the cat: a quantitative study with horse-radish-peroxidase. *Journal of Comparative Neurology* 173, 519–536.

Holmes, W. R., & Woody, C. D. (1989). Effects of uniform and non-uniform synaptic "activation-distributions" on the cable properties of modeled cortical pyramidal neurons. *Brain Research* 505, 12–22.

Hoogland, P. V., Wouterlood, F. G., Welker, E., & van der Loos, H. (1991). Ultrastructure of giant and small thalamic terminals of cortical origin: a study of the projections from the barrel cortex in mice using *Phaseolus vulgaris* leucoagglutinin (PHA-L). *Experimental Brain Research* 87, 159–172.

Horne, M. K., & Butler, E. G. (1995). The role of the cerebello-thalamo-cortical pathway in skilled movement. *Progress in Neurobiology* 46, 199–213.

Horsley, V. (1909). The function of the so-called motor area of the brain. *British Medical Journal* 2, 125–132.

Houser, C. R., Vaughn, J. E., & Barber, R. P. (1980). GABA neurons are the major cell type of the nucleus reticularis thalami. *Brain Research* 200, 341–354.

Hubel, D. (1996). A big step along the visual pathway. *Nature* 380, 197–198.

Hubel, D. H., & Wiesel, T. N. (1961). Integrative action in the cat's lateral geniculate body. *Journal of Physiology* (*London*) 155, 385–398.

Hubel, D. H., & Wiesel, T. N. (1971). Aberrant visual projections in the Siamese cat. *Journal of Physiology* (*London*) 218, 33–62.

Hubel, D. H., & Wiesel, T. N. (1972). Laminar and columnar distribution of geniculo-cortical fibers in the macaque monkey. *Journal of Comparative Neurology* 146, 421–450.

Hubel, D. H., & Wiesel, T. N. (1977). Functional architecture of macaque monkey visual cortex. *Proceedings of the Royal Society of London, Series B, Biological Sciences*, 198, 1–59.

Huber, K. M., Sawtell, N. B., & Bear, M. F. (1998). Effects of the metabotropic glutamate receptor antagonist MCPG on phosphoinositide turnover and synaptic plasticity in visual cortex. *Journal of Neuroscience* 18, 1–9.

Huettner, J. E. (2003). Kainate receptors and synaptic transmission. *Progress in Neurobiology* 70, 387–407.

Hughes, S. W., Cope, D. W., Tóth, T. I., Williams, S. R., & Crunelli, V. (1999). All thalamocortical neurones possess a T-type Ca^{2+} "window" current that enables the expression of bistability-mediated activities. *Journal of Physiology* 517, 805–815.

Huguenard, J. R., & McCormick, D. A. (1992). Simulation of the currents involved in rhythmic oscillations in thalamic relay neurons. *Journal of Neurophysiology* 68, 1373–1383.

Huguenard, J. R., & Prince, D. A. (1992). A novel T-type current underlies prolonged Ca^{2+}-dependent burst firing in GABAergic neurons of rat thalamic reticular nucleus. *Journal of Neuroscience* 12, 3804–3817.

Humphrey, A. L., Sur, M., Uhlrich, D. J., & Sherman, S. M. (1985a). Projection patterns of individual X- and Y-cell axons from the lateral geniculate nucleus to cortical area 17 in the cat. *Journal of Comparative Neurology* 233, 159–189.

Humphrey, A. L., Sur, M., Uhlrich, D. J., & Sherman, S. M. (1985b). Termination patterns of individual X- and Y-cell axons in the visual cortex of the cat: projections to area 18, to the 17–18 border region, and to both areas 17 and 18. *Journal of Comparative Neurology* 233, 190–212.

Hutchins, B., & Updyke, B. V. (1989). Retinotopic organization within the lateral posterior complex of the cat. *Journal of Comparative Neurology* 285, 350–398.

Ichida, J. M., Rosa, M. G. P., & Casagrande, V. A. (2000). Does the visual system of the flying fox resemble that of primates? The distribution of calcium-binding proteins in the primary visual pathway of *Pteropus poliocephalus*. *Journal of Comparative Neurology* 417, 73–87.

Ide, L. S. (1982). The fine structure of the perigeniculate nucleus in the cat. *Journal of Comparative Neurology* 210, 317–334.

Ilinsky, I. A., & Kultas-Ilinsky, K. (1984). An autoradiographic study of topographical relationships between pallidal and cerebellar projections to the cat thalamus. *Experimental Brain Research* 54, 95–106.

Ilinsky, I. A., & Kultas-Ilinsky, K. (1990). Fine structure of the magnocellular subdivision of the ventral anterior thalamic nucleus (VAmc) of *Macaca mulatta*. I. Cell types and synaptology. *Journal of Comparative Neurology* 294, 455–478.

Ilinsky, I. A., Yi, H., & Kultas-Ilinsky, K. (1997). Mode of termination of pallidal afferents to the thalamus: a light and electron microscopic study with anterograde tracers and immunocytochemistry in *Macaca mulatta*. *Journal of Comparative Neurology* 386, 601–612.

Irvin, G. E., Norton, T. T., Sesma, M. A., & Casagrande, V. A. (1986). W-like response properties of interlaminar zone cells in the lateral geniculate nucleus of a primate (*Galago crassicaudatus*). *Brain Research* 362, 254–270.

Irvin, G. E., Casagrande, V. A., & Norton, T. T. (1993). Center/surround relationships of magnocellular, parvocellular, and koniocellular relay cells in primate lateral geniculate nucleus. *Visual Neuroscience* 10, 363–373.

Isu, N., Sakuma, A., Kitahara, M., Watanabe, S., & Uchino, Y. (1989). Extracellular recording of vestibulo-thalamic neurons projecting to the spinal cord in the cat. *Neuroscience Letters* 104, 25–30.

Jack, J. J. B., Noble, D., & Tsien, R. W. (1975). *Electric Current Flow in Excitable Cells*. Oxford University Press, Oxford, England.

Jackson, H. J. (1873). On the anatomical and physiological localization of movements in the brain. *Lancet* 1, 234.

Jahnsen, H., & Llinás, R. (1984a). Electrophysiological properties of guinea-pig thalamic neurones: an *in vitro* study. *Journal of Physiology (London)* 349, 205–226.

Jahnsen, H., & Llinás, R. (1984b). Ionic basis for the electroresponsiveness and oscillatory properties of guinea-pig thalamic neurones *in vitro*. *Journal of Physiology (London)* 349, 227–247.

Jasper, H. H. (2004). Unspecific thalamocortical relations. In *Handbook of Physiology*, Sect. 1, *Neurophysiology*, vol. 2, pp. 1307–1321. American Physiological Society, Bethesda, Md.

Jhaveri, S., Edwards, M. A., & Schneider, G. E. (1991). Initial stages of retinofugal axon development in the hamster: evidence for two distinct modes of growth. *Experimental Brain Research* 87, 371–382.

Jingami, H., Nakanishi, S., & Morikawa, K. (2003). Structure of the metabotropic glutamate receptor. *Current Opinion Neurobiology* 13, 271–278.

Johnson, J. K., & Casagrande, V. A. (1995). Distribution of calcium-binding proteins within the parallel visual pathways of a primate (*Galago crassicaudatus*). *Journal of Comparative Neurology* 356, 238–260.

Johnston, D., Magee, J. C., Colbert, C. M., & Christie, B. R. (1996). Active properties of neuronal dendrites. *Annual Review of Neuroscience* 19, 165–186.

Jones, E. G. (1983). Distribution patterns of individual medial lemniscal axons in the ventrobasal complex of the monkey thalamus. *Journal of Comparative Neurology* 215, 1–16.

Jones, E. G. (1985). *The Thalamus.* Plenum, New York.

Jones, E. G. (1998). Viewpoint: The core and matrix of thalamic organization. *Neuroscience* 85, 331–345.

Jones, E. G. (2001). The thalamic matrix and thalamocortical synchrony. *Trends in Neurosciences* 24, 595–601.

Jones, E. G. (2002a). Thalamic circuitry and thalamocortical synchrony. *Philosophical Transactions of the Royal Society of London, Series B, Biological Sciences* 357, 1659–1673.

Jones, E. G. (2002b). Thalamic organization and function after Cajal. *Progress in Brain Research* 136, 333–357.

Jones, E. G. (2003). Chemically defined parallel pathways in the monkey auditory system. *Annals of the New York Academy of Sciences* 999, 218–233.

Jones, E. G., & Leavitt, R. Y. (1974). Retrograde axonal transport and the demonstration of non-specific projections to the cerebral cortex and striatum from thalamic intralaminar nuclei in the rat, cat and monkey. *Journal of Comparative Neurology* 154, 349–377.

Jones, E. G., & Powell, T. P. (1969). Electron microscopy of synaptic glomeruli in the thalamic relay nuclei of the cat. *Proceedings of the Royal Society of London, Series B, Biological Sciences* 172, 153–171.

Jones, E. G., & Rockel, A. J. (1971). The synaptic organization in the medial geniculate body of afferent fibres ascending from the inferior colliculus. *Zeitschrift für Zellforschung* 113, 44–66.

Josephson, E. M., & Morest, D. K. (2003). Synaptic nests lack glutamate trans-porters in the cochlear nucleus of the mouse. *Synapse* 49, 29–46.

Kaas, J. H. (1995). The evolution of isocortex. *Brain, Behavior and Evolution* 46, 187–196.

Kaas, J. H., & Guillery, R. W. (1973). The transfer of abnormal visual field rep-resentations from the dorsal lateral geniculate nucleus to the visual cortex in Siamese cats. *Brain Research* 59, 61–95.

Kaas, J. H., Guillery, R. W., & Allman, J. M. (1972a). Some principles of organi-zation in the dorsal lateral geniculate nucleus. *Brain, Behavior and Evo-lution* 6, 253–299.

Kaas, J. H., Hall, W. C., Killackey, H. P., & Diamond, I. T. (1972b). Visual cortex of the tree shrew (*Tupaia glis*): architectonic subdivisions and representa-tions of the visual field. *Brain Research* 42, 491–496.

Kaas, J. H., Hackett, T. A., & Tramo, M. J. (1999). Auditory processing in primate cerebral cortex. *Current Opinion in Neurobiology* 9, 164–170.

Kaitz, S. S., & Robertson, R. T. (1981). Thalamic connections with limbic cortex. II. Corticothalamic projections. *Journal of Comparative Neurology* 195, 527–545.

Kakei, S., Na, J., & Shinoda, Y. (2001). Thalamic terminal morphology and dis-tribution of single corticothalamic axons originating from layers 5 and 6 of the cat motor cortex. *Journal of Comparative Neurology* 437, 170–185.

Kalil, R. E., & Chase, R. (1970). Corticofugal influence on activity of lateral geniculate neurons in the cat. *Journal of Neurophysiology* 33, 459–474.

Kandel, E. R., Schwartz, J. H., & Jessell, T. M. (2000). *Principles of Neural Science*. McGraw-Hill, New York.

Kaplan, E. (2004). The M, P, and K pathways of the primate visual system. In *The Visual Neurosciences*, eds. Chalupa, L. M., & Werner, J. S., pp. 481–493. MIT Press, Cambridge, Mass.

Kara, P., Pezaris, J. S., Yurgenson, S., & Reid, R. C. (2002). The spatial recep-tive field of thalamic inputs to single cortical simple cells revealed by the interaction of visual and electrical stimulation. *Proceedings of the National Academy of Sciences of the United States of America* 99, 16261–16266.

Karten, H. J., Hodos, W., Nauta, W. J., & Revzin, A. M. (1973). Neural con-nections of the "visual Wulst" of the avian telencephalon: experimental studies in the piegon (*Columba livia*) and owl (*Speotyto cunicularia*). *Journal of Comparative Neurology* 150, 253–278.

Katz, L. C. (1987). Local circuitry of identified projection neurons in cat visual cortex brain slices. *Journal of Neuroscience* 7, 1223–1249.

Kaufman, E. F. S., & Rosenquist, A. C. (1985). Efferent projections of the tha-lamic intralaminar nuclei in the cat. *Brain Research* 335, 257–279.

Kawajiri, S., & Dingledine, R. (1993). Multiple structural determinants of voltage-dependent magnesium block in recombinant NMDA receptors. *Neuropharmacology* 32, 1203–1211.

Kawano, J. (1998). Cortical projections of the parvocellular laminae C of the dorsal lateral geniculate nucleus in the cat: an anterograde wheat germ agglutinin conjugated to horseradish peroxidase study. *Journal of Com-parative Neurology* 392, 439–457.

Kayama, Y., Shimada, S., Hishikawa, Y., & Ogawa, T. (1989). Effects of stimulating the dorsal raphé nucleus of the rat on neuronal activity in the dorsal lateral geniculate nucleus. *Brain Research* 489, 1–11.

Kelly, L. R., Li, J., Carden, W. B., & Bickford, M. E. (2003). Ultrastructure and synaptic targets of tectothalamic terminals in the cat lateral posterior nucleus. *Journal of Comparative Neurology* 464, 472–486.

Kennedy, H., & Bullier, J. (1985). A double-labeling investigation of the afferent connectivity to cortical areas V1 and V2 of the macaque monkey. *Journal of Neuroscience* 5, 2815–2830.

Kharazia, V. N., & Weinberg, R. J. (1994). Glutamate in terminals of thalamocortical fibers in rat somatic sensory cortex. *Neuroscience Letters* 157, 162–166.

Kidd, F. L., & Isaac, J. T. (2001). Kinetics and activation of postsynaptic kainate receptors at thalamocortical synapses: role of glutamate clearance. *Journal of Neurophysiology* 86, 1139–1148.

Kim, H. G., & Connors, B. W. (1993). Apical dendrites of the neocortex: correlation between sodium- and calcium-dependent spiking and pyramidal cell morphology. *Journal of Neuroscience* 13, 5301–5311.

Kim, U., & McCormick, D. A. (1998). The functional influence of burst and tonic firing mode on synaptic interactions in the thalamus. *Journal of Neuroscience* 18, 9500–9516.

Kimura, A., Donishi, T., Sakoda, T., Hazama, M., & Tamai, Y. (2003). Auditory thalamic nuclei projections to the temporal cortex in the rat. *Neuroscience* 117, 1003–1016.

Koch, C., Poggio, T., & Torre, V. (1982). Retinal ganglion cells: a functional interpretation of dendritic morphology. *Philosophical Transactions of the Royal Society of London* 298, 227–264.

Koerner, F., & Teuber, H. L. (1973). Visual field defects after missile injuries to the geniculo-striate pathway in man. *Experimental Brain Research* 18, 88–113.

Kohonen, T., Lehtiö, P., Rovamo, J., Hyvärinen, J., Bry, K., & Vainio, L. (1977). A principle of neural associative memory. *Neuroscience* 2, 1065–1076.

Kolmac, C. I., & Mitrofanis, J. (1997). Organisation of the reticular thalamic projection to the intralaminar and midline nuclei in rats. *Journal of Comparative Neurology* 377, 165–178.

Koontz, M. A., Rodieck, R. W., & Farmer, S. G. (1985). The retinal projection to the cat pretectum. *Journal of Comparative Neurology* 236, 42–59.

Kölliker, A. (1896). *Handbuch der Gerwebelehre des Menschen. Nervensystemen des Menschen und der Thiere*, 6th ed. Engelmann, Leipzig.

Krubitzer, L. (1998). What can monotremes tell us about brain evolution? *Philosophical Transactions of the Royal Society of London, Series B, Biological Sciences* 353, 1127–1146.

Krubitzer, L. A., & Kaas, J. H. (1992). The somatosensory thalamus of monkeys: cortical connections and a redefinition of nuclei in marmosets. *Journal of Comparative Neurology* 319, 123–140.

Krug, K., Smith, A. L., & Thompson, I. D. (1998). The development of topography in the hamster geniculo-cortical projection. *Journal of Neuroscience* 18, 5766–5776.

Krupa, D. J., Ghazanfar, A. A., & Nicolelis, M. A. (1999). Immediate thalamic sensory plasticity depends on corticothalamic feedback. *Proceedings of the National Academy of Sciences of the United States of America* 96, 8200–8205.

Kudo, M., & Niimi, K. (1980). Ascending projections of the inferior colliculus in the cat: an autoradiographic study. *Journal of Comparative Neurology* 191, 545–556.

Kullmann, D. M. (2001). Presynaptic kainate receptors in the hippocampus: slowly emerging from obscurity. *Neuron* 32, 561–564.

Kultas-Ilinsky, K., & Ilinsky, I. (1991). Fine structure of the ventral lateral nucleus (VL) of the *Macaca mulatta* thalamus: cell types and synaptology. *Journal of Comparative Neurology* 314, 319–349.

Kultas-Ilinsky, K., Reising, L., Yi, H., & Ilinsky, I. A. (1997). Pallidal afferent territory of the *Macaca mulatta* thalamus: neuronal and synaptic organization of the VAdc. *Journal of Comparative Neurology* 386, 573–600.

Kuner, T., & Schoepfer, R. (1996). Multiple structural elements determine subunit specificity of Mg^{2+} block in NMDA receptor channels. *Journal of Neuroscience* 16, 3549–3558.

Kuroda, M., & Price, J. L. (1991). Ultrastructure and synaptic organization of axon terminals from brainstem structures to the mediodorsal thalamic nucleus of the rat. *Journal of Comparative Neurology* 313, 539–552.

Kuroda, M., Lopez-Mascaraque, L., & Price, J. L. (1992a). Neuronal and synaptic composition of the mediodorsal thalamic nucleus in the rat: a light and electron microscopic Golgi study. *Journal of Comparative Neurology* 326, 61–81.

Kuroda, M., Murakami, K., Kishi, K., & Price, J. L. (1992b). Distribution of the piriform cortical terminals to cells in the central segment of the mediodorsal thalamic nucleus of the rat. *Brain Research* 595, 159–163.

Kuroda, M., Yokofujita, J., & Murakami, K. (1998). An ultrastructural study of the neural circuit between the prefrontal cortex and the mediodorsal nucleus of the thalamus. *Progress in Neurobiology* 54, 417–458.

Lachica, E. A., & Casagrande, V. A. (1988). Development of primate retinogeniculate axon arbors. *Visual Neuroscience* 1, 103–123.

Laemle, L. K. (1975). Cell populations of the lateral geniculate nucleus of the cat as determined with horseradish peroxidase. *Brain Research* 100, 650–656.

Lam, Y.-W., & Sherman, S. M. (2005). Mapping by laser photostimulation of connections between the thalamic reticular and ventral posterior lateral nuclei in the rat. *Journal of Neurophysiology*, in press.

Lam, Y.-W., Cox, C. L., Varela, C., & Sherman, S. M. (2005). Morphological correlates of triadic circuitry in the lateral geniculate nucleus of cats and rats. *Journal of Neurophysiology*, 93, 748–757.

Landisman, C. E., & Ts'o, D. Y. (2002a). Color processing in macaque striate cortex: electrophysiological properties. *Journal of Neurophysiology* 87, 3138–3151.

Landisman, C. E., & Ts'o, D. Y. (2002b). Color processing in macaque striate cortex: relationships to ocular dominance, cytochrome oxidase, and orientation. *Journal of Neurophysiology* 87, 3126–3137.

Landisman, C. E., Long, M. A., Beierlein, M., Deans, M. R., Paul, D. L., & Connors, B. W. (2002). Electrical synapses in the thalamic reticular nucleus. *Journal of Neuroscience* 22, 1002–1009.

Landò, L., & Zucker, R. S. (1994). Ca^{2+} cooperativity in neurosecretion measured using photolabile Ca^{2+} chelators. *Journal of Neurophysiology* 72, 825–830.

Lane, R. H., Kaas, J. H., & Allman, J. M. (1974). Visuotopic organization of the superior colliculus in normal and Siamese cats. *Brain Research* 70, 413–430.

Latawiec, D., Martin, K. A. C., & Meskenaite, V. (2000). Termination of the geniculocortical projection in the striate cortex of macaque monkey: a quantitative immunoelectron microscopic study. *Journal of Comparative Neurology* 419, 306–319.

Le Gros Clark, W. E. (1932). The structure and connections of the thalamus. *Brain* 55, 406–470.

LeDoux, J. E., Ruggiero, D. A., & Reis, D. J. (1985). Projections to the subcortical forebrain from anatomically defined regions of the medial geniculate body in the rat. *Journal of Comparative Neurology* 242, 182–213.

Lee, K. H., & McCormick, D. A. (1996). Abolition of spindle oscillations by serotonin and norepinephrine in the ferret lateral geniculate and perigeniculate nuclei in vitro. *Neuron* 17, 309–321.

Lee, K. H., Broberger, C., Kim, U., & McCormick, D. A. (2004). Histamine modulates thalamocortical activity by activating a chloride conductance in ferret perigeniculate neurons. *Proceedings of the National Academy of Sciences of the United States of America* 101, 6716–6721.

Lennie, P. (1980). Perceptual signs of parallel pathways. *Philosophical Transactions of the Royal Society of London, Series B, Biological Sciences* 290, 23–37.

Lenz, F. A., Garonzik, I. M., Zirh, T. A., & Dougherty, P. M. (1998). Neuronal activity in the region of the thalamic principal sensory nucleus (ventralis caudalis) in patients with pain following amputations. *Neuroscience* 86, 1065–1081.

Lesica, N. A., & Stanley, G. B. (2004). Encoding of natural scene movies by tonic and burst spikes in the lateral geniculate nucleus. *Journal of Neuroscience* 24, 10731–10740.

LeVay, S., & Ferster, D. (1977). Relay cell classes in the lateral geniculate nucleus of the cat and the effects of visual deprivation. *Journal of Comparative Neurology* 172, 563–584.

LeVay, S., & Ferster, D. (1979). Proportion of interneurons in the cat's lateral geniculate nucleus. *Brain Research* 164, 304–308.

LeVay, S., & McConnell, S. K. (1982). ON and OFF layers in the lateral geniculate nucleus of the mink. *Nature* 300, 350–351.

Leventhal, A. G. (1979). Evidence that the different classes of relay cells of the cat's lateral geniculate nucleus terminate in different layers of the striate cortex. *Experimental Brain Research* 37, 349–372.

Leventhal, A. G., & Creel, D. J. (1985). Retinal projections and functional architecture of cortical areas 17 and 18 in the tyrosinase-negative albino cat. *Journal of Neuroscience 5*, 795–807.

Leventhal, A. G., Rodieck, R. W., & Dreher, B. (1981). Retinal ganglion cell classes in the old world monkey: morphology and central projections. *Science 213*, 1139–1142.

Leventhal, A. G., Rodieck, R. W., & Dreher, B. (1985). Central projections of cat retinal ganglion cells. *Journal of Comparative Neurology 237*, 216–226.

Levitt, J. B., Yoshioka, T., & Lund, J. S. (1995). Connections between the pulvinar complex and cytochrome oxidase-defined compartments in visual area V2 of macaque monkey. *Experimental Brain Research 104*, 419–430.

Li, J., Guido, W., & Bickford, M. E. (2003a). Two distinct types of corticothalamic EPSPs and their contribution to short-term synaptic plasticity. *Journal of Neurophysiology 90*, 3429–3440.

Li, J. L., Wang, S. T., & Bickford, M. E. (2003b). Comparison of the ultrastructure of cortical and retinal terminals in the rat dorsal lateral geniculate and lateral posterior nuclei. *Journal of Comparative Neurology 460*, 394–409.

Lieberman, A. R. (1973). Neurons with presynaptic perikarya and presynaptic dendrites in the rat lateral geniculate nucleus. *Brain Research 59*, 35–59.

Lieberman, A. R., & Spacek, J. (1997). Filamentous contacts: the ultrastructure and three-dimensional organization of specialized non-synaptic interneuronal appositions in thalamic relay nuclei. *Cell and Tissue Research 288*, 43–57.

Linden, R., & Perry, V. H. (1983). Massive retinotectal projection in rats. *Brain Research 272*, 145–149.

Ling, C. Y., Schneider, G. E., Northmore, D., & Jhaveri, S. (1997). Afferents from the colliculus, cortex, and retina have distinct terminal morphologies in the lateral posterior thalamic nucleus. *Journal of Comparative Neurology 388*, 467–483.

Lisman, J. E. (1997). Bursts as a unit of neural information: making unreliable synapses reliable. *Trends in Neurosciences 20*, 38–43.

Liu, X.-B., Honda, C. N., & Jones, E. G. (1995a). Distribution of four types of synapse on physiologically identified relay neurons in the ventral posterior thalamic nucleus of the cat. *Journal of Comparative Neurology 352*, 69–91.

Liu, X.-B., Warren, R. A., & Jones, E. G. (1995b). Synaptic distribution of afferents from reticular nucleus in ventroposterior nucleus of cat thalamus. *Journal of Comparative Neurology 352*, 187–202.

Liu, X.-B., & Jones, E. G. (1999). Predominance of corticothalamic synaptic inputs to thalamic reticular nucleus neurons in the rat. *Journal of Comparative Neurology 414*, 67–79.

Liu, X.-B., & Jones, E. G. (2003). Fine structural localization of connexin-36 immunoreactivity in mouse cerebral cortex and thalamus. *Journal of Comparative Neurology 466*, 457–467.

Livingstone, M. S., & Hubel, D. H. (1981). Effects of sleep and arousal on the processing of visual information in the cat. *Nature 291*, 554–561.

Livingstone, M. S., & Hubel, D. H. (1984). Anatomy and physiology of a color system in the primate visual cortex. *Journal of Neuroscience* 4, 309–356.

Llinás, R. (1988). The intrinsic electrophysiological properties of mammalian neurons: insights into central nervous system. *Science* 242, 1654–1664.

Llinás, R., & Jahnsen, H. (1982). Electrophysiology of mammalian thalamic neurones *in vitro*. *Nature* 297, 406–408.

Llinás, R. R., & Pare, D. (1991). Of dreaming and wakefulness. *Neuroscience* 44, 521–535.

Lo, F.-S., & Sherman, S. M. (1994). Feedback inhibition in the cat's lateral geniculate nucleus. *Experimental Brain Research* 100, 365–368.

López, D. E., Saldaña, E., Nodal, F. R., Merchán, M. A., & Warr, W. B. (1999). Projections of cochlear root neurons, sentinels of the rat auditory pathway. *Journal of Comparative Neurology* 415, 160–174.

Lorente de Nó, R. (1938). Cerebral cortex: Architecture, intracortical connections, motor projections. In *Physiology of the Nervous System*, ed. Fulton, J., pp. 291–340. Oxford Universitiy Press, Oxford, England.

Lozsádi, D. A. (1995). Organization of connections between the thalamic reticular and the anterior thalamic nuclei in the rat. *Journal of Comparative Neurology* 358, 233–246.

Lozsádi, D. A., Gonzalez-Soriano, J., & Guillery, R. W. (1996). The course and termination of corticothalamic fibres arising in the visual cortex of the rat. *European Journal of Neuroscience* 8, 2416–2427.

Lu, G. W., & Willis, W. D., Jr. (1999). Branching and/or collateral projections of spinal dorsal horn neurons. *Brain Research Reviews* 29, 50–82.

Lu, S.-M., Guido, W., & Sherman, S. M. (1992). Effects of membrane voltage on receptive field properties of lateral geniculate neurons in the cat: contributions of the low threshold Ca^{++} conductance. *Journal of Neurophysiology* 68, 2185–2198.

Lu, S.-M., Guido, W., & Sherman, S. M. (1993). The brainstem parabrachial region controls mode of response to visual stimulation of neurons in the cat's lateral geniculate nucleus. *Visual Neuroscience* 10, 631–642.

Lubke, J. (1993). Morphology of neurons in the thalamic reticular nucleus (TRN) of mammals as revealed by intracellular injections into fixed brain slices. *Journal of Comparative Neurology* 329, 458–471.

Lujan, R., Nusser, Z., Roberts, J. D., Shigemoto, R., & Somogyi, P. (1996). Perisynaptic location of metabotropic glutamate receptors mGluR1 and mGluR5 on dendrites and dendritic spines in the rat hippocampus. *European Journal of Neuroscience* 8, 1488–1500.

Luppino, G., Matelli, M., Carey, R. G., Fitzpatrick, D., & Diamond, I. T. (1988). New view of the organization of the pulvinar nucleus in *Tupaia* as revealed by tectopulvinar and pulvinar-cortical projections. *Journal of Comparative Neurology* 273, 67–86.

Lyon, D. C., Jain, N., & Kaas, J. H. (2003). The visual pulvinar in tree shrews. II. Projections of four nuclei to areas of visual cortex. *Journal of Comparative Neurology* 467, 607–627.

Lysakowski, A., Standage, G. P., & Benevento, L. A. (1988). An investigation of collateral projections of the dorsal lateral geniculate nucleus and other subcortical structures to cortical areas V1 and V4 in the macaque monkey: a double label retrograde tracer study. *Experimental Brain Research* 69, 651–661.

Ma, W., Peschanski, M., & Ralston, H. J. III (1987a). Fine structure of the spinothalamic projections to the central lateral nucleus of the rat thalamus. *Brain Research* 414, 187–191.

Ma, W., Peschanski, M., & Ralston, H. J. III (1987b). The differential synaptic organization of the spinal and lemniscal projections to the ventrobasal complex of the rat thalamus: evidence for convergence of the two systems upon single thalamic neurons. *Neuroscience* 22, 925–934.

Macchi, G. (1983). Old and new anatomo-functional criteria in the subdivision of the thalamic nuclei. In *Somatosensory Integration in the Thalamus*, eds. Macchi, G., Rustioni, A., & Spreafico, R., pp. 3–16. Elsevier, Amsterdam.

Macchi, G. (1993). The intralaminar system revisited. In *Somatosensory Integration in the Thalamus*, eds. Minciacchi, D., Molinari, M., Macchi, G., & Jones, E. G., pp. 175–184. Pergamon Press, Oxford, England.

Macchi, G., & Bentivoglio, M. (1982). The organization of the efferent projections of the thalamic intralaminar nuclei: past, present and future of the anatomical approach. *Italian Journal of Neurological Science* 3, 83–96.

Macchi, G., Bentivoglio, M., Molinari, M., & Minciacchi, D. (1984). The thalamo-caudate versus thalamo-cortical projections as studied in the cat with fluorescent retrograde double labeling. *Experimental Brain Research* 54, 225–239.

MacDermott, A. B., Role, L. W., & Siegelbaum, S. A. (1999). Presynaptic ionotropic receptors and the control of transmitter release. *Annual Review of Neuroscience* 22, 443–485.

Macmillan, N. A., & Creelman, C. D. (1991). *Detection Theory: A User's Guide.* Cambridge University Press, Cambridge, England.

Magee, J., Hoffman, D., Colbert, C., & Johnston, D. (1998). Electrical and calcium signaling in dendrites of hippocampal pyramidal neurons. *Annual Review of Physiology* 60, 327–346.

Majorossy, K., & Kiss, A. (1976). Specific patterns of neuron arrangement and of synaptic articulation in the medial geniculate body. *Experimental Brain Research* 26, 1–17.

Malpeli, J. G., Lee, D., & Baker, F. H. (1996). Laminar and retinotopic organization of the macaque lateral geniculate nucleus: magnocellular and parvocellular magnification functions. *Journal of Comparative Neurology* 375, 363–377.

Manning, K. A., Wilson, J. R., & Uhlrich, D. J. (1996). Histamine-immunoreactive neurons and their innervation of visual regions in the cortex, tectum, and thalamus in the primate *Macaca mulatta. Journal of Comparative Neurology* 373, 271–282.

Marks, G. A., Farber, J., & Roffwarg, H. P. (1981). Phasic influences during REM sleep upon dorsal lateral geniculate nucleus unit activity in the rat. *Brain Research* 222, 388–394.

Martin, K. A. C. (1985). Neuronal circuits in cat striate cortex. *Cerebral Cortex* 2, 241–284.

Mason, R. (1978). Functional organization in the cat's pulvinar complex. *Experimental Brain Research* 31, 51–66.

Massaux, A., & Edeline, J. M. (2003). Bursts in the medial geniculate body: a comparison between anesthetized and unanesthetized states in guinea pig. *Experimental Brain Research* 153, 573–578.

Massaux, A., Dutrieux, G., Cotillon-Williams, N., Manunta, Y., & Edeline, J. M. (2004). Auditory thalamus bursts in anesthetized and non-anesthetized states: contribution to functional properties. *Journal of Neurophysiology* 91, 2117–2134.

Mastronarde, D. N. (1987a). Two classes of single-input X-cells in cat lateral geniculate nucleus. I. Receptive field properties and classification of cells. *Journal of Neurophysiology* 57, 357–380.

Mastronarde, D. N. (1987b). Two classes of single-input X-cells in cat lateral geniculate nucleus. II. Retinal inputs and the generation of receptive-field properties. *Journal of Neurophysiology* 57, 381–413.

Mathers, L. H. (1971). Tectal projection to posterior thalamus of the squirrel monkey. *Brain Research* 35, 357–380.

Mathers, L. H. (1972). The synaptic organization of the cortical projection to the pulvinar of the squirrel monkey. *Journal of Comparative Neurology* 146, 43–60.

Matsuo, S., Hasogai, M., & Nakao, S. (1994). Ascending projections of posterior canal activated excitatory and inhibitory secondary vestibular neurons to the mesodiencephalon in cats. *Experimental Brain Research* 100, 7–17.

Matthews, G. (1996). Neurotransmitter release. *Annual Review of Neuroscience* 19, 219–233.

Matthews, M. R. (1964). Further observations on transneuronal degeneration in the lateral geniculate nucleus of the macaque monkey. *Journal of Anatomy* 98, 255–263.

Maunsell, J. H. R., & Van Essen, D. C. (1983). The connections of the middle temporal visual area (MT) and their relationship to a cortical hierarchy in the macaque monkey. *Journal of Neuroscience* 3, 2563–2586.

Mayer, M. L., & Westbrook, G. L. (1987). The physiology of excitatory amino acids in the vertebrate central nervous system. *Progress in Neurobiology* 28, 197–276.

McCarley, R. W., Benoit, O., & Barrionuevo, G. (1983). Lateral geniculate nucleus unitary discharge in sleep and waking: state- and rate-specific aspects. *Journal of Neurophysiology* 50, 798–818.

McClurkin, J. W., & Marrocco, R. T. (1984). Visual cortical input alters spatial tuning in monkey lateral geniculate nucleus cells. *Journal of Physiology (London)* 348, 135–152.

McClurkin, J. W., Optican, L. M., & Richmond, B. J. (1994). Cortical feedback increases visual information transmitted by monkey parvocellular lateral geniculate nucleus neurons. *Visual Neuroscience* 11, 601–617.

McConnell, S. K., & LeVay, S. (1984). Segregation of on- and off-center afferents in mink visual cortex. *Proceedings of the National Academy of Sciences of the United States of America* 81, 1590–1593.

McCormick, D. A. (1989). Cholinergic and noradrenergic modulation of thalamocortical processing. *Trends in Neurosciences* 12, 215–221.

McCormick, D. A. (1990). Membrane properties and neurotransmitter actions. In *The Synaptic Organization of the Brain,* 3rd ed., ed. Shepherd, G. M., pp. 32–66. Oxford University Press, New York.

McCormick, D. A. (1991a). Cellular mechanisms underlying cholinergic and noradrenergic modulation of neuronal firing in the cat and guinea pig dorsal lateral geniculate nucleus. *Neuroscience* 12, 278–289.

McCormick, D. A. (1991b). Functional properties of a slowly inactivating potassium current in guinea pig dorsal lateral geniculate relay neurons. *Journal of Neurophysiology* 66, 1176–1189.

McCormick, D. A. (1992). Neurotransmitter actions in the thalamus and cerebral cortex and their role in neuromodulation of thalamocortical activity. *Progress in Neurobiology* 39, 337–388.

McCormick, D. A., & Bal, T. (1997). Sleep and arousal: thalamocortical mechanisms. *Annual Review of Neuroscience* 20, 185–215.

McCormick, D. A., & Feeser, H. R. (1990). Functional implications of burst firing and single spike activity in lateral geniculate relay neurons. *Neuroscience* 39, 103–113.

McCormick, D. A., & Huguenard, J. R. (1992). A model of the electrophysiological properties of thalamocortical relay neurons. *Journal of Neurophysiology* 68, 1384–1400.

McCormick, D. A., & Pape, H.-C. (1988). Acetycholine inhibits identified interneurons in the cat lateral geniculate nucleus. *Nature* 334, 246–248.

McCormick, D. A., & Pape, H.-C. (1990a). Properties of a hyperpolarization-activated cation current and its role in rhythmic oscillation in thalamic relay neurones. *Journal of Physiology (London)* 431, 291–318.

McCormick, D. A., & Pape, H.-C. (1990b). Noradrenergic and serotonergic modulation of a hyperpolarization-activated cation current in thalamic relay neurones. *Journal of Physiology (London)* 431, 319–342.

McCormick, D. A., & Prince, D. A. (1986). Acetylcholine induces burst firing in thalamic reticular neurones by activating a potassium conductance. *Nature* 319, 402–405.

McCormick, D. A., & Prince, D. A. (1988) Noradrenergic modulation of firing pattern in guinea-pig and cat thalamic neurons, *in vitro. Journal of Neurophysiology* 59, 978–996.

McCormick, D. A., & Von Krosigk, M. (1992). Corticothalamic activation modulates thalamic firing through glutamate "metabotropic" receptors. *Proceedings of the National Academy of Sciences of the United States of America* 89, 2774–2778.

McCormick, D. A., & Wang, Z. (1991). Serotonin and noradrenaline excite GABAergic neurones in the guinea-pig and cat nucleus reticularis thalami. *Journal of Physiology (London)* 442, 235–255.

McCormick, D. A., & Williamson, A. (1991). Modulation of neuronal firing mode in cat and guinea pig LGNd by histamine: possible cellular mechanisms of histaminergic control of arousal. *Journal of Neuroscience* 11, 3188–3199.

McCrea, R. A., Bishop, G. A., & Kitai, S. T. (1978). Morphological and electrophysiological characteristics of projection neurons in the nucleus interpositus of the cat cerebellum. *Journal of Comparative Neurology* 181, 397–419.

McFarland, N. R., & Haber, S. N. (2002). Thalamic relay nuclei of the basal ganglia form both reciprocal and nonreciprocal cortical connections, linking multiple frontal cortical areas. *Journal of Neuroscience* 22, 8117–8132.

Meeren, H. K., Van Luijtelaar, E. L., & Coenen, A. M. (1998). Cortical and thalamic visual evoked potentials during sleep-wake states and spike-wave discharges in the rat. *Electroencephalography & Clinical Neurophysiology* 108, 306–319.

Merabet, L., Desautels, A., Minville, K., & Casanova, C. (1998). Motion integration in a thalamic visual nucleus. *Nature* 396, 265–268.

Miall, R. C., Price, S., Mason, R., Passingham, R. E., Winter, J. L., & Stein, J. F. (1998). Microstimulation of movements from cerebellar-receiving, but not pallidal-receiving areas of the macaque thalamus under ketamine anaesthesia. *Experimental Brain Research* 123, 387–396.

Miceli, D., Reperant, J., Marchand, L., Ward, R., & Vesselkin, N. (1991). Divergence and collateral axon branching in subsystems of visual cortical projections from the cat lateral posterior nucleus. *Journal für Hirnforschung* 32, 165–173.

Middleton, F. A., & Strick, P. L. (1997). Dentate output channels: motor and cognitive components. *Progress in Brain Research* 114, 553–566.

Miller, R. J. (1998). Presynaptic receptors. *Annual Review of Pharmacology and Toxicology* 38, 201–227.

Milner, A. D., & Goodale, M. A. (1993). Visual pathways to perception and action. *Progress in Brain Research* 95, 317–337.

Minciacchi, D., Granato, A., & Santarelli Macchi, G. (1993). Different weights of subcortical-cortical projections upon primary sensory areas: the thalamic anterior intralaminar system. In *Thalamic Networks for Relay and Modulation*, eds. Minciacchi, D., Molinari, M., Macchi, G., & Jones, E. G., pp. 209–226. Pergamon, Oxford, England.

Minkowski, M. (1914). Experimentelle Untersuchungen über die Beziehungen der Grosshirnrinde und der Netzhaut zu den primären optischen Zentren, besonders zum Corpus geniculatum externum. *Arbeiten Hirnanatomisches Institut Zurich* 7, 259–362.

Mitrofanis, J. (1994). Development of the thalamic reticular nucleus in ferrets with special reference to the perigeniculate and perireticular cell groups. *European Journal of Neuroscience* 6, 253–263.

Mitrofanis, J., & Guillery, R. W. (1993). New views of the thalamic reticular nucleus in the adult and the developing brain. *Trends in Neurosciences* 16, 240–245.

Molinari, M., Leggio, M. G., Dell'Anna, M. E., Giannetti, S., & Macchi, G. (1993). Structural evidence in favour of a relay fnction for the anterior intralaminar nuclei. In *Thalamic Networks for Relay and Modulation*, eds.

Minciacchi, D., Molinari, M., Macchi, G., & Jones, E. G., pp. 197–208. Pergamon, Oxford, England.

Molinari, M., Dell'Anna, M. E., Rausell, E., Leggio, M. G., Hashikawa, T., & Jones, E. G. (1995). Auditory thalamocortical pathways defined in monkeys by calcium-binding protein immunoreactivity. *Journal of Comparative Neurology* 362, 171–194.

Molnar, E., & Isaac, J. T. (2002). Developmental and activity dependent regulation of ionotropic glutamate receptors at synapses. *ScientificWorldJournal* 2, 27–47.

Molnár, Z., Adams, R., & Blakemore, C. (1998). Mechanisms underlying the early establishment of thalamocortical connections in the rat. *Journal of Neuroscience* 18, 5723–5745.

Molotchnikoff, S., Casanova, C., & Cerat, A. (1988). The consequences of the superior colliculus output on lateral geniculate and pulvinar responses. *Progress in Brain Research* 75, 67–74.

Mombaerts, P., Wang, F., Dulac, C., Chao, S. K., Nemes, A., Mendelsohn, M., Edmondson, J., & Axel, R. (1996). Visualizing an olfactory sensory map. *Cell* 87, 675–686.

Montero, V. M. (1986). The interneuronal nature of GABAergic neurons in the lateral geniculate nucleus of the rhesus monkey: a combined HRP and GABA-immunocytochemical study. *Experimental Brain Research* 64, 615–622.

Montero, V. M. (1987). Ultrastructural identification of synaptic terminals from the axon of type 3 interneurons in the cat lateral geniculate nucleus. *Journal of Comparative Neurology* 264, 268–283.

Montero, V. M. (1989). The GABA-immunoreactive neurons in the interlaminar regions of the cat lateral geniculate nucleus: light and electron microscopic observations. *Experimental Brain Research* 75, 497–512.

Montero, V. M. (1991). A quantitative study of synaptic contacts on interneurons and relay cells of the cat lateral geniculate nucleus. *Experimental Brain Research* 86, 257–270.

Montero, V. M., & Guillery, R. W. (1978). Abnormalities of the corticogeniculate pathway in Siamese cats. *Journal of Comparative Neurology* 179, 1–12.

Montero, V. M., & Scott, G. L. (1981). Synaptic terminals in the dorsal lateral geniculate nucleus from neurons of the thalamic reticular nucleus: a light and electron microscope autoradiographic study. *Neuroscience* 6, 2561–2577.

Montero, V. M., & Zempel, J. (1985). Evidence for two types of GABA-containing interneurons in the A-laminae of the cat lateral geniculate nucleus: a double-label HRP and GABA-immunocytochemical study. *Experimental Brain Research* 60, 603–609.

Montero, V. M., Guillery, R. W., & Woolsey, C. N. (1977). Retinotopic organization within the thalamic reticular nucleus demonstrated by a double label autoradiographic technique. *Brain Research* 138, 407–421.

Mooney, D. M., Zhang, L., Basile, C., Senatorov, V. V., Ngsee, J., Omar, A., & Hu, B. (2004). Distinct forms of cholinergic modulation in parallel thalamic sensory pathways. *Proceedings of the National Academy of Sciences of the United States of America* 101, 320–324.

Morest, D. K. (1964). The neuronal architecture of the medial geniculate body of the cat. *Journal of Anatomy (London)* 98, 611–630.

Morest, D. K. (1975). Synaptic relationships of Golgi type II cells in the medial geniculate body of the cat. *Journal of Comparative Neurology* 162, 157–193.

Morrison, J. H., & Foote, S. L. (1986). Noradrenergic and serotoninergic innervation of cortical, thalamic, and tectal visual structures in Old and New World monkeys. *Journal of Comparative Neurology* 243, 117–138.

Mott, D. D., & Lewis, D. V. (1994). The pharmacology and function of central $GABA_B$ receptors. *International Review of Neurobiology* 36, 97–223.

Mountcastle, V. B. (1997). The columnar organization of the neocortex. *Brain* 120 (Pt. 4), 701–722.

Mukhametov, L., & Rizzolatti, G. (1969). Effect of sleep and waking on flash evoked discharges of lateral geniculate units in unrestrained cats. *Brain Research* 13, 404–406.

Mukherjee, P., & Kaplan, E. (1995). Dynamics of neurons in the cat lateral geniculate nucleus: *in vivo* electrophysiology and computational modeling. *Journal of Neurophysiology* 74, 1222–1243.

Munkle, M. C., Waldvogel, H. J., & Faull, R. L. (2000). The distribution of calbindin, calretinin and parvalbumin immunoreactivity in the human thalamus. *Journal of Chemical Neuroanatomy* 19, 155–173.

Murphy, P. C., & Sillito, A. M. (1996). Functional morphology of the feedback pathway from area 17 of the cat visual cortex to the lateral geniculate nucleus. *Journal of Neuroscience* 16, 1180–1192.

Murphy, P. C., Uhlrich, D. J., Tamamaki, N., & Sherman, S. M. (1994). Brainstem modulation of the response properties of cells in the cat's perigeniculate nucleus. *Visual Neuroscience* 11, 781–791.

Murphy, P. C., Duckett, S. G., & Sillito, A. M. (2000). Comparison of the laminar distribution of input from areas 17 and 18 of the visual cortex to the lateral geniculate nucleus of the cat. *Journal of Neuroscience* 20, 845–853.

Nakanishi, S., Nakajima, Y., Masu, M., Ueda, Y., Nakahara, K., Watanabe, D., Yamaguchi, S., Kawabata, S., & Okada, M. (1998). Glutamate receptors: brain function and signal transduction. *Brain Research Reviews* 26, 230–235.

Nakano, K. (2000). Neural circuits and topographic organization of the basal ganglia and related regions. *Brain & Development* 22(Suppl. 1), S5–S16.

Nakayasu, H., Kimura, H., & Kuriyama, K. (1995). Cerebral $GABA_A$ and $GABA_B$ receptors: structure and function. *Annals of the New York Academy of Sciences* 757, 516–527.

Négyessy, L., Hámori, J., & Bentivoglio, M. (1998). Contralateral cortical projection to the mediodorsal thalamic nucleus: origin and synaptic organization in the rat. *Neuroscience* 84, 741–753.

Nelson, J. I., Salin, P. A., Munk, M. H. J., Arzi, M., & Bullier, J. (1992). Spatial and temporal coherence in cortico-cortical connections: a cross-correlation study in areas 17 and 18 in the cat. *Visual Neuroscience* 9, 21–37.

Nelson, R., & Kolb, H. (2004). ON and OFF pathways in the vertebrate retina and visual system. In *The Visual Neurosciences*, eds. Chalupa, L. M., & Werner, J. S., pp. 260–278. MIT Press, Cambridge, Mass.

Nelson, S. B., & LeVay, S. (1985). Topographic organization of the optic radiation of the cat. *Journal of Comparative Neurology* 240, 322–330.

Nicolelis, M. A., Baccala, L. A., Lin, R. C., & Chapin, J. K. (1995). Sensorimotor encoding by synchronous neural ensemble activity at multiple levels of the somatosensory system. *Science* 268, 1353–1358.

Nicolelis, M. A. L., & Fanselow, E. E. (2002). Dynamic shifting in thalamocortical processing during different behavioural states. *Philosophical Transactions of the Royal Society of London, Series B, Biological Sciences* 357, 1753–1758.

Nicoll, R. A. (1988). The coupling of neurotransmitter receptors to Ion channels in the brain. *Science* 241, 545–551.

Nicoll, R. A., Malenka, R. C., & Kauer, J. A. (1990). Functional comparison of neurotransmitter receptor subtypes in mammalian central nervous system. *Physiological Reviews* 70, 513–565.

Niimi, K., Ono, K., & Kusunose, M. (1984). Projections of the medial geniculate nucleus to layer 1 of the auditory cortex in the cat traced with horseradish peroxidase. *Neuroscience Letters* 45, 223–228.

Niimi, K., Yamazaki, Y., Matsuoka, H., Kusunose, M., Imataki, T., & Ono, K. (1985). Thalamic projections to the posterior suprasylvian gyrus and the ventrally adjacent cortex in the cat traced with horseradish peroxidase. *Journal für Hirnforschung* 26, 497–508.

Nissl, F. (1913). Die Grosshirnanteile des Kanninchens. *Archiv für Psychiatrie und Nervenkrankheiten* 52, 867–953.

Norton, T. T., Casagrande, V. A., Irvin, G. E., Sesma, M. A., & Petry, H. M. (1988). Contrast-sensitivity functions of W-, X-, and Y-like relay cells in the lateral geniculate nucleus of bush baby, *Galago crassicaudatus*. *Journal of Neurophysiology* 59, 1639–1656.

Ogren, M. P., & Hendrickson, A. E. (1979). The morphology and distribution of striate cortex terminals in the inferior and lateral subdivisions of the Macaca monkey pulvinar. *Journal of Comparative Neurology* 188, 179–199.

Ohara, P. T. (1988). Synaptic organization of the thalamic reticular nucleus. *Journal of Electron Microscopy Technique* 10, 283–292.

Ohara, P. T., & Havton, L. A. (1994). Preserved features of thalamocortical projection neuron dendritic architecture in the somatosensory thalamus of the rat, cat and macaque. *Brain Research* 648, 259–264.

Ohara, P. T., & Lieberman, A. R. (1981). Thalamic reticular nucleus: anatomical evidence that cortico-reticular axons establish monosynaptic contact with reticulo-geniculate projection cells. *Brain Research* 207, 153–156.

Ohara, P. T., & Lieberman, A. R. (1985). The thalamic reticular nucleus of the adult rat: experimental anatomical studies. *Journal of Neurocytology* 14, 365–411.

Ohara, P. T., Chazal, G., & Ralston, H. J. III (1989). Ultrastructural analysis of GABA-immunoreactive elements in the monkey thalamic ventrobasal complex. *Journal of Comparative Neurology* 283, 541–558.

Ojima, H. (1994). Terminal morphology and distribution of corticothalamic fibers originating from layers 5 and 6 of cat primary auditory cortex. *Cerebral Cortex* 4, 646–663.

Ojima, H., Murakami, K., & Kishi, K. (1996). Dual termination modes of corticothalamic fibers originating from pyramids of layers 5 and 6 in cat visual cortical area 17. *Neuroscience Letters* 208, 57–60.

Olausson, B., Shyu, B. C., & Rydenhag, B. (1989). Projection from the thalamic intralaminar nuclei on the isocortex of the rat: a surface potential study. *Experimental Brain Research* 75, 543–554.

Olavarria, J., & Montero, V. M. (1984). Relation of callosal and striate-extrastriate cortical connections in the rat: morphological definition of extrastriate visual areas. *Experimental Brain Research* 54, 240–252.

Olavarria, J., & Montero, V. M. (1989). Organization of visual cortex in the mouse revealed by correlating callosal and striate-extrastriate connections. *Visual Neuroscience* 3, 59–69.

O'Regan, J. K., & Noë, A. (2001). A sensorimotor account of vision and visual consciousness. *Behavioral and Brain Sciences* 24, 939–973.

Otani, S., Daniel, H., Roisin, M. P., & Crepel, F. (2003). Dopaminergic modulation of long-term synaptic plasticity in rat prefrontal neurons. *Cerebral Cortex* 13, 1251–1256.

Ozawa, S., Kamiya, H., & Tsuzuki, K. (1998). Glutamate receptors in the mammalian central nervous system. *Progress in Neurobiology* 54, 581–618.

Ozen, G., Augustine, G. J., & Hall, W. C. (2000). Contribution of superficial layer neurons to premotor bursts in the superior colliculus. *Journal of Neurophysiology* 84, 460–471.

Pallas, S. L., Hahm, J., & Sur, M. (1994). Morphology of retinal axons induced to arborize in a novel target, the medial geniculate nucleus. I. Comparison with arbors in normal targets. *Journal of Comparative Neurology* 349, 343–362.

Pallas, S. L., & Sur, M. (1994). Morphology of retinal axon arbors induced to arborize in a novel target, the medial geniculate nucleus. II. Comparison with axons from the inferior colliculus. *Journal of Comparative Neurology* 349, 363–376.

Pandya, D. N., & Rosene, D. L. (1993). Laminar termination patterns of thalamic, callosal, and association afferents in the primary auditory area of the rhesus monkey. *Experimental Neurology* 119, 220–234.

Pape, H.-C., Budde, T., Mager, R., & Kisvárday, Z. F. (1994). Prevention of Ca^{2+}-mediated action potentials in GABAergic local circuit neurones of rat thalamus by a transient K^+ current. *Journal of Physiology (London)* 478, 403–422.

Pape, H.-C., & Mager, R. (1992). Nitric oxide controls oscillatory activity in thalamocortical neurons. *Neuron* 9, 441–448.

Pape, H.-C., & McCormick, D. A. (1989). Noradrenaline and serotonin selectively modulate thalamic burst firing by enhancing a hyperpolarization-activated cation current. *Nature* 340, 715–718.

Pape, H.-C., & McCormick, D. A. (1995). Electrophysiological and pharmacological properties of interneurons in the cat dorsal lateral geniculate nucleus. *Neuroscience* 68, 1105–1125.

Paré, D., Hazrati, L. N., Parent, A., & Steriade, M. (1990). Substantia nigra pars reticulata projects to the reticular thalamic nucleus of the cat: a morphological and electrophysiological study. *Brain Research* 535, 139–146.

Parra, P., Gulyas, A. I., & Miles, R. (1998). How many subtypes of inhibitory cells in the hippocampus? *Neuron* 20, 983–993.

Patel, N. C., & Bickford, M. E. (1997). Synaptic targets of cholinergic terminals in the pulvinar nucleus of the cat. *Journal of Comparative Neurology* 387, 266–278.

Patel, N. C., Carden, W. B., & Bickford, M. E. (1999). Synaptic targets of cholinergic terminals in the cat lateral posterior nucleus. *Journal of Comparative Neurology* 410, 31–41.

Paus, T., Collins, D. L., Evans, A. C., Leonard, G., Pike, B., & Zijdenbos, A. (2001). Maturation of white matter in the human brain: a review of magnetic resonance studies. *Brain Research Bulletin* 54, 255–266.

Pearson, J. C., & Haines, D. E. (1980). Somatosensory thalamus of a prosimian primate (*Galago senegalensis*). II. An HRP and Golgi study of the ventral posterolateral nucleus (VPL). *Journal of Comparative Neurology* 190, 559–580.

Penny, G. R., Itoh, K., & Diamond, I. T. (1982). Cells of a different sizes in the ventral nuclei project to different layers of the somatic cortex in the cat. *Brain Research* 242, 55–65.

Penny, G. R., Fitzpatrick, D., Schmechel, D. E., & Diamond, I. T. (1983). Glutamic acid decarboxylase-immunoreactive neurons and horseradish peroxidase-labeled projection neurons in the ventral posterior nucleus of the cat and *Galago senegalensis*. *Journal of Neuroscience* 3, 1868–1887.

Perkel, D. H., Gerstein, G. L., & Moore, G. P. (1967). Neuronal spike trains and stochastic point processes. II. Simultaneous spike trains. *Biophysical Journal* 7, 419–440.

Perry, V. H., & Cowey, A. (1984). Retinal ganglion cells that project to the superior colliculus and pretectum in the macaque monkey. *Neuroscience* 12, 1125–1137.

Peruzzi, D., Bartlett, E., Smith, P. H., & Oliver, D. L. (1997). A monosynaptic GABAergic input from the inferior colliculus to the medial geniculate body in rat. *Journal of Neuroscience* 17, 3766–3777.

Peschanski, M., Lee, C. L., & Ralston, H. J. III (1984). The structural organization of the ventrobasal complex of the rat as revealed by the analysis of physiologically characterized neurons injected intracellularly with horseradish peroxidase. *Brain Research* 297, 63–74.

Peters, A., & Palay, S. L. (1966). The morphology of laminae A and A1 of the dorsal nucleus of the lateral geniculate body of the cat. *Journal of Anatomy* 100, 451–486.

Peters, A., Palay, S. L., & Webster, H. d. (1991). *The Fine Structure of the Nervous System*. Oxford University Press, New York.

Pfrieger, F. W., & Barres, B. A. (1996). New views on synapse–glia interactions. *Current Opinion in Neurobiology* 6, 615–621.

Pin, J. P., & Bockaert, J. (1995). Get receptive to metabotropic glutamate receptors. *Current Opinion in Neurobiology* 5, 342–349.

Pin, J. P., & Duvoisin, R. (1995). The metabotropic glutamate receptors: structure and functions. *Neuropharmacology* 34, 1–26.

Pinault, D., & Deschênes, M. (1998a). Anatomical evidence for a mechanism of lateral inhibition in the rat thalamus. *European Journal of Neuroscience* 10, 3462–3469.

Pinault, D., & Deschênes, M. (1998b). Projection and innervation patterns of individual thalamic reticular axons in the thalamus of the adult rat: a three-dimensional, graphic, and morphometric analysis. *Journal of Comparative Neurology* 391, 180–203.

Pinault, D., Bourassa, J., & Deschênes, M. (1995a). Thalamic reticular input to the rat visual thalamus: a single fiber study using biocytin as an anterograde tracer. *Brain Research* 670, 147–152.

Pinault, D., Bourassa, J., & Deschênes, M. (1995b). The axonal arborization of single thalamic reticular neurons in the somatosensory thalamus of the rat. *European Journal of Neuroscience* 7, 31–40.

Pinault, D., Smith, Y., & Deschênes, M. (1997). Dendrodendritic and axoaxonic synapses in the thalamic reticular nucleus of the adult rat. *Journal of Neuroscience* 17, 3215–3233.

Polyak, S. (1957). *The Vertebrate Visual System*. University of Chicago Press, Chicago.

Powell, T. P. S., & Cowan, W. M. (1956). A study of thalamo-striate relations in the monkey. *Brain* 79, 364–390.

Power, B. D., Kolmac, C. I., & Mitrofanis, J. (1999). Evidence for a large projection from the zona incerta to the dorsal thalamus. *Journal of Comparative Neurology* 404, 554–565.

Power, B. D., & Mitrofanis, J. (2001). Zona incerta: substrate for contralateral interconnectivity in the thalamus of rats. *Journal of Comparative Neurology* 436, 52–63.

Power, B. D., & Mitrofanis, J. (2002). Ultrastructure of afferents from the zona incerta to the posterior and parafascicular thalamic nuclei of rats. *Journal of Comparative Neurology* 451, 33–44.

Powers, R. K., Sawczuk, A., Musick, J. R., & Binder, M. D. (1999). Multiple mechanisms of spike-frequency adaptation in motoneurones. *Journal de Physiologie* (Paris) 93, 101–114.

Preuss, T. M., & Goldman-Rakic, P. S. (1987). Crossed corticothalamic and thalamocortical connections of macaque prefrontal cortex. *Journal of Comparative Neurology* 257, 269–281.

Price, J. L. (1986). Subcortical projections from the amygdaloid complex. *Advances in Experimental Medicine and Biology* 203, 19–33.

Purves, D., Augustine, G. J., Fitzpatrick, D., Katz, L. C., Lamantia, A.-S., & McNamara, J. O. (1997). *Neuroscience*. Sinauer, Sunderland, Mass.

Qian, A., & Johnson, J. W. (2002). Channel gating of NMDA receptors. *Physiology & Behavior* 77, 577–582.

Raczkowski, D., & Fitzpatrick, D. (1989). Organization of cholinergic synapses in the cat's dorsal lateral geniculate and perigeniculate nuclei. *Journal of Comparative Neurology* 288, 676–690.

Raczkowski, D., Hamos, J. E., & Sherman, S. M. (1988). Synaptic circuitry of physiologically identified W-cells in the cat's dorsal lateral geniculate nucleus. *Journal of Neuroscience* 8, 31–48.

Radhakrishnan, V., Tsoukatos, J., Davis, K. D., Tasker, R. R., Lozano, A. M., & Dostrovsky, J. O. (1999). A comparison of the burst activity of lateral thalamic neurons in chronic pain and non-pain patients. *Pain* 80, 567–575.

Rafols, J. A., & Valverde, F. (1973). The structure of the dorsal lateral geniculate nucleus in the mouse: a Golgi and electron microscopic study. *Journal of Comparative Neurology* 150, 303–332.

Rall, W. (1977). Core conductor theory and cable properties of neurons. In *Handbook of Physiology: The Nervous System I*, eds. Kandel, E., & Geiger, S., pp. 39–97. American Physiological Society, Bethesda, Md.

Ralston, H. J., III (1971). Evidence for presynaptic dendrites and a proposal for their mechanism of action. *Nature* 230, 585–587.

Ralston, H. J., III (1969). The synaptic organization of lemniscal projections to the ventrobasal thalamus of the cat. *Brain Research* 14, 99–116.

Ralston, H. J., III, & Herman, M. M. (1969). The fine structure of neurons and synapses in ventrobasal thalamus of the cat. *Brain Research* 14, 77–97.

Ramcharan, E. J., Gnadt, J. W., & Sherman, S. M. (2000). Burst and tonic firing in thalamic cells of unanesthetized, behaving monkeys. *Visual Neuroscience* 17, 55–62.

Ramcharan, E. J., Gnadt, J. W., & Sherman, S. M. (2005). Higher order thalamic relays burst more than do first order relays. *Proceedings of the National Academy of Sciences of the United States of America*, in press.

Rapisardi, S. C., & Miles, T. P. (1984). Synaptology of retinal terminals in the dorsal lateral geniculate nucleus of the cat. *Journal of Comparative Neurology* 223, 515–534.

Rausell, E., Bae, C. S., Vinuela, A., Huntley, G. W., & Jones, E. G. (1992). Calbindin and parvalbumin cells in monkey VPL thalamic nucleus: distribution, laminar cortical projections, and relations to spinothalamic terminations. *Journal of Neuroscience* 12, 4088–4111.

Rausell, E., & Jones, E. G. (1991). Chemically distinct compartments of the thalamic VPM nucleus in monkeys relay principal and spinal trigeminal pathways to different layers of the somatosensory cortex. *Journal of Neuroscience* 11, 226–237.

Reale, R. A., & Imig, T. J. (1980). Tonotopic organization in auditory cortex of the cat. *Journal of Comparative Neurology* 192, 265–291.

Recasens, M., & Vignes, M. (1995). Excitatory amino acid metabotropic receptor subtypes and calcium regulation. *Annals of the New York Academy of Sciences* 757, 418–429.

Reichova, I., & Sherman, S. M. (2004). Somatosensory corticothalamic projections: Distinguishing drivers from modulators. *Journal of Neurophysiology* 92, 2185–2197.

Reid, R. C., & Alonso, J. M. (1995). Specificity of monosynaptic connections from thalamus to visual cortex. *Nature* 378, 281–284.

Reid, R. C., & Alonso, J. M. (1996). The processing and encoding of information in the visual cortex. *Current Opinion in Neurobiology* 6, 475–480.

Reid, S. N. M., Romano, C., Hughes, T., & Daw, N. W. (1997). Developmental and sensory-dependent changes of phosphoinositide-linked metabotropic glutamate receptors. *Journal of Comparative Neurology* 389, 577–583.

Reinagel, P., Godwin, D. W., Sherman, S. M., & Koch, C. (1999). Encoding of visual information by LGN bursts. *Journal of Neurophysiology* 81, 2558–2569.

Reuter, H. (1996). Diversity and function of presynaptic calcium channels in the brain. *Current Opinion in Neurobiology* 6, 331–337.

Richard, D., Gioanni, Y., Kitsikis, A., & Buser, P. (1975). A study of geniculate unit activity during cryogenic blockade of the primary visual cortex in the cat. *Experimental Brain Research* 22, 235–242.

Riedel, G., Platt, B., & Micheau, J. (2003). Glutamate receptor function in learning and memory. *Behavioural Brain Research* 140, 1–47.

Riggs, L. A., Ratliff, F., Cornsweet, J. C., & Cornsweet, T. N. (1953). The disappearance of steadily fixated visual test objects. *Journal of the Optical Society of America, A, Optics and Image Science* 43, 495–501.

Rinvik, E., & Grofova, I. (1974a). Light and electron microscopical studies of the normal nuclei ventralis lateralis and ventralis anterior thalami in the cat. *Anatomy and Embryology* 146, 57–93.

Rinvik, E., & Grofova, I. (1974b). Cerebellar projections to the nuclei ventralis lateralis and ventralis anterior thalami: experimental electron microscopical and light microscopical studies in the cat. *Anatomy and Embryology* 146, 95–111.

Rittenhouse, C. D., Shouval, H. Z., Paradiso, M. A., & Bear, M. F. (1999). Monocular deprivation induces homosynaptic long-term depression in visual cortex. *Nature* 397, 347–350.

Rivadulla, C., Rodriguez, R., Martinez-Conde, S., Acuña, C., & Cudeiro, J. (1996). The influence of nitric oxide on perigeniculate GABAergic cell activity in the anaesthetized cat. *European Journal of Neuroscience* 8, 2459–2466.

Rizzolatti, G., & Luppino, G. (2001). The cortical motor system. *Neuron* 31, 889–901.

Robertson, R. T., & Cunningham, T. J. (1981). Organization of corticothalamic projections from the parietal cortex in the cat. *Journal of Comparative Neurology* 199, 569–585.

Robson, J. A. (1983). The morphology of corticofugal axons to the dorsal lateral geniculate nucleus in the cat. *Journal of Comparative Neurology* 216, 89–103.

Robson, J. A., & Hall, W. C. (1977a). The organization of the pulvinar in the grey squirrel (*Sciurus carolinensis*). I. Cytoarchitecture and connections. *Journal of Comparative Neurology* 173, 355–388.

Robson, J. A., & Hall, W. C. (1977b). The organization of the pulvinar in the grey squirrel (*Sciurus carolinensis*). II. Synaptic organization and comparisons with the dorsal lateral geniculate nucleus. *Journal of Comparative Neurology* 173, 389–416.

Rockel, A. J., Hiorns, R. W., & Powell, T. P. S. (1980). The basic uniformity in structure of the neocortex. *Brain* 103, 221–244.

Rockland, K. S. (1989). Bistratified distribution of terminal arbors of individual axons projecting from area V1 to middle temporal area (MT) in the macaque monkey. *Visual Neuroscience* 3, 155–170.

Rockland, K. S. (1996). Two types of corticopulvinar terminations: round (type 2) and elongate (type 1). *Journal of Comparative Neurology* 368, 57–87.

Rockland, K. S. (1998). Convergence and branching patterns of round, type 2 corticopulvinar axons. *Journal of Comparative Neurology* 390, 515–536.

Rockland, K. S., & Knutson, T. (2000). Feedback connections from area MT of the squirrel monkey to areas V1 and V2. *Journal of Comparative Neurology* 425, 345–368.

Rockland, K. S., & Pandya, D. N. (1979). Laminar origins and terminations of cortical connections of the occipital lobe in the rhesus monkey. *Brain Research* 179, 3–20.

Rockland, K. S., & Virga, A. (1989). Terminal arbors of individual "feedback" axons projecting from area V2 to V1 in the macaque monkey: a study using immunohistochemistry of anterogradely transported *Phaseolus vulgaris*-leucoagglutinin. *Journal of Comparative Neurology* 285, 54–72.

Rockland, K. S., Andresen, J., Cowie, R. J., & Robinson, D. L. (1999). Single axon analysis of pulvinocortical connections to several visual areas in the macaque. *Journal of Comparative Neurology* 406, 221–250.

Rodieck, R. W. (1998). *The First Steps in Seeing*. Sinauer, Sunderland, Mass.

Rodieck, R. W., & Brening, R. K. (1983). Retinal ganglion cells: properties, types, genera, pathways and trans-species comparisons. *Brain, Behavior and Evolution* 23, 121–164.

Rogawski, M. A. (1985). The A-current: How ubiquitous a feature of excitable cells is it? *Trends in Neurosciences* 8, 214–219.

Romanski, L. M., Tian, B., Fritz, J., Mishkin, M., Goldman-Rakic, P. S., & Rauschecker, J. P. (1999). Dual streams of auditory afferents target multiple domains in the primate prefrontal cortex. *Nature Neuroscience* 2, 1131–1136.

Rose, J. E. (1952). The cortical connections of the reticular complex of the thalamus. *Association for Nervous and Mental Disorders* 30, 455–479.

Rose, J. E., & Woolsey, C. N. (1948). Structure and relations of limbic cortex and anterior thalamic nuclei in rabbit and cat. *Journal of Comparative Neurology* 89, 79–347.

Rose, J. E., & Woolsey, C. N. (1949). The relations of thalamic connections, cellular structure and evocable electrical activity in the auditory region of the cat. *Journal of Comparative Neurology* 91, 441–466.

Rose, J. E., & Woolsey, C. N. (1958). Cortical connections and functional organization of the thalamic auditory system of the cat. In *Biological and Bio-*

chemical Bases of Behavior, eds. Harlow, H. F., & Woolsey, C. N., pp. 127–150. University of Wisconsin Press, Madison.

Rouiller, E. M., & Welker, E. (2000). A comparative analysis of the morphology of corticothalamic projections in mammals. *Brain Research Bulletin 53*, 727–741.

Royce, G. J. (1983). Cells of origin of corticothalamic projections upon the centromedian and parafascicular nuclei in the cat. *Brain Research 258*, 11–21.

Royce, G. J., & Mourey, R. J. (1985). Efferent connections of the centromedian and parafascicular thalamic nuclei: an autoradiographic investigation in the cat. *Journal of Comparative Neurology 235*, 277–300.

Royce, G. J., Bromley, S., Gracco, C., & Beckstead, R. M. (1989). Thalamocortical connections of the rostral intralaminar nuclei: an autoradiographic analysis in the cat. *Journal of Comparative Neurology 288*, 555–582.

Sáez, J. A., Palomares, J. M., Vives, F., Domínguez, I., Villegas, I., Montes, R., Price, D. J., & Ferrer, J. M. (1998). Electrophysiological and neurochemical study of the rat geniculo-cortical pathway: evidence for glutamatergic neurotransmission. *European Journal of Neuroscience 10*, 2790–2801.

Sakai, S. T., Inase, M., & Tanji, J. (1996). Comparison of cerebellothalamic and pallidothalamic projections in the monkey (*Macaca fuscata*): a double anterograde labeling study. *Journal of Comparative Neurology 368*, 215–228.

Salin, P.-A., & Bullier, J. (1995). Corticocortical connections in the visual system: structure and function. *Physiological Reviews 75*, 107–154.

Salt, T. E. (2002). Glutamate receptor functions in sensory relay in the thalamus. *Philosophical Transactions of the Royal Society of London, Series B, Biological Sciences 357*, 1759–1766.

Salt, T. E., & Eaton, S. A. (1996). Functions of ionotropic and metabotropic glutamate receptors in sensory transmission in the mammalian thalamus. *Progress in Neurobiology 48*, 55–72.

Sanchez-Gonzalez, M. A., Garcia-Cabezas, M. A., Rico, B., & Cavada, C. (2005). The primate thalamus is a key target for brain dopamine. *Journal of Neuroscience 25*, 6076–6083.

Sanchez-Vives, M. V., Bal, T., Kim, U., Von Krosigk, M., & McCormick, D. A. (1996). Are the interlaminar zones of the ferret dorsal lateral geniculate nucleus actually part of the perigeniculate nucleus? *Journal of Neuroscience 16*, 5923–5941.

Sanchez-Vives, M. V., & McCormick, D. A. (1997). Functional properties of perigeniculate inhibition of dorsal lateral geniculate nucleus thalamocortical neurons *in vitro*. *Journal of Neuroscience 17*, 8880–8893.

Sanderson, K. J. (1971). The projection of the visual field to the lateral geniculate and medial interlaminar nuclei in the cat. *Journal of Comparative Neurology 143*, 101–118.

Sanderson, K. J., Bishop, P. O., & Darian-Smith, I. (1971). The properties of the binocular receptive fields of lateral geniculate neurons. *Experimental Brain Research 13*, 178–207.

Schall, J. D., Ault, S. J., Vitek, D. J., & Leventhal, A. G. (1988). Experimental induction of an abnormal ipsilateral visual field representation in the geniculocortical pathway of normally pigmented cats. *Journal of Neuroscience* 8, 2039–2048.

Schambra, U. B., Lauder, J. M., & Silver, J. (1992). *Atlas of the Prenatal Mouse Brain*. Academic Press, San Diego, Calif.

Scharfman, H. E., Lu, S.-M., Guido, W., Adams, P. R., & Sherman, S. M. (1990). N-methyl-D-aspartate (NMDA) receptors contribute to excitatory postsynaptic potentials of cat lateral geniculate neurons recorded in thalamic slices. *Proceedings of the National Academy of Sciences of the United States of America* 87, 4548–4552.

Scheibel, M. E., & Scheibel, A. B. (1966). The organization of the nucleus reticularis thalami: a Golgi study. *Brain Research* 1, 43–62.

Schiller, J., Schiller, Y., Stuart, G., & Sakmann, B. (1997). Calcium action potentials restricted to distal apical dendrites of rat neocortical pyramidal neurons. *Journal of Physiology* 505, 605–616.

Schiller, P. H., & Malpeli, J. G. (1977). Properties and tectal projections of monkey retinal ganglion cells. *Journal of Neurophysiology* 40, 428–445.

Schiller, P. H., & Malpeli, J. G. (1978). Functional specificity of lateral geniculate nucleus laminae of the rhesus monkey. *Journal of Neurophysiology* 41, 788–797.

Schiller, P. H., & Tehovnik, E. J. (2001). Look and see: how the brain moves your eyes about. *Progress in Brain Research* 134, 127–142.

Schmidt, M. (1996). Neurons in the cat pretectum that project to the dorsal lateral geniculate nucleus are activated during saccades. *Journal of Neurophysiology* 76, 2907–2918.

Schmielau, F., & Singer, W. (1977). The role of visual cortex for binocular interactions in the cat lateral geniculate nucleus. *Brain Research* 120, 354–361.

Schneider, G. E. (1969). Two visual systems. *Science* 163, 895–902.

Schwartz, M. L., Dekker, J. J., & Goldman-Rakic, P. S. (1991). Dual mode of corticothalamic synaptic termination in the mediodorsal nucleus of the rhesus monkey. *Journal of Comparative Neurology* 309, 289–304.

Sefton, A. J., & Burke, W. (1966). Mechanisms od recurrent inhibition in the lateral geniculate nucleur of the cat. *Nature* 211, 1276–1278.

Shapley, R., & Lennie, P. (1985). Spatial frequency analysis in the visual system. *Annual Reviews in Neuroscience* 8, 547–583.

Sharma, J., Angelucci, A., & Sur, M. (2000). Induction of visual orientation modules in auditory cortex. *Nature* 404, 841–847.

Shatz, C. J. (1994). Role for spontaneous neural activity in the patterning of connections between retina and LGN during visual system development. *International Journal of Developmental Neuroscience* 12, 531–546.

Shatz, C. J. (1996). Emergence of order in visual system development. *Proceedings of the National Academy of Sciences of the United States of America* 93, 602–608.

Shatz, C. J., & LeVay, S. (1979). Siamese cat: altered connections of visual cortex. *Science* 204, 328–330.

Sherman, S. M. (1985). Functional organization of the W-, X-, and Y-cell pathways in the cat: a review and hypothesis. In *Progress in Psychobiology and*

Physiological Psychology, vol. 11, eds. Sprague, J. M., & Epstein, A. N., pp. 233–314. Academic Press, Orlando, Fla.

Sherman, S. M. (1996). Dual response modes in lateral geniculate neurons: mechanisms and functions. *Visual Neuroscience* 13, 205–213.

Sherman, S. M. (2001). Tonic and burst firing: dual modes of thalamocortical relay. *Trends in Neurosciences* 24, 122–126.

Sherman, S. M. (2004). Interneurons and triadic circuitry of the thalamus. *Trends in Neurosciences* 27, 670–675.

Sherman, S. M., & Friedlander, M. J. (1988). Identification of X versus Y properties for interneurons in the A-laminae of the cat's lateral geniculate nucleus. *Experimental Brain Research* 73, 384–392.

Sherman, S. M., & Guillery, R. W. (1996). The functional organization of thalamocortical relays. *Journal of Neurophysiology* 76, 1367–1395.

Sherman, S. M., & Guillery, R. W. (1998). On the actions that one nerve cell can have on another: Distinguishing "drivers" from "modulators." *Proceedings of the National Academy of Sciences of the United States of America* 95, 7121–7126.

Sherman, S. M., & Guillery, R. W. (2001). *Exploring the Thalamus.* Academic Press, San Diego, Calif.

Sherman, S. M., & Guillery, R. W. (2004). Thalamus. In *Synaptic Organization of the Brain,* ed. Shepherd, G. M., pp. 311–359. Oxford University Press, Oxford, England.

Sherman, S. M., & Koch, C. (1986). The control of retinogeniculate transmission in the mammalian lateral geniculate nucleus. *Experimental Brain Research* 63, 1–20.

Sherman, S. M., & Spear, P. D. (1982). Organization of visual pathways in normal and visually deprived cats. *Physiological Reviews* 62, 738–855.

Shibata, H. (1998). Organization of projections of rat retrosplenial cortex to the anterior thalamic nuclei. *European Journal of Neuroscience* 10, 3210–3219.

Shinoda, Y., Futami, T., Mitoma, H., & Yokota, J. (1988). Morphology of single neurones in the cerebello-rubrospinal system. *Behavioural Brain Research* 28, 59–64.

Shipp, S. (2001). Corticopulvinar connections of areas V5, V4, and V3 in the macaque monkey: A dual model of retinal and cortical topographies. *Journal of Comparative Neurology* 439, 469–490.

Shipp, S. (2003). The functional logic of cortico-pulvinar connections. *Philosophical Transactions of the Royal Society of London, Series B, Biological Sciences* 358, 1605–1624.

Shipp, S., & Zeki, S. (1989a). The organization of connections between areas V5 and V1 in macaque monkey visual cortex. *European Journal of Neuroscience* 1, 309–332.

Shipp, S., & Zeki, S. (1989b). The organization of connections between areas V5 and V2 in macaque monkey visual cortex. *European Journal of Neurosciences* 1, 333–354.

Shore, S. E., & Moore, J. K. (1998). Sources of input to the cochlear granule cell region in the guinea pig. *Hearing Research* 116, 33–42.

Shosaku, A. (1985). A comparison of receptive field properties of vibrissa neurons between the rat thalamic reticular and ventro-basal nuclei. *Brain Research* 347, 36–40.

Shosaku, A., Kayama, Y., & Sumitomo, I. (1984). Somatopic organization in the rat thalamic reticular nucleus. *Brain Research* 311, 57–63.

Sidibe, M., Bevan, M. D., Bolam, J. P., & Smith, Y. (1997). Efferent connections of the internal globus pallidus in the squirrel monkey. I. Topography and synaptic organization of the pallidothalamic projection. *Journal of Comparative Neurology* 382, 323–347.

Sillito, A. M., & Jones, H. E. (2002). Corticothalamic interactions in the transfer of visual information. *Philosophical Transactions of the Royal Society of London, series B, Biological Sciences* 357, 1739–1752.

Sillito, A. M., Jones, H. E., Gerstein, G. L., & West, D. C. (1994). Feature-linked synchronization of thalamic relay cell firing induced by feedback from the visual cortex. *Nature* 369, 479–482.

Silver, R. A., Cull-Candy, S. G., & Takahashi, T. (1996). Non-NMDA glutamate receptor occupancy and open probability at a rat cerebellar synapse with single and multiple release sites. *Journal of Physiology* 494 (Pt. 1), 231–250.

Sincich, L. C., Park, K. V., Wohlgemuth, MN. J., & Horton, J. C. (2004). Bypassing V1: a direct geniculate input to area MT. *Nature Neuroscience* 7, 1123–1128.

Singer, W. (1977). Control of thalamic transmission by corticofugal and ascending reticular pathways in the visual system. *Physiological Reviews* 57, 386–420.

Singer, W., & Gray, C. M. (1995). Visual feature integration and the temporal correlation hypothesis. *Annual Reviews in Neuroscience* 18, 555–586.

Sirota, M. G., Swadlow, H. A., & Beloozerova, I. N. (2005). Three channels of corticothalamic communication during locomotion. *Journal of Neuroscience* 25, 5915–5925.

Smith, G. D., & Sherman, S. M. (2002). Detectability of excitatory versus inhibitory drive in an integrate-and-fire-or-burst thalamocortical relay neuron model. *Journal of Neuroscience* 22, 10242–10250.

Smith, G. D., Cox, C. L., Sherman, S. M., & Rinzel, J. (2000). Fourier analysis of sinusoidally-driven thalamocortical relay neurons and a minimal integrate-and-fire-or-burst model. *Journal of Neurophysiology* 83, 588–610.

Smith, G. D., Cox, C. L., Sherman, S. M., & Rinzel, J. (2001). A firing-rate model of spike-frequency adaptation in sinusoidally-driven thalamocortical relay neurons. *Thalamus* 1, 135–156.

So, Y.-T., & Shapley, R. (1981). Spatial tuning of cells in and around lateral geniculate nucleus of the cat: X and Y relay cells and perigeniculate interneurons. *Journal of Neurophysiology* 45, 107–120.

Sohal, V. S., & Huguenard, J. R. (2003). Inhibitory interconnections control burst pattern and emergent network synchrony in reticular thalamus. *Journal of Neuroscience* 23, 8978–8988.

Sohal, V. S., Keist, R., Rudolph, U., & Huguenard, J. R. (2003). Dynamic GABA$_A$ receptor subtype-specific modulation of the synchrony and duration of thalamic oscillations. *Journal of Neuroscience* 23, 3649–3657.

Somogyi, G., Hajdu, F., & Tömböl, T. (1978). Ultrastructure of the anterior ventral and anterior medial nuclei of the cat thalamus. *Experimental Brain Research* 31, 417–431.

Spillane, J. D. (1981). *The Doctrine of the Nerves.* Oxford University Press, New York.

Sprague, J. M. (1966). Interaction of cortex and superior colliculus in mediation of visually guided behavior in the cat. *Science* 153, 1544–1547.

Spreafico, R., Hayes, N. L., & Rustioni, A. (1981). Thalamic projections to the primary and secondary somatosensory cortices in cat: single and double retrograde tracer studies. *Journal of Comparative Neurology* 203, 67–90.

Spreafico, R., De Curtis, M., Frassoni, C., & Avanzini, G. (1988). Electrophysiological characteristics of morphologically identified reticular thalamic neurons from rat slices. *Neuroscience* 27, 269–238.

Spreafico, R., Battaglia, G., & Frassoni, C. (1991). The reticular thalamic nucleus (RTN) of the rat: cytoarchitectural, Golgi, immunocytochemical, and horseradish peroxidase study. *Journal of Comparative Neurology* 304, 478–490.

Stackman, R. W., & Taube, J. S. (1998). Firing properties of rat lateral mamillary single units: head direction, head pitch and angular head velocity. *Journal of Neuroscience* 18, 9020–9037.

Stanford, L. R., Friedlander, M. J., & Sherman, S. M. (1983). Morphological and physiological properties of geniculate W-cells of the cat: a comparison with X- and Y-cells. *Journal of Neurophysiology* 50, 582–608.

Stanton, G. B. (1980). Topographical organization of ascending cerebellar projections from the dentate and interposed nuclei in *Macaca mulatta*: an anterograde degeneration study. *Journal of Comparative Neurology* 190, 699–731.

Stanton, G. B. (2001). Organization of cerebellar and area "y" projections to the nucleus reticularis tegmenti pontis in macaque. *Journal of Comparative Neurology* 432, 169–183.

Stent, G. S. (1978). *Paradoxes of Progress.* W. H. Freeman, San Francisco.

Steriade, M., & Contreras, D. (1995). Relations between cortical and thalamic cellular events during transition from sleep patterns to paroxysmal activity. *Journal of Neuroscience* 15, 623–642.

Steriade, M., & Deschênes, M. (1984). The thalamus as a neuronal oscillator. *Brain Research Reviews* 8, 1–63.

Steriade, M., & Llinás, R. (1988). The functional states of the thalamus and the associated neuronal interplay. *Physiological Reviews* 68, 649–742.

Steriade, M., & McCarley, R. W. (1990). *Brainstem Control of Wakefulness and Sleep.* Plenum, New York.

Steriade, M., Deschênes, M., Domich, L., & Mulle, C. (1985). Abolition of spindle oscillations in thalamic neurons disconnected from nucleus reticularis thalami. *Journal of Neurophysiology* 54, 1473–1497.

Steriade, M., Jones, E. G., & Llinás, R. (1990). *Thalamic Oscillations and Signalling.* Wiley, New York.

Steriade, M., Contreras, D., Curró Dossi, R., & Nuñez, A. (1993a). The slow (<1 Hz) oscillation in reticular thalamic and thalamocortical neurons: scenario of sleep rhythm generation in interacting thalamic and neocortical networks. *Journal of Neuroscience* 13, 3284–3299.

Steriade, M., McCormick, D. A., & Sejnowski, T. J. (1993b). Thalamocortical oscillations in the sleeping and aroused brain. *Science* 262, 679–685.

Sterling, P. (2004). How retinal circuits optimize the transfer of visual information. In *The Visual Neurosciences*, eds. Chalupa, L. M., & Werner, J. S., pp. 234–259. MIT Press, Cambridge, Mass.

Storm, J. F. (1990). Potassium currents in hippocampal pyramidal cells. *Progress in Brain Research* 83, 161–187.

Stratford, K. J., Tarczy-Hornoch, K., Martin, K. A. C., Bannister, N. J., & Jack, J. J. B. (1996). Excitatory synaptic inputs to spiny stellate cells in cat visual cortex. *Nature* 382, 258–261.

Strick, P. L. (1988). Anatomical organization of multiple motor areas in the frontal lobe: implications for recovery of function. *Advances in Neurology* 47, 293–312.

Stryker, M. P., & Zahs, K. R. (1983). On and off sublaminae in the lateral geniculate nucleus of the ferret. *Journal of Neuroscience* 3, 1943–1951.

Stuart, G., Schiller, J., & Sakmann, B. (1997a). Action potential initiation and propagation in rat neocortical pyramidal neurons. *Journal of Physiology* 505, 617–632.

Stuart, G., Spruston, N., Sakmann, B., & Hausser, M. (1997b). Action potential initiation and backpropagation in neurons of the mammalian CNS. *Trends in Neurosciences* 20, 125–131.

Sur, M., & Sherman, S. M. (1982). Linear and nonlinear W-cells in C-laminae of the cat's lateral geniculate nucleus. *Journal of Neurophysiology* 47, 869–884.

Sur, M., Esguerra, M., Garraghty, P. E., Kritzer, M. F., & Sherman, S. M. (1987). Morphology of physiologically identified retinogeniculate X- and Y-axons in the cat. *Journal of Neurophysiology* 58, 1–32.

Sur, M., Garraghty, P. E., & Roe, A. W. (1988). Experimentally induced visual projections into auditory thalamus and cortex. *Science* 242, 1437–1441.

Suzuki, H., & Kato, H. (1966). Binocular interaction at cat's lateral geniculate body. *Journal of Neurophysiology* 29, 909–920.

Swadlow, H. A., & Gusev, A. G. (2001). The impact of "bursting" thalamic impulses at a neocortical synapse. *Nature Neuroscience* 4, 402–408.

Swadlow, H. A., Gusev, A. G., & Bezdudnaya, T. (2002). Activation of a cortical column by a thalamocortical impulse. *Journal of Neuroscience* 22, 7766–7773.

Szentágothai, J. (1963). The structure of the synapse in the lateral geniculate nucleus. *Acta Anatomica* 55, 166–185.

Tamamaki, N., Uhlrich, D. J., & Sherman, S. M. (1994). Morphology of physiologically identified retinal X and Y axons in the cat's thalamus and midbrain as revealed by intra-axonal injection of biocytin. *Journal of Comparative Neurology* 354, 583–607.

Taube, J. S. (1995). Head direction cells recorded in the anterior thalamic nuclei of freely moving rats. *Journal of Neuroscience* 15, 70–86.

Tehovnik, E. J., Slocum, W. M., & Schiller, P. H. (2002). Differential effects of laminar stimulation of V1 cortex on target selection by macaque monkeys. *European Journal of Neuroscience* 16, 751–760.

Thach, W. T., Goodkin, H. P., & Keating, J. G. (1992). The cerebellum and the adaptive coordination of movement. *Annual Review of Neuroscience* 15, 403–442.

Thomas, U. (2002). Modulation of synaptic signalling complexes by Homer proteins. *Journal of Neurochemistry* 81, 407–413.

Thompson, S. M., Capogna, M., & Scanziani, M. (1993). Presynaptic inhibition in the hippocampus. *Trends in Neurosciences* 16, 222–227.

Thomson, A. M. (2000a). Facilitation, augmentation and potentiation at central synapses. *Trends in Neurosciences* 23, 305–312.

Thomson, A. M. (2000b). Molecular frequency filters at central synapses. *Progress in Neurobiology* 62, 159–196.

Thomson, A. M., & Deuchars, J. (1994). Temporal and spatial properties of local circuits in neocortex. *Trends in Neurosciences* 17, 119–126.

Thomson, A. M., & Deuchars, J. (1997). Synaptic interactions in neocortical local circuits: dual intracellular recordings *in vitro*. *Cerebral Cortex* 7, 510–522.

Thomson, A. M., & West, D. C. (2003). Presynaptic frequency filtering in the gamma frequency band: dual intracellular recordings in slices of adult rat and cat neocortex. *Cerebral Cortex* 13, 136–143.

Tömböl, T. (1967). Short neurons and their synaptic relations in the specific thalamic nuclei. *Brain Research* 3, 307–326.

Tömböl, T. (1969). Two types of short axon (Golgi 2nd) interneurons in the specific thalamic nuclei. *Acta Morphologica Academiae Scientiarium Hungaricae* 17, 285–297.

Tong, L., & Spear, P. D. (1986). Single thalamic neurons project to both lateral suprasylvian visual cortex and area 17: a retrograde fluorescent double-labeling study. *Journal of Comparative Neurology* 246, 254–264.

Torrealba, F., Guillery, R. W., Eysel, U. T., Polley, E. H., & Mason, C. A. (1982). Studies of retinal representations within the cat's optic tract. *Journal of Comparative Neurology* 211, 377–396.

Tóth, T. I., Hughes, S. W., & Crunelli, V. (1998). Analysis and biophysical interpretation of bistable behaviour in thalamocortical neurons. *Neuroscience* 87, 519–523.

Towns, L. C., Tigges, J., & Tigges, M. (1990). Termination of thalamic intralaminar nuclei afferents in visual cortex of squirrel monkey. *Visual Neuroscience* 5, 151–154.

Trevelyan, A. J., & Thompson, I. D. (1995). Neonatal monocular enucleation and the geniculo-cortical system in the golden hamster: shrinkage in dorsal lateral geniculate nucleus and area 17 and the effects on relay cell size and number. *Visual Neuroscience* 12, 971–983.

Tsukahara, N., Toyama, K., & Kosaka, K. (1967). Electrical activity of red nucleus neurons investigated with intracellular microelectrodes. *Experimental Brain Research* 4, 18–33.

Tsumoto, T., Creutzfeldt, O. D., & Legendy, C. R. (1978). Functional organization of the cortifugal system from visual cortex to lateral geniculate nucleus in the cat. *Experimental Brain Research* 32, 345–364.

Tsumoto, T., & Suda, K. (1980). Three groups of cortico-geniculate neurons and their distribution in binocular and monocular segments of cat striate cortex. *Journal of Comparative Neurology* 193, 223–236.

Turner, J. P., & Salt, T. E. (1998). Characterization of sensory and corticothalamic excitatory inputs to rat thalamocortical neurones *in vitro*. *Journal of Physiology* 510, 829–843.

Tusa, R. J., & Palmer, L. A. (1980). Retinotopic organization of areas 20 and 21 in the cat. *Journal of Comparative Neurology* 193, 147–164.

Tusa, R. J., Palmer, L. A., & Rosenquist, A. C. (1978). The retinotopic organization of area 17 (striate cortex) in the cat. *Journal of Comparative Neurology* 177, 213–236.

Tusa, R. J., Rosenquist, A. C., & Palmer, L. A. (1979). Retinotopic organization of areas 18 and 19 in the cat. *Journal of Comparative Neurology* 185, 657–678.

Uchizono, K. (1965). Characteristic of excitatory and inhibitory synapses in the central nervous system of the cat. *Nature* 207, 642–643.

Uhlrich, D. J., Cucchiaro, J. B., & Sherman, S. M. (1988). The projection of individual axons from the parabrachial region of the brainstem to the dorsal lateral geniculate nucleus in the cat. *Journal of Neuroscience* 8, 4565–4575.

Uhlrich, D. J., Cucchiaro, J. B., Humphrey, A. L., & Sherman, S. M. (1991). Morphology and axonal projection patterns of individual neurons in the cat perigeniculate nucleus. *Journal of Neurophysiology* 65, 1528–1541.

Uhlrich, D. J., Manning, K. A., & Pienkowski, T. P. (1993). The histaminergic innervation of the lateral geniculate complex in the cat. *Visual Neuroscience* 10, 225–235.

Uhlrich, D. J., Manning, K. A., & Xue, J. T. (2002). Effects of activation of the histaminergic tuberomammillary nucleus on visual responses of neurons in the dorsal lateral geniculate nucleus. *Journal of Neuroscience* 22, 1098–1107.

Uhlrich, D. J., Manning, K. A., & Feig, S. L. (2003). Laminar and cellular targets of individual thalamic reticular nucleus axons in the lateral geniculate nucleus in the prosimian primate *Galago*. *Journal of Comparative Neurology* 458, 128–143.

Ullan, J. (1985). Cortical topography of thalamic intralaminar nuclei. *Brain Research* 328, 333–340.

Updyke, B. V. (1975). The patterns of projection of cortical areas 17, 18, and 19 onto the laminae of the dorsal lateral geniculate nucleus in the cat. *Journal of Comparative Neurology* 163, 377–396.

Updyke, B. V. (1977). Topographic organization of the projections from cortical areas 17, 18, and 19 onto the thalamus, pretectum and superior colliculus in the cat. *Journal of Comparative Neurology* 173, 81–122.

Updyke, B. V. (1979). A Golgi study of the class V cell in the visual thalamus of the cat. *Journal of Comparative Neurology* 186, 603–620.

Updyke, B. V. (1981). Projections from visual areas of the middle suprasylvian sulcus onto the lateral posterior complex and adjacent thalamic nuclei in cat. *Journal of Comparative Neurology* 201, 477–506.

Updyke, B. V. (1983). A reevaluation of the functional organization and cytoarchitecture of the feline lateral posterior complex, with observations on adjoining cell groups. *Journal of Comparative Neurology* 219, 143–181.

Usrey, W. M., Reppas, J. B., & Reid, R. C. (1998). Paired-spike interactions and synaptic efficacy of retinal inputs to the thalamus. *Nature* 395, 384–387.

Usrey, W. M., Reppas, J. B., & Reid, R. C. (1999). Specificity and strength of retinogeniculate connections. *Journal of Neurophysiology* 82, 3527–3540.

Valdivia, O. (1971). Methods of fixation and the morphology of synaptic vesicles. *Journal of Comparative Neurology* 142, 257–273.

Van Essen, D. C. (1979). Visual areas of the mammalian cerebral cortex. *Annual Reviews in Neuroscience* 2, 227–263.

Van Essen, D. C. (1985). Functional organization of primate visual cortex. In *Cerebral Cortex*, vol. 3, eds. Peters, A., & Jones, E. G., pp. 259–329. Plenum, New York.

Van Essen, D. C. (2005). Cortico-cortical and thalamo-cortical information flow in the primate visual system. *Progress in Brain Research* 149, 173–185.

Van Essen, D. C., & Maunsell, J. H. R. (1983). Hierarchical organization and functional streams in the visual cortex. *Trends in Neurosciences* 6, 370–375.

Van Essen, D. C., Anderson, C. H., & Felleman, D. J. (1992). Information processing in the primate visual system: an integrated systems perspective. *Science* 255, 419–423.

Van Hooser, S. D., Heimel, J. A. F., & Nelson, S. B. (2003). Receptive field properties and laminar organization of lateral geniculate nucleus in the gray squirrel (*Sciurus carolinensis*). *Journal of Neurophysiology* 90, 3398–3418.

Van Hooser, S. D., Heimel, J. A., & Nelson, S. B. (2005). Functional cell classes and functional architecture in the early visual system of a highly visual rodent, in *Cortical Function: A view from the Thalamus*, eds. Casagrande, V. A., Guillery, R. W., & Sherman, S. M. *Progress in Brain Research* 149, 127–145.

Van Horn, S. C., & Sherman, S. M. (2004). Differences in projection patterns between large and small corticothalamic terminals. *Journal of Comparative Neurology* 475, 406–415.

Van Horn, S. C., Hamos, J. E., & Sherman, S. M. (1986). Ultrastructure of the intrageniculate axon collateral of a projection neuron in the cat. *Abstracts—Society for Neuroscience* 12, 1037.

Van Horn, S. C., Erişir, A., & Sherman, S. M. (2000). The relative distribution of synapses in the A-laminae of the lateral geniculate nucleus of the cat. *Journal of Comparative Neurology* 416, 509–520.

Vaney, D. I., Peichl, L., Wässle, H., & Illing, R.-B. (1981). Almost all ganglion cells in the rabbit retina project to the superior colliculus. *Brain Research* 212, 447–453.

Vann, S. D., Honey, R. C., & Aggleton, J. P. (2003). Lesions of the mammillothalamic tract impair the acquisition of spatial but not nonspatial contextual conditional discriminations. *European Journal of Neuroscience* 18, 2413–2416.

Varela, C., & Sherman, S. M. (2004) A further difference between first and higher order thalamic relays in response to cholinergic input. *Abstnacts—Society for Neuroscience.* Program No. 528.16.

Vetter, D. E., Saldana, E., & Mugnaini, E. (1993). Input from the inferior colliculus to the medial olivocochlear neurons in the rat: a double label study with PHA-L and cholera toxin. *Hearing Research* 70, 173–186.

Vidnyanszky, Z., & Hamori, J. (1994). Quantitative electron microscopic analysis of synaptic input from cortical areas 17 and 18 to the dorsal lateral geniculate nucleus in cats. *Journal of Comparative Neurology* 349, 259–268.

Vidnyánszky, Z., Borostyánkoi, Z., Görcs, T. J., & Hámori, J. (1996). Light and electron microscopic analysis of synaptic input from cortical area 17 to the lateral posterior nucleus in cats. *Experimental Brain Research* 109, 63–70.

Vitten, H., & Isaacson, J. S. (2001). Synaptic transmission: exciting times for presynaptic receptors. *Current Biology* 11, R695–R697.

von Gudden, B. (1874). Ueber die Kreuzung der Fasern im Chiasma Nervorum Opticorum. *Albrecht von Graefe's Archiv für Klinische Experimenten in Ophthalmologie* 20(II), 249–268.

Von Krosigk, M., Bal, T., & McCormick, D. A. (1993). Cellular mechanisms of a synchronized oscillation in the thalamus. *Science* 261, 361–364.

Von Melchner, L., Pallas, S. L., & Sur, M. (2000). Visual behaviour mediated by retinal projections directed to the auditory pathway. *Nature* 404, 871–876.

von Monakow, C. (1895). Experimentelle und pathologisch-anatomische Untersuchungen über die Haubenregion, Sehhügel und die Regio subthalamica, nebst Beiträgen zur Kenntnis früh erworbener Groß- und Kleihirndefekten. *Archiv für Psychiatrie und Nervenkrankheiten* 27, 1–128.

Wagner, S., Castel, M., Gainer, H., & Yarom, Y. (1997). GABA in the mammalian suprachiasmatic nucleus and its role in diurnal rhythmicity. *Nature* 387, 598–603.

Walker, A. E. (1938). *The Primate Thalamus.* University of Chicago Press, Chicago.

Wall, J. T., Symonds, L. L., & Kaas, J. H. (1982). Cortical and subcortical projections of the middle temporal area (MT) and adjacent cortex in galagos. *Journal of Comparative Neurology* 211, 193–214.

Walls, G. L. (1953). The lateral geniculate nucleus and visual histophysiology. *University of California Publications Physiology*, pp. 1–100. Berkeley, Calif.

Walsh, C., & Polley, E. H. (1985). The topography of ganglion cell production in the cat's retina. *Journal of Neuroscience* 5, 741–750.

Walshe, F. M. R. (1948). *Critical Studies in Neurology.* Livingstone, London.

Wang, S., Bickford, M. E., Van Horn, S. C., Erişir, A., Godwin, D. W., & Sherman, S. M. (2001). Synaptic targets of thalamic reticular nucleus terminals in the visual thalamus of the cat. *Journal of Comparative Neurology* 440, 321–341.

Wang, S., Eisenback, M. A., & Bickford, M. E. (2002a). Relative distribution of synapses in the pulvinar nucleus of the cat: implications regarding the "driver/modulator" theory of thalamic function. *Journal of Comparative Neurology* 454, 482–494.

Wang, S., Eisenback, M., Datskovskaia, A., Boyce, M., & Bickford, M. E. (2002b). GABAergic pretectal terminals contact GABAergic interneurons in the cat dorsal lateral geniculate nucleus. *Neuroscience Letters* 323, 141–145.

Wang, S., Van Horn, S. C., & Sherman, S. M. (2003) Synaptic distribution in the somatosensory thalamic nuclei of the cat. *Abstracts—Society for Neuroscience.* Program No. 699.20.

Warren, R. M., & Warren, R. P. (1968). *Helmholtz on Perception: Its Physiology and Development.* Wiley, New York.

Wässle, H., & Illing, R.-B. (1980). The retinal projection to the superior colliculus in the cat: a quantitative study with HRP. *Journal of Comparative Neurology* 190, 333–356.

Weber, A. J., Kalil, R. E., & Behan, M. (1989). Synaptic connections between corticogeniculate axons and interneurons in the dorsal lateral geniculate nucleus of the cat. *Journal of Comparative Neurology* 289, 156–164.

Weliky, M., & Katz, L. C. (1999). Correlational structure of spontaneous neuronal activity in the developing lateral geniculate nucleus in vivo. *Science* 285, 599–604.

Welker, W. (1987). Comparative study of cerebellar somatosensory representations. In *Cerebellum and Neuronal Plasticity*, eds. Glickstein, M., Yeo, C., & Stein, J., pp. 109–118. Plenum, New York.

Whitley, J. M., & Henkel, C. K. (1984). Topographical organization of the inferior collicular projection and other connections of the ventral nucleus of the lateral lemniscus in the cat. *Journal of Comparative Neurology* 229, 257–270.

Wiesel, T. N., & Hubel, D. H. (1963). Effects of visual deprivation on morphology and physiology of cells in the cat's lateral geniculate body. *Journal of Neurophysiology* 26, 978–993.

Williamson, A. M., Ohara, P. T., & Ralston, H. J. III. (1993). Electron microscopic evidence that cortical terminals make direct contact onto cells of the thalamic reticular nucleus in the monkey. *Brain Research* 631, 175–179.

Williamson, A. M., Ohara, P. T., Ralston, D. D., Milroy, A. M., & Ralston, H. J., III. (1994). Analysis of gamma-aminobutyric acidergic synaptic contacts in the thalamic reticular nucleus of the monkey. *Journal of Comparative Neurology* 349, 182–192.

Wilson, J. R. (1986). Synaptic connections of relay and local circuit neurons in the monkey's dorsal lateral geniculate nucleus. *Neuroscience Letters* 66, 79–84.

Wilson, J. R., Friedlander, M. J., & Sherman, S. M. (1984). Fine structural morphology of identified X- and Y-cells in the cat's lateral geniculate nucleus. *Proceedings of the Royal Society of London, Series B, Biological Sciences* 221, 411–436.

Wilson, J. R., Forestner, D. M., & Cramer, R. P. (1996). Quantitative analyses of synaptic contacts of interneurons in the dorsal lateral geniculate nucleus of the squirrel monkey. *Visual Neuroscience* 13, 1129–1142.

Wilson, J. R., Manning, K. A., Forestner, D. M., Counts, S. E., & Uhlrich, D. J. (1999). Comparison of cholinergic and histaminergic axons in the lateral geniculate complex of the macaque monkey. *Anatomical Record* 255, 295–305.

Wilson, P. D., Rowe, M. H., & Stone, J. (1976). Properties of relay cells in cat's lateral geniculate nucleus: a comparison of W-cells with X- and Y-cells. *Journal of Neurophysiology* 39, 1193–1209.

Winckler, B., & Mellman, I. (1999). Neuronal polarity: controlling the sorting and diffusion of membrane components. *Neuron* 23, 637–640.

Winer, J. A. (1985). The medial geniculate body of the cat. *Advances in Anatomy, Embryology, and Cell Biology* 86, 1–97.

Winer, J. A., & Larue, D. T. (1988). Anatomy of glutamic acid decarboxylase immunoreactive neurons and axons in the rat medial geniculate body. *Journal of Comparative Neurology* 278, 47–68.

Winer, J. A., & Morest, D. K. (1983). The neuronal architecture of the dorsal division of the medial geniculate body of the cat: a study with the rapid golgi method. *Journal of Comparative Neurology* 221, 1–30.

Wong, R. O. L., Chernjavsky, A., Smith, S. J., & Shatz, C. J. (1995). Early functional neural networks in the developing retina. *Nature* 374, 716–718.

Wong-Riley, M. T. T. (1979). Changes in the visual system of monocularly sutured or enucleated cats demonstrable with cytochrome oxidase histochemistry. *Brain Research* 171, 11–28.

Wu, L. G., & Saggau, P. (1997). Presynaptic inhibition of elicited neurotransmitter release. *Trends in Neurosciences* 20, 204–212.

Wu, L. G., Borst, J. G., & Sakmann, B. (1998). R-type Ca^{2+} currents evoke transmitter release at a rat central synapse. *Proceedings of the National Academy of Sciences of the United States of America* 95, 4720–4725.

Xu-Friedman, M. A., & Regehr, W. G. (2003). Ultrastructural contributions to desensitization at cerebellar mossy fiber to granule cell synapses. *Journal of Neuroscience* 23, 2182–2192.

Yen, C.-T., Conley, M., Hendry, S. H. C., & Jones, E. G. (1985a). The morphology of physiologically identified GABAergic neurons in the somatic sensory part of the thalamic reticular nucleus in the cat. *Journal of Neuroscience* 5, 2254–2268.

Yen, C.-T., Conley, M., & Jones, E. G. (1985b). Morphological and functional types of neurons in cat ventral posterior thalamic nucleus. *Journal of Neuroscience* 5, 1316–1338.

Yeterian, E. H., & Pandya, D. N. (1997). Corticothalamic connections of extrastriate visual areas in rhesus monkeys. *Journal of Comparative Neurology* 378, 562–585.

Yukie, M., & Iwai, E. (1981). Direct projection from the dorsal lateral geniculate nucleus to the prestriate cortex in macaque monkeys. *Journal of Comparative Neurology* 201, 81–97.

Zahs, K. R., & Stryker, M. P. (1988). Segregation of ON and OFF afferents to ferret visual cortex. *Journal of Neurophysiology* 59, 1410–1429.

Zeki, S. (1993). *A Vision of the Brain*, pp. 1–366. Blackwell Scientific Publications, Oxford, England.

Zeki, S., & Shipp, S. (1988). The functional logic of cortical connections. *Nature* 335, 311–317.

Zeki, S. M. (1969). Representation of central visual fields in prestriate cortex of monkey. *Brain Research* 14, 271–291.

Zhan, X. J., Cox, C. L., Rinzel, J., & Sherman, S. M. (1999). Current clamp and modeling studies of low threshold calcium spikes in cells of the cat's lateral geniculate nucleus. *Journal of Neurophysiology* 81, 2360–2373.

Zhan, X. J., Cox, C. L., & Sherman, S. M. (2000). Dendritic depolarization efficiently attenuates low threshold calcium spikes in thalamic relay cells. *Journal of Neuroscience* 20, 3909–3914.

Zhang, L. M., & Jones, E. G. (2004). Corticothalamic inhibition in the thalamic reticular nucleus. *Journal of Neurophysiology* 91, 759–766.

Zhou, Q., Godwin, D. W., O'Malley, D. M., & Adams, P. R. (1997). Visualization of calcium influx through channels that shape the burst and tonic firing modes of thalamic relay cells. *Journal of Neurophysiology* 77, 2816–2825.

Zhu, J. J., & Heggelund, P. (2001). Muscarinic regulation of dendritic and axonal outputs of rat thalamic interneurons: a new cellular mechanism for uncoupling distal dendrites. *Journal of Neuroscience* 21, 1148–1159.

Zhu, J. J., Uhlrich, D. J., & Lytton, W. W. (1999). Burst firing in identified rat geniculate interneurons. *Neuroscience* 91, 1445–1460.

Index

Page numbers followed by "f" refer to figures.